Feeling Dis-ease in Modern History

History of Emotions

Series Editors:
Peter N. Stearns, University Professor in the Department of History at George Mason University, USA
Susan J. Matt, Presidential Distinguished Professor of History at Weber State University, USA

Editorial Board:
Rob Boddice, Senior Research Fellow, Academy of Finland Centre of Excellence in the History of Experiences, Tampere University, Finland
Charles Zika, University of Melbourne & Chief Investigator for the Australian Research Council's Centre for the History of Emotions, Australia
Pia Campeggiani, University of Bologna, Italy
Angelika Messner, Kiel University, Germany
Javier Moscoso, Centro de Ciencias Humanas y Sociales, Madrid, Spain

The History of Emotions offers a new and vital approach to the study of the past. The field is predicated on the idea that human feelings change over time, and they are the product of culture as well as of biology. Bloomsbury's History of Emotions series seeks to publish state-of-the-art scholarship on the history of human feelings and emotional experience from antiquity to the present day, and across all seven continents. With a commitment to a greater thematic, geographical and chronological breadth, and a deep commitment to interdisciplinary approaches, it will offer new and innovative titles which convey the rich diversity of emotional cultures.

Published:
Fear in the German Speaking World, 1600–2000, edited by Thomas Kehoe and Michael Pickering (2020)
Feelings and Work in Modern History, edited by Agnes Arnold-Forster and Alison Moulds (2022)

Forthcoming:
Emotions in the Ottoman Empire, Nil Tekgül
The Business of Emotions in Modern History, edited by Andrew Popp and Mandy Cooper
The Renaissance of Feeling, Kirk Essary
Emotional Histories in the Fight to End Prostitution, Michele Greer

Feeling Dis-ease in Modern History

Experiencing Medicine and Illness

Edited by
Rob Boddice and Bettina Hitzer

BLOOMSBURY ACADEMIC
LONDON • NEW YORK • OXFORD • NEW DELHI • SYDNEY

BLOOMSBURY ACADEMIC
Bloomsbury Publishing Plc
50 Bedford Square, London, WC1B 3DP, UK
1385 Broadway, New York, NY 10018, USA
29 Earlsfort Terrace, Dublin 2, Ireland

BLOOMSBURY, BLOOMSBURY ACADEMIC and the Diana logo are
trademarks of Bloomsbury Publishing Plc

First published in Great Britain 2022
This paperback edition published 2023

Copyright © Rob Boddice and Bettina Hitzer, 2022

Rob Boddice and Bettina Hitzer have asserted their right under the Copyright,
Designs and Patents Act, 1988, to be identified as Editors of this work.

For legal purposes the Acknowledgements on p. x constitute an
extension of this copyright page.

Cover image: Benjavisa/iStock

All rights reserved. No part of this publication may be reproduced or transmitted in
any form or by any means, electronic or mechanical, including photocopying,
recording, or any information storage or retrieval system, without prior
permission in writing from the publishers.

Bloomsbury Publishing Plc does not have any control over, or responsibility for, any
third-party websites referred to or in this book. All internet addresses given in this
book were correct at the time of going to press. The author and publisher regret any
inconvenience caused if addresses have changed or sites have ceased to exist, but
can accept no responsibility for any such changes.

A catalogue record for this book is available from the British Library.

Library of Congress Cataloging-in-Publication Data

Names: Boddice, Rob, editor. | Hitzer, Bettina, editor.
Title: Feeling dis-ease in modern history : experiencing medicine and
illness / edited by Rob Boddice and Bettina Hitzer.
Description: London ; New York : Bloomsbury Academic, 2022. |
Series: History of emotions | Includes bibliographical references and index.
Identifiers: LCCN 2021053439 | ISBN 9781350228375 (hardback) |
ISBN 9781350228405 (paperback) | ISBN 9781350228382 (pdf) |
ISBN 9781350228399 (epub)
Subjects: LCSH: Sick–Psychology. | Diseases–Social aspects.
Classification: LCC R726.5 .F44 2022 | DDC 610.1/9–dc23/eng/20220121
LC record available at https://lccn.loc.gov/2021053439

ISBN: HB: 978-1-3502-2837-5
PB: 978-1-3502-2840-5
ePDF: 978-1-3502-2838-2
eBook: 978-1-3502-2839-9

Series: History of Emotions

Typeset by Newgen KnowledgeWorks Pvt. Ltd., Chennai, India

To find out more about our authors and books visit www.bloomsbury.com
and sign up for our newsletters.

Contents

List of figures	vii
Notes on contributors	viii
Acknowledgements	x

Introduction

Emotion and experience in the history of medicine: Elaborating a theory and seeking a method   3
    Rob Boddice and Bettina Hitzer

Lived epidemic
Commentary   21

1. Feeling the dis-ease of Ebola: An invisible war   25
    Emmanuel King Urey Yarkpawolo
2. Ebola *wahala*: Breaching experiments in a Sierra Leonean border town   43
    Luisa Enria and Angus Fayia Tengbeh
3. History before corona: Memory, experience and emotions   61
    Bettina Hitzer

Datafication and knowledge production
Commentary   85

4. The binary logic of emotion in the sensorium of virtual health: The case of Happify   87
    Kirsten Ostherr
5. Third person: Narrating dis-ease and knowledge in psychiatric case histories   103
    Marietta Meier

Dis-ease narratives: Making and listening
Commentary   121

6. Feeling (and falling) ill: Finding a language of illness   125
    Franziska Gygax

7 Beyond symptomology: Listening to how Palestinians conceive of
their own suffering and well-being   141
Heidi Morrison

Expertise, authority, emotion
Commentary   155

8 Forensic sense: Sexual violence, medical professionals and the senses   157
Joanna Bourke
9 The concept of 'Leidensdruck' in West German criminal therapy,
1960–85   175
Marcel Streng

Construction and contingency of experience
Commentary   193

10 The efficacy of Arcadia: Constructing emotions of nature in the
pained body through landscape imagery, c.1945–present   195
Brenda Lynn Edgar
11 'Fashionable' diseases in Georgian Britain: Medical theory, cultural
meanings and lived experience   215
James Kennaway

Material, objects, feelings
Commentary   235

12 From a patient's point of view: A sensual-perceptual approach to
bed treatment   237
Monika Ankele
13 *Feeling* Penfield   255
Annmarie Adams

Select bibliography   273
Index   277

Figures

10.1	Photographic installations by David Carlier and Studiobivouac, La Tour Hospital, Geneva, Switzerland, 2017	196
10.2	Room at Hammersmith Hospital, London, used for psilocybin trials, 2016	202
12.1	Room drawn from the perspective of a hospital bed by Bernhard(t) B., Breitenau psychiatric hospital, 1932	238
12.2	Sick ward using bed treatment at the Waldau psychiatric hospital near Bern, drawn by Léon Alphonse Kropf	248
13.1	Exterior view of the MNI	258
13.2	MNI lobby view	259
13.3	Fold-out diagram of the MNI lobby	262
13.4	Menu for the inauguration of Montreal Neurological Institute dinner with handwriting, 27 September 1934	269

Contributors

Annmarie Adams is Stevenson Chair in the History and Philosophy of Science, including Medicine at the Department of Social Studies of Medicine, McGill University, Canada.

Monika Ankele is Wissenschaftliche Mitarbeiterin at the Organizational Unit Ethics, Collections and History of Medicine (Josephinum) at the Medical University of Vienna, Austria.

Rob Boddice is Senior Research Fellow, Academy of Finland Centre of Excellence in the History of Experiences, Tampere University, Finland.

Joanna Bourke is Professor of History, Department of History, Classics and Archaeology, and Director of Sexual Harms and Medical Encounters (SHaME), Birkbeck, University of London, UK.

Brenda Lynn Edgar is Research Associate at the Institute for Ethics, History, and the Humanities, Faculty of Medicine, University of Geneva, Switzerland.

Luisa Enria is Assistant Professor in the Department of Global Health and Development, London School of Hygiene and Tropical Medicine, UK.

Franziska Gygax is Professor Emerita at the Department of Languages and Literatures, University of Basel, Switzerland.

Bettina Hitzer is Wissenschaftliche Mitarbeiterin (Heisenberg Position) at the Hannah-Arendt-Institut für Totalitarismusforschung, Technische Universität, Dresden, Germany.

James Kennaway is a historian of medicine at the University of Groningen, Netherlands.

Marietta Meier is Titularprofessorin in Modern History, Universität Zürich, Switzerland.

Heidi Morrison is Associate Professor of History at the University of Wisconsin, La Crosse, United States.

Kirsten Ostherr is Gladys Louise Professor of English and Director of Medical Humanities at Rice University, United States.

Marcel Streng is Lecturer at the Institut für Geschichte, Theorie und Ethik der Medizin der Heinrich-Heine-Universität Düsseldorf, Germany.

Angus Fayia Tengbeh is Health Portfolio Consultant, the World Bank, Sierra Leone.

Emmanuel King Urey Yarkpawolo is President of the Salvation Army Polytechnic, Monrovia, Liberia.

Acknowledgements

Rob Boddice would like to thank all the participants to the Feeling Dis/Ease conference at the Max Planck Institute for Human Development, Berlin, in January 2020 – which now feels like the before times – and particularly Bettina Hitzer for the invitation to participate in it, and subsequently to join her in this project. The conference was everything a conference should be and a reminder, now, of so much that has been lost. For the time and freedom to pursue the work involved in writing for and editing this book, thanks go to the Academy of Finland Centre of Excellence in the History of Experiences, Tampere University Finland. The entire span of time that this book has been in the works has been one of dis-ease, whether of geography, health or general uncertainty, and thanks go to Stephanie Olsen and Sébastien for sharing and easing the load.

Bettina Hitzer's thanks go to the Max Planck Society that supported her research on 'Emotions and Illness. Histories of an Intricate Relationship', a research group that she led from 2014 to 2020 at the Berlin-based Max Planck Institute for Human Development. This research profited enormously from discussions within its Center for the History of Emotions. The Feeling Dis/Ease conference would not have been possible without Karola Rockmann's dedicated and circumspect support in planning and organizing everything. It was staged as a concluding conference and ended up being the beginning of further thinking about the connection between emotion, experience and illness, not least through the ongoing discussions with Rob Boddice while working on this book in times of a global pandemic. Having Christoph, Felix, Carlotta and Henrietta at my side has been a constant source of feeling at ease.

Thanks from both of us to Abigail Lane, Peter Stearns and Susan Matt for steering the project so efficiently through the process with Bloomsbury.

Introduction

Emotion and experience in the history of medicine: Elaborating a theory and seeking a method

Rob Boddice and Bettina Hitzer

Dis-ease

What does it mean to write about feelings – senses and emotions – and experiences of disease, medicine, illness and health? For many, the key question would revolve around the *who* of historical inquiry: is it to be patient-centred or doctor-centred?[1] Do we look at experience from the top down or from the bottom up? Many works have thrown their lot on one side or the other, but a more successful approach, for our purposes, has focused on the dynamics, inherently political, of the encounter. In the encounter, the experience of disease, or of medicine, is seen as a process, or as a series of interconnected and intersubjective practices, framed by cultural scripts of authority and expectation and a conceptual repertoire of diagnostic categories, symptomologies and prescriptions for relief. The dynamic encounter, in many respects, captures the process of matching or failing to match the lived experience of disease or ill health with the conceptual framework of the medical field, embodied in the figure of the medical authority, be they doctor, nurse, midwife, therapist or the like. It is replete with satisfactions of the feeling of being heard and treated, salved and succoured by the acknowledgement that a complaint conforms to the medical understanding of what is real and what is possible; it is also replete with dissatisfactions, of the feeling of being ignored

---

[1] See, for examples of both, Courtney E. Thompson, 'Finding Deborah: Centering Patients and Placing Emotion in the History of Disease', *Isis*, 111 (2020): 826–9; Michael Brown, 'Surgery, Identity and Embodied Emotion: John Bell, James Gregory and the Edinburgh "Medical War"', *History*, 104 (2019): 19–41.

or misunderstood, of the frustration that an experience cannot be shoehorned into medical categories of disease or illness. Perhaps the latter is the more common: a mismatch of expectations, concepts, feelings, senses and language. The experience of each individual in a space – a doctor's office, a hospital bed, a healing ritual or ceremony, a missionary vaccination station, an analyst's couch – is their own, but the experience of the whole, of the encounter itself, is more complex, difficult to render in words, frayed at the edges, messy at its core, political through and through. Is it this untidy whole that, in fact, we should try to capture? And if so, how?

It is not simply that doctors and other medical figures bring to bear one set of feelings and concepts and their patients bring another. Individual medical authorities also embody different medical schools and other cultural formations – religion, class, gender, race, age, nationality and so on – that intersect with the culture of their specific expertise and practices of administering it. Likewise, a patient is never reducible to the complaint presented to the medical authority, but rather that complaint is formed in their own bioculturally constructed intersectional fabric, which may include the medical authority. As Bonea, Dickson, Shuttleworth and Wallis have shown, anxiety, overpressure and stress – archetypal complaints of urban modernity – were themselves driven by medical anxiety and fears that modernity might produce them: a perfectly circular biocultural configuration of affective experience as cause and effect.[2] These observations have the effect of drawing our gaze away from the encounter, away from the specific moment in which the experience of disease is mediated in the balance of a meeting of worlds, to the cultures and bodies that lead to this moment, and to the cultures and bodies that go on after this moment. And they also lead away from the specifics of discrete medical complaints – from *disease* – to the ways in which people think about, feel about, experience their bodies in illness and health in a general and ongoing way. Our attention is drawn to the fears that accompany the idea that one *might* be unwell, or that attend an epidemic disease that has not yet touched us directly, but which is nonetheless *out there*. Our attention is drawn to the lay understanding of illness, the precautions that might be taken or the anxieties they might produce. And our attention is drawn to the ways in which knowledge about health and disease is produced, disseminated and disrupted. Many more focal points could be enumerated, which encompass social, cultural and intellectual formations, but

---

[2] Amelia Bonea, Melissa Dickson, Sally Shuttleworth and Jennifer Wallis, *Anxious Times: Medicine and Modernity in Nineteenth-Century Britain* (Pittsburgh, PA: University of Pittsburgh Press, 2019).

they amount to a focus on the feelings, highly situated, always mediated, of *disease* that attend the very notion of disease.

In search of a method

This represents something of a departure, insofar as we are attempting to collapse the distinction between biology and culture, or at least to avoid explanatory devices that make use of one or the other when it suits the argument. While historians of medicine have, for many years, pursued the cultural construction of illness, and the inscription of illness upon bodies, there remains an implicit sense (at least, for some) in which bodies themselves are biologically static, to be written upon, yes, but writing nothing in return. Our reformulation is subtle, on the face of it, but in its substitution of a biocultural model in place of a biology-culture model, we suggest the possibility of substantial historiographical revision. Olivia Weisser's *Ill Composed*, for example, begins with the claim that 'illness, then as now, is not only a sequence of biological processes but also a complex social event defined by prevailing norms and behaviors'.[3] *Not only … but also*. It is this that we collapse, meaning that prevailing norms and behaviours are both formational of body-minds as well as being formed by body-minds in a continuously unstable dynamic process. The body is not merely a site for the performance of 'culturally defined roles, norms, and ideals that are propagated by our society' that we 'unknowingly adhere to', but the body actively and knowingly makes the culture which in turn writes to the body, just as the body is made by the culture that, also in some ways knowingly and politically, writes to it.[4] This takes us some distance from medical histories that appeal to a grand 'we', or to 'the peculiar features of being human', or to 'basic aspects of human existence' that endure across time and space.[5] We grant the possibilities of continuity and radical change over time, but such possibilities are always framed by situated biocultural particularities, which we have encouraged our contributors to this book to pursue. Having recourse to some kind of fundamental substrate of humanness, to be mined from under all the cultural muck, strikes us as a

---

[3] Olivia Weisser, *Ill Composed: Sickness, Gender, and Belief in Early Modern England* (New Haven, CT: Yale University Press, 2015), 2.
[4] Weisser, *Ill Composed*, 2.
[5] Christopher Milnes, *A History of Euphoria: The Perception and Misperception of Health and Well-Being* (New York: Routledge, 2019), 4–5.

dangerous fantasy that delivers history, however unwittingly, into the hands of evolutionary psychology.

This throws us into an avenue of investigation that, up to now, historians of emotion have been reluctant to pursue, despite the attention given to precisely this problem in some formative works in the field: collective experience. The problem lies in two preoccupations that seem to block an elaborate theorization of how collective emotions have been formed and changed in situated contexts. First, historians have been attracted to the subject, to modern Western liberal notions of the subjective experience, of the first-person agentic *I*. Of course, this is a valid and important vein of research, but it is both highly situated and distinctly limited. How does one parlay what one knows about the modern subject into an analysis of an aggregate of subjects, whose feelings and experiences do not seem, on the face of it, to emerge from any one of them individually, but rather to be an unstable product of the whole? Second, historians have been overwhelmingly persuaded by the idea, first coined by Barbara Rosenwein, in turn riffing on Benedict Anderson, of 'emotional communities'.[6] Rosenwein's original definition of this idea was that emotional communities were like what we regularly think of as communities, insofar as they could be big or small, local or national, connected to class or religion, but had specifically to do with commonalities of emotional *expression*. Later, the dynamics of feeling were incorporated into these communities such that historians were no longer mining the mere outward expression of emotions but looking for situated emotional styles hitched to group identity and formation.[7] In more recent times, 'emotional community' has come to stand in for seemingly any kind of connection between people, including those who have never actually met in person and who do not inhabit a common space. The problem, which has not really been broached at all, is what to do with collective experience that is poorly described by the word 'community'.[8]

Does a collective awareness of or apprehension of smallpox amount to a community? Do the practices of those avoiding the Spanish flu amount to community? On the contrary, it is at these moments of widespread fear that

---

[6] Barbara Rosenwein, 'Worrying about Emotions in History', *American Historical Review*, 107 (2002): 821–45; Benedict Anderson, *Imagined Communities: Reflections on the Origin and Spread of Nationalism* (London: Verso, 1983).

[7] Benno Gammerl, 'Emotional Styles – Concepts and Challenges', *Rethinking History*, 16 (2012): 161–75.

[8] Sociologists and social psychologists are more familiar with the problem. For an attempt to use their insights and apply them to an historical example, see Piroska Nagy and Xavier Biron-Ouellet, 'A Collective Emotion in Medieval Italy: The Flagellant Movement of 1260', *Emotion Review*, 12 (2020): 135–45.

we see the typical components of what is usually understood as community fall apart, and yet the collective is, nevertheless, experiencing something together, in common to a certain extent. They may be disunited in practice, and yet united in experience.

Experience

What is meant here by experience? Without wanting to ignore a centuries-old philosophical debate about this term, a more pragmatic approach to 'experience' will be taken here – in the spirit of the historian as omnivore, as it is often said half reproachfully, half appreciatively on the part of philosophy.[9] 'Experience' has different layers. As epidemics in particular bring to mind, prior to narration and even before perception, there is a precipitating 'event', an original 'experience' in the world.[10] Experience thereafter comprises what could be described as processes in response to this 'event': a set of occurrences that affect a group or society as a whole without necessarily affecting them in the same way. When a disease like the plague of Athens or the corona pandemic occurs, the 'event' initiates a process that affects groups, societies or maybe even the whole world. A number of differentiations can then be made that distinguish the common experience ever more finely. It matters whether or not I experience the corona pandemic in a country with a well-developed healthcare system; what measures governments take; what financial resources I have at my disposal (and thus what options for retreat to the home office, for example); what beliefs I have with regard to the body, the immune system and the effectiveness of vaccinations; and so on. This example illustrates that while the experience of the initial event may be common to groups or societies at some level, a 'shared experience' cannot be inferred from it without further ado. It also illustrates that there are no obvious 'lessons' to draw from shared memories of past 'events', however attractive

---

[9] The centuries-old debate can be found in Martin Jay, *Songs of Experience: Modern American and European Variations on a Universal Theme* (Berkeley: University of California Press, 2005). We take some inspiration here from Paul Stenner, *Liminality and Experience: A Transdisciplinary Approach to the Psychosocial* (Houndmills: Palgrave Macmillan, 2017), and find some sympathy with Thomas Fuchs, *Ecology of the Brain: The Phenomenology and Biology of the Embodied Brain* (Oxford: Oxford University Press, 2018).

[10] For a recasting of what we typically mean by an historical 'event', see Rob Boddice and Mark Smith, *Emotion, Sense, Experience* (Cambridge: Cambridge University Press, 2020), 50–1; see also Joanna Bourke on pain as an 'event': *The Story of Pain: From Prayer to Painkillers* (Oxford: Oxford University Press, 2014). The precipitating 'event' in this case is prior to meaningful experience and involves historical practice on a different, ecological level, with the human decentred. See Dominic LaCapra, *History and Its Limits: Human, Animal, Violence* (Ithaca, NY: Cornell University Press, 2009).

reductive similarities might seem.¹¹ Moreover, what is considered 'shared' is also dependent on the perspective of the person relating this experience or investigating it as an historian, and adopting this or that degree of differentiation with regard to the experience of such an event.

Nevertheless, being affected by an event in common is an important dimension of experience, and especially with regard to the experience of dis-ease. Epidemics and pandemics as well as other forms of illness can create a common framework of experience, which exerts influence on the people who live within it, who, for example, are confronted with the diagnosis of a serious mental illness and possibly have to submit to a therapeutic regime in a special space for a certain time (or forever). However, a shared experience does not necessarily follow from this. We should be careful not to jump automatically from one to the other. Nevertheless, the disease 'event' that affects many in common is an important reference point in the experiential history of dis-ease. Historical engagement with experience, then, begins before engagement with what constitutes shared experience. It begins with a careful reconstruction of what characterizes the 'event' and what is common to it at different levels for different societies or groups.

In the narration of history, such an 'event' often becomes the overarching frame of reference. Societies, groups or individuals use these 'events' to pattern their narration of time, without necessarily giving rise to a sense of community. For – as Martin Jay, for example, has rightly pointed out – historical action is always experienced from 'a partial point of view': the storming of the Bastille represented a fundamentally different event for the assailants than for the defenders who were ultimately defeated.¹² And yet, both experiences are bound together in the historical moment of the storming of the Bastille and served as a reference for both groups in their respective futures. Something similar applies, for example, to a group of patients who underwent a similar therapy at the same time and possibly even in the same place.

Such a common experience can become a shared experience in two ways. First, it is possible that all those who lived through the same pivotal event or the same prolonged crisis (or period of transformation) define themselves as a group through this experience, even if they may have experienced this event or crisis

---

[11] Guillaume Lachenal and Gaëtan Thomas, 'COVID-19: When History Has No Lessons', *History Workshop Features*, 30 March 2020, https://www.historyworkshop.org.uk/covid-19-when-history-has-no-lessons/; cf. Erica Charters and Richard A. McKay, 'The History of Science and Medicine in the Context of COVID-19', *Centaurus*, 62 (2020): 223–33.

[12] Martin Jay, Review of David Carr, 'Experience and History: Phenomenological Perspectives and the Historical World', *Journal of the Philosophy of History*, 10 (2016): 325–31, 329.

in different ways. It is therefore possible that today's generation of young people will later perceive themselves as Generation Corona. Second, shared experience arises when an event is perceived by a specific group in a similar way, all individual differences in experience notwithstanding. This allows commonalities to emerge that were already present but unrecognized, or else creates new commonalities through new shared conditions or circumstances. This applies, for example, to self-help groups, blogs or even just the self-perception as 'survivors' made by people having suffered from cancer, as well as, of course, to many other seriously or chronically ill people.

We often associate this kind of shared experience exclusively with crisis events: epidemics, disturbing diagnoses, traumas caused by violence. Our gaze then often turns to the way crisis splinters order and expectation. As it is already inscribed into our concept of crisis, we tend to recognize the transformative and disruptive in the crisis. And indeed, it is not uncommon for crises to accelerate, intensify or discontinue developments or to help previously marginalized positions to gain dominance. In this case, we usually explain the connection between illness and experience by reference to fear, shame and disgust, playing out at a societal level but in highly situated terms. These moments of crisis should give us pause: the same forces are at work when there is no crisis. There is a context, a collective understanding, a sense of reality, a felt experience, that exists among people, despite their being otherwise mutually disconnected from each other. A 'crisis' may reveal what was there all along. Crises are, as Erica Charters and Richard A. McKay have written with regard to epidemics like Covid-19, 'stunning tips of icebergs' that suddenly make us see what has been out of sight for so long.[13] This broad experience, which comprises bodies, minds, knowledges (formal and vernacular), beliefs and all manner of cultural intersections, scripts and politics, is the fundamental *scene* – the landscape, if you will – which is brought to bear in the moment of the encounter. We cannot understand the latter without the former. We need an approach to the collective experience that goes beyond what we currently have.

Context

The answer lies in the careful reconstruction of context, which sits at the core of our method. The specifics of individual, intersubjective or collective experience

---

[13] Charters and McKay, 'History of Science and Medicine in the Context of COVID-19', 225.

and practice will elude us, in their distinct historical configurations, if we fail to pay attention first and foremost to the rich tapestry of context, to the techniques and practices that frame experience and to the structures of power that create or delimit that frame. All of this can be recoverable from the archive. In order to understand situated experiences of dis-ease, that is, of embrained, embodied and encultured thoughts and feelings about medicine, medical authorities, illness and health, we must first know about the situated context of possibilities. We know that we can access the given conceptual repertoire, the range of expressions and gestures, the accepted assemblage of meanings attached to cultural symbols. All these and more colour the canvass upon which the specifics of lived experience are painted. They help us understand the feelings of satisfaction, frustration, fear, anxiety, transgression and conformity that attend not just the medical encounter but also the very idea of medicine, as people strive to preserve their sense of well-being, to safeguard their health, to embrace or fail to accept their weaknesses, disabilities or chronic conditions, to resolve or fail to resolve their illnesses.

It is important at this juncture to pack away any historiographical ambitions to tie up historical experiences of medicine and (ill) health in any kind of neat way. We are, in this introduction and throughout this book, dealing with contexts of possibility that are always unstable, in processes of change and disruption. Experience is messy, disjointed, potentially framed by access to many different cultural repertoires at once. Events, especially in times of war, epidemic, violence and shifting legal frameworks, often rapidly overtake historical actors. We should expect people to have doubts, to be bewildered, to not know how to think-feel. We should scour the historical record not only for their expressions, for their conformity and orthodoxy in utterance and gesture, but also for their silences, the blankness of their features, their speaking of something while they are alluding covertly to something different, the constitutional aporia that attaches itself to uncertain states of mental and physical ill health and disease. We should be prepared to encounter people who have endured traumatic experiences and who might not be able to create consistent narratives or 'claim' their experience at all, as Cathy Caruth had pointed out.[14] We should expect to find people who do not know how to read cultural scripts – about emotion, about sensation – and who are confronted by medical treatment or medical politics as if by an alien being. Such experiences

---

[14] Cathy Caruth, *Unclaimed Experience: Trauma, Narrative, and History* (Baltimore, MD: Johns Hopkins University Press, 1996).

might be difficult to recover for they are difficult to record, but we can surely tease them from the historical record, through the absences and silences, if not directly. Many of these testimonies are not the most obvious, the ones that come to us first when we ask how dis-ease was felt. That is why it is important to discern whose experiences were heard and whose cultural scripts were dominant. In order not to reproduce the cultural politics of emotions that were influential at a given time, we need actively to search for other experiences, to make 'feeling differently' the programme of our research, or at least to include it in our considerations.[15] A crucial way to do this is to reconstruct the context that allows us to recognize and possibly fill in the absences, silences, breaches and evasions. The historian of experience, at least in this iteration of experience, must be prepared to explicate situated meaning, rather than assume any kind of easy translation or connection to it.

Recovering the body

To feel fear, for example, is always to feel fear in context. There is therefore no point, no value, in referring to fear *itself* as an explanatory for experience, or of locating fear in some part of the brain or claiming for it a timelessness that inheres in bodily processes.[16] Only the situated meaning of *this* fear, in *this* moment, in *this* situation, in *this* body and brain is relevant, and it takes skill and depth of historical understanding to convey the experience of it. Emotions, sensations and experiences cannot be essentialized or reduced to some fundamental aspect or component, to adopt the psychomechanical metaphor, of the biological or physiological human.[17] The last decade has taken many historians away from Dror Wahrman's suggestion, in 2008, that we return to some form of corporeal essentialism, based partly on Lyndal Roper and partly on Daniel Lord Smail, which was coupled with the lament

---

[15] Sara Ahmed, *The Cultural Politics of Emotion* (2nd edition, Edinburgh: Edinburgh University Press, 2014); Benno Gammerl, Jan Simon Hutta and Monique Scheer, 'Feeling Differently: Approaches and Their Politics', *Emotion, Space and Society*, 25 (2017): 87–94.

[16] There is a convergence of agreement, with wrinkles, across disciplinary lines. See Ruth Leys, 'How Did Fear Become a Scientific Object and What Kind of Object Is It?', *Representations*, 110 (2010): 66–104; Lisa Feldman Barrett, 'Seeing Fear: It's All in the Eyes?', *Trends in Neurosciences*, 41 (2018): 559–63.

[17] There are key differences of opinion about how, in practice, we do the history of experience and what it might entail, but the leaders in the field agree strongly on this point. See Javier Moscoso, 'Emotional Experiences', *History of Psychology*, 24 (2021): 136–41; Juan M. Zaragoza Bernal, 'A Change of Pace: The History of (Emotional) Experiences', *History of Psychology*, 24 (2021): 130–5.

that 'historians do not really have critical tools to assess the knowledge coming from these biological fields'. It was not entertained at that point that historians might acquire such tools and be able to work in a critical cross-disciplinary space, where we do not merely borrow from the 'latest "science"' but aim to contribute something to it.[18]

To say that the body is historical does not necessarily reduce it to a cultural formation. If the cultural history of medicine has sometimes erased corporeality in its discursive preoccupations, that does not mean that the reintroduction of the body must have us accede to 'perennial patterns in the wiring of human bodies and minds, and in the ways in which that wiring can short-circuit', as Philippa Carter recently put it.[19] Rather, in thinking bioculturally, we can explore the relation of brain-body development and the production of meaningful sensation, emotion and experience to culturally situated conceptual repertoires. Significant sections of the biological sciences are, through the consideration of multiple forms and expressions of plasticity – neuro, visceral, epigenetic, predictive processing and so on – grappling with the ghosts of corporeal essentialism in their own disciplines. Those historians who defend and endorse an increasingly outmoded metaphor of universal mechanical wiring or programming will remain out of touch, still unable to critically engage with the sciences. As Margaret Lock and Gisli Palsson put it, science is not equipped to answer the nature versus nurture problem and neither are the humanities.[20] The question preserves a binary that should be collapsed. Attempts to trace boundaries are doomed.

Instead, we should take seriously this notion, now supported across the disciplines by a formidable, if only loosely connected, group of social

---

[18] Dror Wahrman, 'Change and the Corporeal in Seventeenth- and Eighteenth-Century Gender History: Or, Can Cultural History Be Rigorous?', *Gender & History*, 20 (2008): 584–602. Specifically, Wahrman was conjuring with Roper's claim that 'it does not endanger the status of the historical to concede that there are aspects of human nature which are enduring, just as there are aspects of human physiology which are constitutional', pointing at the overemphasis of the culturally constructed body (598) and Smail's description of 'nature and culture', 'locked in a *pas de deux*' (600). Roper's claims, which practically if not intellectually align with Lynn Hunt's, have been thoroughly overtaken by the findings of social psychology, social neuroscience, cultural anthropology and the history of emotions, working (however unwittingly) in tandem on the question of the situated, local brain-body. Smail's retention of a nature/culture binary have since given way to a more dynamic model. See Lynn Hunt, 'The Experience of Revolution', *French Historical Studies*, 32 (2009): 671–8; Rob Boddice and Daniel Lord Smail, 'Neurohistory', *Debating New Approaches to History*, ed. Peter Burke and Marek Tamm (London: Bloomsbury, 2018); Jeremy Burman, 'History from Within? Contextualizing the New Neurohistory and Seeking Its Methods', *History of Psychology*, 15 (2012): 84–99; Larry McGrath, 'Historiography, Affect, and the Neurosciences', *History of Psychology*, 20 (2017): 129–47.
[19] Philippa Carter, 'Childbirth, "Madness", and Bodies in History', *History Workshop Journal*, 91 (2021): 3.
[20] Margaret Lock and Gisli Palsson, *Can Science Solve the Nature/Nurture Debate?* (Cambridge: Polity, 2016).

neuroscientists, social psychologists, cultural psychiatrists, neurophilosophers, anthropologists, social theorists and historians such as ourselves and other historians of medicine, emotion and experience, that humans are biocultural beings, plastic in development and formation, but also in disintegration and decay, according to the dynamic situation of bodies and minds in specific cultural and conceptual worlds.[21] This includes the corporal dimension, but the biocultural approach means we do not have to, indeed *cannot*, wrestle with the limits of culture and the presence of biology. There is no dividing line, no place to parcel off these categories. People are of the times and places and other intersections in which their lives play out. We cannot hope to access their experiences without first reconstructing those contexts that provided the framework, the atmosphere and the style that delimited and coloured that experience, and the conceptual (linguistic and non-linguistic – we include expression in this) repertoire that provided not only the vocabulary of experience but also the meaningful perception of situated reality.

Key questions

It may seem that the emphasis on the situatedness of experience lived by bioculturally formed human beings should lead us to make finer and finer distinctions until we finally end up with highly particular experiences, made in specific situations, felt by a unique person. But the biocultural focus must keep the collective – humans at the level of situated culture – in view, even if there is always a tension between it and the situated self, however that self is historically configured. Such observations and tensions raise two fundamental questions: first, what is the theoretical underpinning and ultimately political significance of such a form of historiography? And second, what is its significance and scope?

To begin with the first question: the form of historiography we present here seems to align itself with philosophical and political discussions that fundamentally renounce all notions of universalism. Instead of a universal canon

---

[21] This is perhaps best represented by the compendious multidisciplinary volume, *Culture, Mind, and Brain: Emerging Concepts, Models, and Applications*, ed. Laurence J. Kirmayer et al. (Cambridge: Cambridge University Press, 2020), but see Boddice and Smith, *Emotion, Sense, Experience*, 34–57, for a review and further references. On disintegration, and for an exemplary model of the approach we describe, see Todd Meyers and Stefanos Geroulanos, *The Human Body in the Age of Catastrophe: Brittleness, Integration, Science, and the Great War* (Chicago: University of Chicago Press, 2018).

of values, there are only particular values that can be traced back to particular identities. In Lynn Hunt's history of human rights, the inventors of universalism emphasized the equality of human beings rooted in their universal bodies, with universal feelings that trumped any particularities.[22] It had a profound effect, but what if we mark it as a situated historical construction? What happens to the interpretation of it if we, as historians of emotions and experiences, no longer consider the body merely as a representation but nevertheless postulate its biocultural plasticity and the situatedness of its experiences? Does this not remove any foundation for connecting people to humanity through their feelings and experiences?

In fact, little of the assumed essence of body and feeling remains here that could bind human experience together as a universal. Ultimately, the essence here can only be seen in the fundamental ability of the human body to feel and to experience, which encompasses all human senses as well as cognition. But this does not at all mean a withdrawal into the particular and the identitarian. For even if we as human beings are not connected to each other through the universality of our bodies and their sensations, we are connected through the contexts and spaces in which we move and experience. While these contexts are extraordinarily diverse, they are not self-enclosed. Thus, every human experience takes place in a context, which must be carefully reconstructed in its specific form in order to make the experience comprehensible and understandable. At the same time, however, this specific context refers beyond itself. First – scaled according to the micro-, meso- or macro-perspective of the historian – as a context shared by people. But then also as a context that in many of its elements links to other contexts, shares them, adopts them, translates them and appropriates them. Through this interconnectedness of experience, commonality originates just as much as through the shared and interconnected spaces of experience. Universality thus emerges, even without the assumption of universal bodies and sensibilities, through the existence of a multitude of contexts that connect us to ever different groups of people in different ways. In a globalized world, whose future seems to depend on the tenuousness or tenacity of its ecosystem, there are no humans (and other living beings) with whom nothing connects, even if we acknowledge that all bodies are bioculturally shaped and that experience is always situated experience.

And it is precisely to this insight that the answer to the second question about the meaningfulness and scope of such a form of historiography finally

---

[22] Lynn Hunt, *Inventing Human Rights: A History* (New York: W. W. Norton, 2007).

ties in. In this book the contributors' level of focus varies, from single rooms or pieces of furniture, and from tightly delimited temporal ranges, to national cultures and global interconnections over long periods. What is the ideal approach to get at the situated experience of dis-ease? Do microhistorical and macrohistorical approaches share something in common? The evidence of these chapters suggests that they do. The microhistorical approach is valueless without a thoroughgoing understanding of the broader context of meaning in which the situated study takes place. And the macro-level approach is equally useless without granular exemplification, nuance, detail. Both, ultimately, rely on context and specifics, though they play out in different narrative styles. And both depend upon an understanding of the ways in which contexts intersect and the ways in which body-minds inhabit multiple contexts at the same time. This reveals two things: first, situatedness is not synonymous with adopting a microhistorical perspective, possibly even narrowed down to an individual biography. Rather, it is vital that scale and situatedness refer directly to each other and do not fall back on the universality of an essentialized body in order to reduce the complexity of the situatedness of experience.[23] But second, since contexts refer to other contexts often of a different scope, microhistorical and macrohistorical perspectives must be set in relation to each other.[24] Microhistory in the sense of Carlo Ginzburg was concerned with the reconstruction of a complex micromechanics of experience, power and *Eigen-Sinn*, which is not primarily tied back to the macro-perspective through spatial entanglements, but through the assumption that large historical processes are revealed here on a microscopic scale.[25] Global history has undertaken to rethink such microhistorical concepts, initially using the instruments already introduced in global history. It has pointed to translations, circulations, travelling and intersections. More recently, however, the idea of the relationality of places and contexts has been increasingly emphasized. These approaches have been further developed in the concepts of *translocality*, of a *microhistory of the global* and of a *micro-spatial perspective*.[26] They indicate ways in which the

---

[23] See also the discussions in Sebouh David Aslanian, Joyce E. Chaplin, Ann McGrath and Kristin Mann, 'How Size Matters: The Question of Scale in History', *American Historical Review*, 118 (2013): 1431–72.

[24] See Boddice and Smail, 'Neurohistory'.

[25] Carlo Ginzburg, *The Cheese and the Worms: The Cosmos of a Sixteenth-Century Miller* (Baltimore, MD: Johns Hopkins University Press, 1992); also Giovanni Levi, *Inheriting Power: The Story of an Exorcist* (Chicago: University of Chicago Press, 1988). For an explanation of *Eigen-Sinn*, see Alf Lüdtke, *The History of Everyday Life: Reconstructing Historical Experiences and Ways of Life* (Princeton, NJ: Princeton University Press, 1995), 313–14.

[26] Ulrike Freitag and Achim von Oppen (eds), *Translocality: The Study of Globalising Processes from a Southern Perspective* (Leiden: Brill, 2010) ; Angelika Epple, 'Globale Mikrogeschichte. Auf dem

history of situated experiences and emotions we envision here can be written by combining micro- and macro-perspectives.

Norms, frames, scripts

Regardless of the question of scale, it is important here to emphasize process and duration, insofar as we have no intention to freeze moments in time. As E. P. Thompson noted, experience is lost if we attempt to 'stop history'.[27] 'Snapshots' or 'freezeframes' miss the instability that is at the heart of historical experience. If we want to show how change (and continuity) over time occurs, freezing moments in time seems antithetical to the ambition. Rather, we see historical change as part of the dynamic relation of body-minds in worlds, where sensory and emotional and cognitive experiences are both the result of occurrences in the world but also causative of events. We have to allow for the experience of time, for the experience of uncertainty, for the experience of working out how to feel, or of being frustrated in working out how to feel. All of these processes take place in relational exchanges that disappear if frozen. This is true for any experience of illness, as well as for negotiations (individual or collective) of experience of normality or wellness, categories that are all the more political for having their politics rendered invisible. The experience of an incurable or chronic illness or pain puts even greater emphasis on longer-time processes of meaning making, memory, moral economies of hope and despair, engagement with social institutions and welfare and the politics of *invalidity* and exclusion.[28]

Weg zu einer Geschichte der Relationen', *Im Kleinen das Große suchen. Mikrogeschichte in Theorie und Praxis*, ed. Ewald Hieb and Ernst Langthaler (Innsbruck: Studienverlag, 2012), 37–47; Romain Bertrand and Guillaume Calafat, 'La microhistoire globale: affaire(s) à suivre', *Annales. Histoire, Sciences Sociales*, 73 (2018): 1–18; John-Paul A. Ghobrial, 'Introduction: Seeing the World Like a Microhistorian', *Past & Present*, 242, Supplement 14 (2019): 1–22; Jan de Vries, 'Playing with Scales: The Global and the Micro, the Macro and the Nano', *Past & Present*, 242, Supplement 14 (2019): 23–36; Christian G. De Vito, 'History without Scale: The Micro-Spatial Perspective', *Past & Present*, 242, Supplement 14 (2019): 348–72.

[27] E. P. Thompson, *The Making of the English Working Class* (London: Pelican, 1968), 11. This is perhaps the limit of our agreement with Thompson's approach to experience. For all that Thompson built context, experience of dis-ease was deterministically linked to economic conditions and therefore readily accessible through the historian's imagination. Hence we find, in Thompson's interpretation of historical experience, more of Thompson than of history. See, for example, his reference to 'some subterranean alteration of mood' (127), to 'deep sources of feeling' (157), to 'violent mass hysteria' (418) and to the 'psychic processes of counter-revolution' (419).

[28] See Rob Boddice, 'Hurt Feelings?', *Pain and Emotion in Modern History*, ed. Rob Boddice (Houndmills: Palgrave Macmillan, 2014); Javier Moscoso, 'Exquisite and Lingering Pains: Facing Cancer in Early Modern Europe', *Pain and Emotion in Modern History*, ed. Boddice; Bourke, *Story of Pain*, esp. 131–58; Keith Wailoo, *Pain: A Political History* (Baltimore, MD: Johns Hopkins University

These kinds of experience, which are not so much breaches in normality but a challenge to the very notion of normality, can be lived as prolonged acts of resistance as well as of suffering, as challenges to systematic norms and meaning-making scripts. Nonetheless, our focus on instability, change, navigation and negotiation does not discount less mutable phenomena in the history of feeling dis-ease that we equally have to take into account. The experience of dis-ease is deeply engrained by more stable though not immobile norms about what is normal, healthy, beneficial or morally sound.[29] Diseases, disorders and conditions are named and framed.[30] These framings draw on medical and social knowledge and thought styles, techniques and technologies of observation and treatment, institutional or spatial settings as well as moral evaluations of all kinds. All of these categories are often more persistent and do not change very quickly. As Rosenberg has argued, the crucial moment where framing comes into play is the moment of diagnosis.[31] But the experience of dis-ease is not resolved in that very moment. The diagnosis is preceded by discomfort, suspicion, queries for the interpretation of symptoms, or sometimes it comes out of the blue, without premonition. And the experience of dis-ease does not end with the diagnosis. Receiving a diagnosis is only the beginning of a further complex process of negotiation. This process does not only follow a timeline; it is frequently experienced following specific temporal structures establishing chronological order, causal relations, accelerations, slowdowns, ruptures, periods of crisis. We may find these timelines of dis-ease experience in narrations that might be in constant flux (over the course of a disease as well as when looking back on past experiences). Nevertheless, they make use of, alter or shatter former narrative scripts. And scripts we find also on the level of feeling itself. Since emotions and sensory perceptions are not universal but learned by a bioculturally constructed mind-body, feeling is embedded into scripts that may vary according to the emotional style a particular situation may preset, without ever predetermining the actual felt experience in a strict sense. Norms, frames and scripts as more

---

Press, 2014), esp. 131–67; Bill Hughes, *A Historical Sociology of Disability: Human Validity and Invalidity from Antiquity to Early Modernity* (New York: Routledge, 2019); Emily K. Abel, *Sick and Tired. An Intimate History of Fatigue* (Chapel Hill: University of North Carolina Press, 2021); Bettina Hitzer, *Cancer and the Emotions in 20th-Century Germany* (Oxford: Oxford University Press, forthcoming).

[29] See Laurent Berlant, 'Slow Death (Sovereignty, Obesity, Lateral Agency)', *Critical Inquiry*, 33 (2007): 754–80.

[30] Charles E. Rosenberg, 'Introduction. Framing Disease: Illness, Society, and History', *Framing Disease: Studies in Cultural History*, ed. Charles E. Rosenberg and Janet Golden (New Brunswick: Rutgers University Press, 1992), xiii–xxvi.

[31] Rosenberg, 'Introduction', xviii.

stable phenomena are thus part of a context within which situated experience takes place, without this context equalling the experience itself. They provide an embodiment for alternative perceptions and meaning-making structures that might otherwise be suppressed.

Similarly, historically situated instances of mental trauma for which there was no recognized script might manifest through 'orthodox' expressions of illness – bodily complaints and verbal utterances – that gain medical attention for an illness in an oblique way that in turn colours the experience of that illness. Late-nineteenth-century hysteria is a classic case in point, but there are others: self harm, eating disorders and so on.[32] In all cases, the body can act as a refuge for the kind of emotions, senses and feelings that are ordinarily given no forum or recognition for expression. As such, these kinds of experiences can be drivers of change. This kind of change can occur on different levels, and we should be prepared to look for these changes in the history and presence of feeling dis-ease. It might be that these previously non-recognized feelings were involved in the emergence of a formerly unknown 'fashionable' disease. It might be that they created novel forms of narrating a disease like cancer. It might be that they alert us to the necessity of developing new diagnostic understandings for a trauma like that experienced by Palestinians. It might be that those previously unrecognized feelings coming from a different context alter the experience of an illness, as in the case of the Ebola epidemic in Liberia. And it might be that those digital tools currently designed for capturing the experience of dis-ease will not only transform our experience of dis-ease but also lead to the non-recognition of what has constituted the feeling of dis-ease so far. The experience of feeling dis-ease cannot be assumed to be static, and if we want to represent it then we have to incorporate the dynamic processes that comprise it into our analysis, finding a methodology so to do. To navigate the experience of an illness, as with the navigation of all feelings, is a situated, political but also a temporal process.

By showing how feelings of dis-ease, of the experience of medicine and illness, are constructed always in context, we hope to reveal, obliquely, the ways in which

---

[32] Rob Boddice, 'Hysteria or Tetanus? Ambivalent Embodiments and the Authenticity of Pain', *Emotional Bodies*, ed. Dolores Martín Moruno and Beatriz Pichel (Urbana-Champaign: University of Illinois Press, 2019); J. J. Brumberg, *Fasting Girls: The Emergence of Anorexia Nervosa as a Modern Disease* (Cambridge, MA: Harvard University Press, 1988); Susan Bordo, *Unbearable Weight: Feminism, Western Culture, and the Body* (new edition, Berkeley: University of California Press, 2003); Deborah Padfield, *Perceptions of Pain* (London: Dewi Lewis, 2003); for a general approach, see Deborah Lupton, *Medicine as Culture: Illness, Disease and the Body* (3rd edition, London: Sage, 2012).

current experiences of disease are constructed and seamlessly naturalized. Be it in times of a pandemic or not, historicism reveals the structures through which experience is framed, politicized, mediated and delimited. It offers a tool for asking probing questions of our own times, but it does not make any claims, a priori, for the value of any particular historical example in making sense of ourselves.

Lived epidemic

Commentary

In this book we explore the lived experience of illness, broadly construed. It is not simply an account of the emotional and sensory disruptions that attend diseases, mental illnesses or traumas; it is also an account of how medical practitioners, experts, lay authorities and the public at large felt about such disruptions, as well as the perceived absence of such disruptions in the experience of health. Instead of summarizing each chapter in a general introduction, we present a set of critical commentaries that draw out common or competing threads in each thematic section. We highlight the intersection of intellectual history and medical knowledge; of institutional atmospheres, built environments and technological practicalities; and of emotional and sensory experience, in order to present a complex *affective* account of feeling well and of feeling ill. We are especially interested in the ways in which dynamics of power and authority have either validated or discounted dis-eased feelings, probing the politics of medical expertise to better understand situated expressions of illness and their reception, as well as their social, cultural and moral valuation. The contributors draw heavily on methodologies from the history of emotions, the history of the senses, the history of science and knowledge, the medical humanities and the social history of medicine, to give an account of how it felt to *undergo* illness, as patient, victim, survivor, consumer, doctor, expert, witness, community or society: a complex range of feelings that we capture in the phrase *feeling dis-ease*.

In light of the Covid-19 pandemic, this work has assumed a sense of urgency and immediacy. Making connections with other pandemics and epidemics, we have striven to present a volume that addresses this urgency directly, with implications not just for historical study and critical inquiry but with a general purchase on the affective register of scientific and medical communication, and on the politics of contagion, falling ill and keeping well. In this first section, the connection to current concerns is explicit.

The volume is framed by first-person narratives. It begins with a first-person account of the Ebola epidemic in Liberia. Historians often call upon such narratives as sources, but rarely do they seek and publish such narratives as critical elements in the production of knowledge about the lived experience of medicine and disease. The departure point, for Emmanuel King Urey Yarkpawolo, was his involvement with a documentary film being made by Gregg Mitman, which was overtaken by the Ebola outbreak. Here, Urey Yarkpawolo recounts his specific experience within a broader context of the experience and memory of civil war, through which Ebola becomes but another front in a longer story of social, economic and political dis-ease. The epidemic is a framing event for the telling of a life, of a culture and of corruption and suffering. Ebola, in this account, comes to embody fear, but it is a fear that is deeply embedded in *longue-durée* structural problems that the disease acutely revealed and escalated.

As a foil for the opening chapter, Luisa Enria and Angus Fayia Tengbeh's chapter on the Ebola epidemic in Sierra Leone explores precisely the ways in which a disease makes visible the latent social context, challenging the notion of disease as cause of social crisis. The chapter adds theoretical heft, to examine epidemic disease as a breaching experiment, revealing underlying structures of the everyday. Both chapters, ultimately, speak obliquely to the unfolding of events around us all. They highlight the imperative of understanding disease in the context of its experience, according to the sociocultural and political conditions of that context. While there is a clear impetus to provide a general theoretical approach, it is to the specifics of time and place that we are alerted.

And this is the way in which Bettina Hitzer caps this section, with a reflection on the (lack of) cultural memory of epidemics in Western society – particularly, influenza epidemics in the twentieth century – and the relation of this to the Covid-19 pandemic beginning in 2020. At its heart is the politics of communication – strategies of informing and not informing the public – about the presence of disease, and the connection of these politics to preparedness, both in medical terms and in socio-emotional terms. Hitzer reminds us, as our introduction suggests, of the need to put disease 'events' into broader temporal experiential context and, at the same time, into specific local and microhistorical political context. What a disease is from the point of view of a society undergoing it (i.e. a society not necessarily universally infected with a specific virus but 'infected' with a specific idea or perception of its presence) cannot be reduced to the disease 'itself' but must be weighed in the balance of previous experiences, decisions and indecisions of the past, that comprise not simply a cultural frame but a biocultural disposition, on a social level. All these chapters, taken together, demonstrate that to talk about the fear of disease (or its absence) is not simply to talk about an unchanging emotion – *fear* – with a changeable object – *disease* – but rather about a range of experiences that tend to be bracketed under the label 'fear'.

1

Feeling the dis-ease of Ebola: An invisible war

Emmanuel King Urey Yarkpawolo

Introduction

'He was shot! If you are trying to save people from Ebola, and you turn around, you're shooting them, I don't know what is the difference. You are trying to save people from dying from of a sickness, then you are physically shooting them.'[1] These were the words I uttered after watching breathtaking footage of a shooting that took place in West Point, a densely populated slum community in Monrovia, during the height of the 2014 Ebola outbreak.[2] Professor Gregg Mitman showed the footage to me and my wife in our Madison apartment. Seeing the footage took me by surprise.[3] I had just returned from Liberia with Joseph, our second eldest son, on 29 July 2014. Bobby and Lloyd, two of our sons, had stayed behind due to difficulties obtaining visas, and my wife Vivian and I were very worried about them. I followed the news closely. Both the local and international media were not encouraging as the number of Ebola cases continued to increase. The US Centers for Disease Control and Prevention (CDC) had predicted that 1.4 million people would be infected by January 2015 without a serious international response to curb the spread of the disease.[4]

I first met Gregg in 2011 when I was a graduate student at the University of Wisconsin-Madison. Gregg had started a research project that focused on a

---

[1] For more information on when and how I made this statement watch *In the Shadow of Ebola* by Gregg Mitman and Sarita Seigel.
[2] Population estimates of West Point range from 29,000 to 75,000. See *Monrovia City Corporation's Slum Initiative* by City Alliance (n.d.).
[3] Professor Gregg Mitman is a Professor of History of Science, Medical History, and Environmental Studies at the University of Wisconsin-Madison. He was the lead producer of the documentary *In the Shadow of Ebola*.
[4] On the grim number of EBV cases, see *WHO, CDC Publish Grim New Ebola Projections*, 23 September 2014. Retrieved 17 December 2021, from https://www.science.org/content/article/who-cdc-publish-grim-new-ebola-projections.

1926 Harvard scientific expedition to Liberia, comprised of an eight-member team of scientists led by Dr Richard Strong, head of Harvard University's Department of Tropical Medicine. The expedition travelled through the interior of Liberia, collecting plants and animals, as well as blood samples from Liberia's indigenous peoples, in the name of American science, medicine and empire. Parts of the documentary evidence that Gregg had gathered included two-and-a-half hours of footage and over six hundred photographs taken by the expedition in 1926. The footage and photographs depict various aspects of life (including diseases such as smallpox and schistosomiasis) found on the coast and in the interior of Liberia at the very moment that Firestone Tire & Rubber Company was granted a lease by the Liberian government for up to one million acres of land to grow an American source of rubber.[5] Gregg showed me the footage and some of the photographs. I was overwhelmed with joy when I saw the pictures. I had lived through thirteen-year civil wars that destroyed every fabric of the Liberian society including historical institutions such as the archives and museums. This was an eye-opener, and I immediately told Gregg we needed to repatriate the materials to Liberia, a proposal he agreed with.

As part of the repatriation process we decided to produce a documentary called *The Land Beneath Our Feet* and build a public history website (www.liberianhistory.org) where we would make the materials available.[6] We made a number of trips between the United States and Liberia between 2012 and 2016, retracing the expedition journey and conducting oral history interviews. We were in Monrovia on one of these trips in June 2014 when the West African Ebola virus (EBV) hit the city. Uncertain about where the outbreak was headed, we decided to pause work on the historical documentary and follow the outbreak on the ground in Liberia and in the United States as it unfolded over the course of six months. The work resulted in the completion of a short documentary (*In the Shadow of Ebola*), which offers an intimate story of my family and Liberia in combatting the worst Ebola outbreak in history.[7]

The emergence of EBV in a city of more than one million residents in a country that had suffered political and economic instabilities for more than a quarter century was a perfect storm. Years of civil wars, corruption and lack of

---

[5] See www.liberianhistory.org.
[6] *The Land Beneath Our Feet* is a documentary that follows me as I retraced the journey of a Harvard expedition trip to Liberia in 1926. This is a never-before-seen footage of Liberia's past. The uncovered footage was embraced as a national treasure. For more information, see www.thelandbeneathourfeet.com.
[7] For more information, see www.intheshadowofebola.com.

trust in the governing system of the country laid the foundation for what was to come in the wake of the EBV. I was born and grew up in Liberia. I lived through the civil wars and knew fear: fear of being conscripted as a child soldier; fear of seeing the blood of murdered people; fear of being killed. The civil wars had killed more than 250,000 people and displaced more than one million people. The EBV – an invisible war with microscopic warriors – would take a share of the carnage, and of the fear and anxiety of Liberians.

Gregg and Sarita Siegel, co-producer and co-director of *In the Shadow of Ebola*, captured a few scenes of me as I struggled to obtain visas for my children, who were in Liberia. I did not want to leave them behind in the face of this deadly disease. As the disease spread quickly, both Sarita and Gregg departed Liberia and our Liberian cinematographer, Alex Wiaplah, and I stayed on. Alex captured various scenes of the suffering of people as the EBV spread like wildfire. In July 2014, I departed with Joseph for the United States and Alex stayed in Liberia to continue shooting various scenes.

In Madison, Gregg called and indicated that he and his team wanted to show me something. I agreed and we scheduled. Apparently, Alex had captured a shooting that took place in West Point and emailed the footage to Gregg. Gregg wanted to show me this footage and capture my reaction. A few days later Gregg and a film team arrived at our apartment. My wife and I sat next to each other as we watched the footage on a laptop. The scene opened with a group of soldiers heavily armed with AR-15 rifles, dressed in military-style uniforms, on one side and a group of young people on the other side of what seemed to be a barricade. Earlier, I had read in the news that the government had decided to use a school in West Point as an Ebola treatment centre and that the people of West Point had resisted. There was also news that some Liberians were planning to overthrow the government as it had failed to protect the Liberian people in the face of this deadly virus. Rumours indicated that West Point would be the base for the attack. In response, the security apparatus of the Liberian government barricaded West Point during the night hours. On 20 August 2014, West Pointers woke up and realized the main entry to their community had been blocked.

In the midst of this, the police decided to evacuate the township commissioner of West Point. The young people resisted the evacuation. This led to a commotion between the young people and the military. Within seconds of starting to watch the footage, we heard a loud noise. It was the sound of a gun. A sixteen-year-old boy, who we later identified as Shaki Kamara, was shot and his leg was shattered. Shaki died later that day from blood loss.

I was not prepared for this. How could government efforts to save people from Ebola involve shooting them? I expressed this on camera. At first, my head rose, I felt chilled, and became afraid. Next came frustration, hopelessness and anger.

I had lived through the first few months of the outbreak in Liberia. Our camera crew had captured the scene of a pregnant woman apparently dead by the sidewalk. Another middle-aged woman explained to us that the corpse had been there from the morning hours until midday and that the Ebola Burial Team did not arrive on time to save 'moving child life' in the woman. She continued, 'This is a curse to the nation. To see a pregnant woman die and the child in her stomach struggles until it dies too, this is a curse to the nation.'[8] The emergency section of the John F. Kennedy (JFK) Memorial Hospital, the largest referral hospital in Liberia, which was turned into an Ebola Treatment Unit (ETU), was already overrun with Ebola patients. We saw a yellow taxi carrying some Ebola patients and upon arrival at the JFK, the ETU was closed. There were already many sick people sitting outside the gate. With an angry mob outside of the gate, we saw a few ETU workers all dressed in space-like suits opening the gate and a grey Hyundai SUV was driving outside the fence. But with the commotion outside, the vehicle backed up into the fence and the security closed the gate. Angry men were yelling and kicking the gate.

At the Clay Junction, the main highway connecting southwestern part of Liberia to Monrovia, security forces enforced a government-imposed quarantine and blocked the road, preventing travel and food from reaching population centres. Market women appealed that the road should be opened so that they could pass to sell their goods. They complained of a lack of food and of hunger killing their children, in addition to the burden of the EBV. But the shooting of Shaki Kamara was a totally different experience for me. It brought back fresh memories of the many civil wars I had lived through. It speaks to the underlying social and political forces that influence the experience of dis-ease during the epidemic.

When EBV entered Liberia, the country was not prepared to deal with a disease of such virulent nature. The country's health infrastructure was completely destroyed. The civil wars were the result of inequalities enabled by corruption in a succession of governments. Poor public-service deliveries and constant unfulfilled promises had created an information vacuum within the Liberian population, with many people not trusting the government, setting the stage for the perfect storm. Here I explore how the personal and the economic,

---

[8] See *In the Shadow of Ebola* by Gregg Mitman and Sarita Seigel.

social and political forces of a nation shaped the anxieties, fears and actions that motivated my family and me during the Ebola epidemic, just one of the many wars I have lived through.

A country at war

The new Gomue village. On a scorching sunny day in February 2013, our camera crew arrived. Inquisitive people, young and old, mostly farmers, gathered. Among them were two of my sisters and our aging father who was little over one hundred years old. Our camera crew set up their cameras. For the past year we had been travelling through Liberia, documenting oral histories, mostly of the elderly, and at the same time retracing the path of the 1926 Harvard expedition to Liberia. It was time for my share of the interview and to capture my story. The producers had thought it wise to select Gomue, a village situated near the Guinea border about 214 kilometres north of Monrovia, as a fitting venue.

Gomue is a small village with just ten houses. I refer to it as the new Gomue because it was established after the first Liberian civil war which lasted from 1989 to1997. I was born in the old Gomue village, roughly the same size of the new Gomue. We deserted the old Gomue village in 1994 after the rebel faction of the United Liberation Movement of Liberia for Democracy (ULIMO) invaded Bong County.[9] It was looted and eventually destroyed by the rebels. When peace was negotiated in 1996, followed by presidential and general elections that brought the ex-rebel leader-turned-politician Charles Taylor to power in 1997, we returned from exile and established the new Gomue.

Facing Gregg, who sat sideways to the camera, I began to narrate the story of the war. Fresh memories of pains, confusion, hopelessness and anger came back to me as I started to speak.

We were in Gomue village on Christmas Eve in 1989. Everything for the Christmas celebration was set. Aunt Nyamah had already bought my Christmas clothes. Like other parents, she hid them from me. She would not reveal the gifts until early Christmas morning. After a long day's work, our father usually sat under

---

[9] The invasion of Liberia by the National Patriotic Front of Liberia (NPFL) or Charles Taylor rebel forces sought to eliminate the Krahn (President Samuel Doe Tribe) and the Mandingo ethnic groups. Many people in these two ethnic groups fled the country and sought refuge in neighbouring Sierra Leone and Guinea. Ex-Armed Forces of Liberia (AFL), who were predominantly from the Krahn and Mandingo ethnic groups, combined forces and formed the United Liberation Movement of Liberia for Democracy (ULIMO) and launched attack against the NPFL. Bong County was their focus as Taylor was based in Gbarnga, the county capital of Bong County.

the orange trees near our small soccer field and played his radio. We played soccer and listened to the traditional music played on the radio. As we were playing, the Kpelle announcer on the Radio Gbarnga said that some rebel groups had entered Nimba County from the Ivory Coast. At eight years old I was still too young to understand the news about war but the adults did not seem to take it too seriously either.

The following day was Christmas. We got up very early in the morning to check our traps. Any catch would be added to the chickens and the goats that would be used as meat for the celebration. Every household cooked. There were different kinds of soups. Some cooked palm butter with snails, some fried rice and others cooked water greens. My favourite was the fried potato greens with fried chicken. By midday, we wore our Christmas clothes and moved around in groups to visit our friends. During the evening hours, we sat around the soccer field and watched the bigger boys play as we cheered them on.

As 1989 concluded, there were many stories. We heard on the radio that some of the rebels were captured and were confessing how they were recruited to fight. One storyline indicated that recruitment in Charles Taylor's rebel forces was the result of the economic hardship that many young people, especially young men, faced in Liberia. A secret recruiter would tell a potential recruit that there were lots of jobs in the Ivory Coast – that the Ivorian government and other employers were recruiting people across the Liberian border. The recruiter would tell the potential recruit that he was willing to lend some money to pay transportation costs and, once in Ivory Coast, the recruit would work and reimburse the recruiter. Once they arrived in the Ivory Coast, they would make their way to either Burkina Faso or Libya, where Charles Taylor had his training bases. The recruits were told that they were in training to return and save Liberia from the hands of President Samuel Doe.[10]

The rumours of war continued in the new year. We heard that Mother Dukuly, founder of the Faith Healing Temple, had prophesied that a 'rain' was coming.[11] The rain was deadly and would kill anybody with a single drop. Some people interpreted this prophesy as the civil war.

Gomue was surrounded by orange and grapefruit trees. We picked and sold oranges in Naama, a town in Bong County where President Doe had his stronghold military barracks. My elder sister, Garmei, was in a relationship with Mr Sando, a

---

[10] Samuel Doe was the twenty-first president of Liberia who ruled from 1980 to 1990 when he was captured and killed by Independent National Patriotic Front of Liberia (INPFL), a breakaway faction of the NPFL.

[11] Mother Dukuly made several prophecies including a warning to President Tubman to attend a clinic in London (where he eventually died), and that President Tolbert would not be succeeded by a vice president (Tolbert was killed by Doe).

military officer of Camp Naama. We usually left Gomue on Wednesday morning and, after a whole day's walk with bags of oranges, we arrived in Naama during the evening hours. Sometimes we stayed overnight at Garmei and her husband's apartment in the barracks. On Thursday, which was market day, soldiers were loaded on military trucks and headed to Nimba where the fighting was ongoing. The soldiers would be singing and sometimes bystanders would join in the celebration. Many times, these trucks returned during night hours with fewer men and in total silence. Back in Gomue, we continued our usual work, setting traps, clearing the scrub, felling the trees, burning the fields and removing the debris to make way for the women to plant the rice. It was during one of these activities that the rebels, wearing red head ties, arrived on our farm. My sisters were planting rice. I was driving birds when we heard a group of men shouting, 'Do not move, stay where you are and put your hands up in the air.' We fell in total silence. We had heard about the rebels. We had heard about the suffering of people in Nimba. Now we were finally in their hands. They assembled us around the farm kitchen and asked if we had any Doe soldiers among us. They asked if we had any weapons. Our father told them we did not have any soldiers and we had no weapons as we were just farmers with machetes to produce food.

The rebels explained that they were fighting to remove Doe from power and to save Liberia, that they were not harming people but fighting for people. Anyone interested and willing to join them was welcome. After asking for chicken and taking some rice, they asked that our sisters accompany them to the barracks.

'Looking back, I realized that three of our beautiful sisters were captured, and unexpectedly became the wives of rebel forces. In essence, they were raped,' I explained with tears dropping from my eyes as I looked at my sisters, who were standing by to watch the interview.

We continued our usual farming activities but we were now under the authority of Charles Taylor, who had captured nearly 90 per cent of the country and had declared himself President of what he called 'Greater Liberia'. His soldiers would arrive in the village unexpectedly to arrest and conscript young men and women into their fighting forces, the National Patriotic Front of Liberia (NPFL). We had to be on alert and in hiding all the time. We would go to the farm and stay the entire day working and looking over our shoulders and would return late in the night to the village. Usually, two or three men would be on guard. Our guard post on the main entry was on the top of a hill where one would see people in the distance. If a guard saw strange people from a distance, he would throw a sign to another person who would run to inform us that strange people were coming and for all the young men and women to hide.

On one occasion, two rebels entered the village and killed my dog. They fired at the dog with a gun, while it was under the table where our father was sitting. It was my first time hearing gunshots very close, as I was just behind the house picking some oranges. First, I rushed to the bush behind the orange trees to hide but hearing only the voices of the rebels, I thought they had killed our father, who I had left on the porch with the dog. After a few minutes of confusion and fear, I decided to come out of hiding and see what had happened. From behind the house, one of the rebels saw me and with his gun pointed at me commanded that I take the dog and put it in a bag. I was relieved when I saw our father standing by quietly. I hurried and put the dog in the bag and after a few minutes, they told me to take the dog and follow them to the bigger town where many of the rebels were staying.

We trekked about an hour and arrived in Shankpallai, a bigger town in Zota District where we own a family house. Upon arrival, I saw the blood of a man who had just been killed. I cannot remember exactly the story leading to his killing but it was my first time seeing human blood flowing on the ground. The town was quiet and fearful. I was scared and my stomach started boiling, as if I wanted to use the toilet. With the rebels behind me and a bag of dead dog on my head, I had to keep moving. We finally arrived at our house where I cleaned and butchered the dog and roasted its skin. The rebels took their meat and returned the intestines to me, which I later threw away.

After several failed peace negotiations, the war finally climaxed in 1996 with an election that saw Charles Taylor elected as President. But this peace time was short-lived as ethnic groups (mainly the Krahn and Mandingoes), who were killed in large numbers during the war, regrouped in neighbouring Guinea and Sierra Leone and launched another attack against President Taylor. The Liberians United for Reconciliation and Democracy (LURD) rebel group attacked from the west-northern border of Liberia with Guinea. We heard the story of this new war but many people did not believe it in the city. Like the rumour of the first civil war, some people thought that Taylor was finding the means to get money from the international community.

At this time I lived with my uncle in Belefanai, a town situated along the Gbarnga-Voinjama highway. As in 1990, we saw trucks full of jubilant soldiers heading to the battlefield. Sometimes a week or two later those trucks passed by during the night hours, usually empty and quiet.

Awarded a scholarship by The Salvation Army Church, I moved to Monrovia in August 2000 to continue my high school education. On 29 November 2000, I decided to walk along the beach from 17th Street towards central Monrovia. After walking for a few minutes, I arrived behind the Palm African Plaza. I saw a group of children playing in the distance but to get to the other side of the beach I needed to pass behind the Executive Mansion. I did not know that walking behind the Mansion was forbidden. As I walked, two Anti-Terrorist Unit (ATU) guards, an elite security unit of Taylor, shouted, 'Hey, stop.' One raised his voice: 'Do not move and put your hands up.' Trembling with fear, I stopped and raised my hands in the air. 'With your hands in the air walk straight here', they commanded. I proceeded with my hands raised up in the air. Realizing that I had no weapon, they ordered me to take off my shirt, my trousers, and sneakers and follow them. One was in front of me and the other was behind. As we walked to the Executive Mansion fence, I saw no gate but layers of bricks stacked on the wall of the fence. We stepped on the bricks and climbed the fence of the Executive Mansion and jumped inside.

As we continued to walk, I started crying and begging for help. I told the soldiers that I did not know that nobody was allowed to walk behind the Mansion. My crying fell on deaf ears as the ATU officers repeatedly told me that I was a spy and that they had a rule that no one ever goes over the fence and returns. We arrived at the prison unit where I was thrown in jail. The jail was partially dark. I saw a group of people, mostly young men, inside. 'Who just came?', a person describing himself as the 'boss' of the jail asked. 'Do you have an offering?', he continued.[12] 'The rule for this house is that every new prisoner needs to give an offering and if there is no offering he receives 50 lashes as an introduction to this jail compound', he warned me. I said I had no money. My shirt, trousers and sneakers had been left outside and I was only in boxers. He commanded his men to flog me. Just as they were about to whip me, I got a call that the ATU Commander was calling me. They took me outside and, after facing a series of questions, he ordered my release.

In June 2003, the story of war that began in Lofa finally became a reality in the eyes of Monrovians. Monrovia was under attack. The rebels entered from Bomi highway. After a few days, they captured the Freeport of Monrovia. With the two bridges connecting central Monrovia fortified by Charles Taylor militants, the rebels resorted to bombing the city from across the bridges. It is difficult to describe the assault on the city in words. Many people thought that the Gray Stone compound near the US embassy was a safe haven as it was under US embassy control. They moved into the compound in numbers. But it was not safe. No part of central Monrovia was safe. The bombs dropped everywhere, in any place. Bombs landing in the Gray Stone compound killed many people and left many more wounded.

---

[12] I was told that the rule of jail was for a newcomer to give money as an offering to the 'jail commander' or the head prisoner.

The war finally ended in August 2003 with the forced departure of Charles Taylor from Liberia. A National Transitional Government was installed to lead the country for two years. The election of 2005 brought in the Ellen Johnson (first female president of an African country) administration in 2006. The international community spent millions of dollars trying to reform the governing system, rebuilding the military and police. What no one expected was another war, the war of the deadly EBV, which I call the invisible war.

Invisible war

25 May 2014. We arrived in Monrovia to continue shooting our documentary film, *The Land Beneath Our Feet*. A few days prior to travelling to Monrovia from the United States, we heard about Ebola in Lofa.[13] Coincidentally, the disease started at the border of Lofa with Guinea, the same location where the second civil war started.[14] Monrovia was peaceful, as people did not believe the news of this strange disease, just as they had not believed news of the second rebel invasion from Lofa. Some people believed that the rumours of a strange disease were a lie, a plot invented by the government to steal money from the donor community. We went on with our usual business of shooting scenes of Providence Island from the eight-storey old Ducor Palace Hotel, overlooking the Atlantic Ocean and the Borough of West Point, as well as viewing and shooting scenes from Broad Street.

Days later, the rumours of a strange disease that had started in Lofa became a reality to us when the first Ebola cases were discovered at the Redemption Hospital, the second largest government hospital in Monrovia, situated in the heavily populated Borough of New Kru Town, west of the city. Within a few weeks, several nurses and a Ugandan medical doctor contracted the disease and died. The hospital became chaotic. Some people still doubted the existence of this highly infectious and deadly disease. This doubt became a major factor in the spreading of the disease.

The more than twenty-five years of political instabilities had destroyed every functional system in the country including the country's healthcare systems. The

---

[13] The EBV disease was first reported on 30 March 2014: https://www.ncbi.nlm.nih.gov/pmc/articles/PMC4734504/#R1.
[14] The second Liberian civil war started in 1999 against the Charles Taylor-led government and lasted until 2003, when Taylor was forced to leave office on 11 August. The first Liberian civil war brought by Taylor started in 1989 and ended in 1996, after which Taylor was elected president in 1997. There was a brief period of peace from 1996 to 1998 before another insurrection in 1999.

World Health Organization (WHO) estimated that countries hardest hit by the EBV had only one to two doctors available to treat 100,000 people.[15] Liberia had one doctor per 100,000 Liberians; Sierra Leone had two. Compare this to the United States, which had just one case of Ebola with 245 doctors per 100,000 people.[16] Liberia had few functional hospitals and only one biomedical research centre. Years of political instability, corruption and weak government had presented a situation where the majority of citizens did not trust the government. With Monrovia, a city of more than one million people, being one of the first urban centres for the EBV outbreak, it felt certain that we were in trouble.[17]

The Liberia Institute for Biomedical Research (LIBR), the one (ill-equipped) research centre, did not have any testing equipment for Ebola.[18] Initial samples were sent out of the country for testing. This made contact tracing difficult as results took days to confirm. Compounding the problem were the symptoms of Ebola (EBV), which are similar to other diseases that are common in Liberia. For example, the WHO indicated that if one contracted EBV, it took 2–21 days for the person to show symptoms of the disease.[19] Only people with symptoms could spread the disease to non-infected people through blood or bodily fluids, by direct contact or by touching an object that had been contaminated by the blood or bodily fluid of an infected person. The WHO further stated that the symptoms included fever, fatigue, muscle pain, headache, sore throat, vomiting, diarrhoea and so on. These are the symptoms of malaria, which accounts for about 33 per cent of inpatient deaths in healthcare facilities in Liberia.[20] This made distinguishing EBV from other diseases difficult.

As the EBV was new to Liberia, so were the prevention mechanisms for healthcare workers. Since the symptoms of EBV were indistinguishable from

---

[15] See *Unprecedented Number of Medical Staff Infected with Ebola*: Ebola situation assessment published on 25 August 2014 by WHO. https://apps.who.int/mediacentre/news/ebola/25-august-2014/en/index.html.

[16] On the doctor-to-population ratios, see *Physician Density in West African Countries Suffering from the 2014 Ebola Outbreak*, by Statista. https://www.statista.com/statistics/320288/doctors-density-in-west-african-countries-suffering-from-ebola/.

[17] On the subject of Monrovia as being one of the first urban centres for Ebola outbreak, see Tolbert G. Nyenswah et al., 'Ebola and Its Control in Liberia, 2014–2015', *Emerging Infectious Diseases*, 22 (2016): 169–77.

[18] LIBR only started testing EBV in July when the US National Institute of Health provided some support. See Nyenswah et al., 'Ebola'; M. Allison Arwady et al., 'Evolution of Ebola Virus Disease from Exotic Infection to Global Health Priority, Liberia, Mid-2014', *Emerging Infectious Diseases*, 21 (2015): 578–84.

[19] WHO Briefing Note, 'Ebola Virus Disease: Occupational Safety and Health', 5 September 2014. https://www.who.int/occupational_health/publications/joint_who_ilo_ebola_briefingnote_5sept2014.pdf.

[20] On the prevalence of malaria in Liberia, see the 2011 malaria indicator survey report. https://dhsprogram.com/pubs/pdf/MIS12/MIS12.pdf.

other diseases, healthcare workers had to treat every sick person as a suspected EBV case until proven negative through laboratory testing. Healthcare workers had to dress in astronaut-like suits, a type of dress that many people were not familiar with in Liberia. Additionally, this personal protective equipment (PPE) and general PPE such as gloves and other protective gear were in short supply at healthcare facilities, including the Redemption Hospital. In an ill-prepared country, with a limited number of healthcare service providers, with limited protective gear, nurses and doctors became afraid to touch incoming patients. Whether these incoming patients were Ebola carriers or carriers of other treatable diseases, who knew? In the uncertainty, the sick had become objects to be feared.

Following the discovery of EBV cases at the Redemption Hospital, I read in the news in July that a senior medical doctor at the JFK Memorial Hospital had contracted the disease and had died. The hospital had closed down its emergency section because the hospital had been overrun by sick people.[21] I had visited this section of the hospital several times, and it had always been busy with emergency cases ranging from accidents from motor vehicles to acute diseases. Now, the door was shut. I did not know where we were heading.

Almost a week after the closure of the JFK emergency section, I heard the news that four nurses and a doctor from the Phebe Hospital in Bong County, central Liberia, had presented symptoms of Ebola and were headed to Monrovia for testing. My best friend's wife was a nurse and worked at Phebe. My fear increased. I called her: no response. I called her husband but he was deep in the forest of south-eastern Liberia and out of phone coverage. Was she one of the suspected cases? I broke down in tears. After four trying hours, she finally picked up my call and said she was not one of the suspected cases but that she was worried, as she had interacted with some of the nurses who were symptomatic and her blood sample was collected for testing in Monrovia. She was even afraid to nurse her baby. Her test proved negative the following day and this brought some relief.

All of the four nurses and the doctor tested positive and before long three of the nurses were dead. Phebe hospital was a ghost town. Patients discharged themselves and left. Nurses were no longer going to work because they did not have protective gear. New patients were afraid to go to hospitals. Patients

---

[21] Jonathan Paye-Layleh, 'Ebola Outbreak Kills Senior Liberian Doctor', *Record-Courier*, 28 July 2014. Retrieved 17 December 2021, from https://medicalxpress.com/news/2014-07-ebola-liberian-doctor-americans-infected.html.

became untouchable. A case in point was my friend's daughter. Suddenly she had a fever and was acutely sick. My friend took her to a hospital but the health workers were afraid to touch her. Again, there was no testing equipment at this facility and health workers did not have protective gear. The teenager suffered all by herself for two and a half hours and died. Samples taken from her body finally proved negative of Ebola but positive for chronic malaria.

I had planned to spend only one month in Liberia (25 May–25 June), but the living conditions of my children and grandma were not good. The heavy rainfall in June had flooded our apartment. I stayed for another month to find another apartment for them while making an effort to obtain visas for our three boys to take them with me to the United States. I did not have a vehicle, and I had to take public transport, usually a shared 1.6 Nissan Sunny cab. This vehicle is designed to take at most five people (three passengers in the back seat, one front passenger and a driver) but in Liberia four passengers are crammed in the back seat overloading the vehicle to six people. I was so afraid because they told us that an infected person's body fluids, including blood and sweat, should not touch an uninfected person. How could I manage as the scorching sun and humidity caused us to perspire? There was no way that four people crammed in a three-seater taxi could not touch one another. The minibuses were no different.

If lack of protective gear for health workers, poor infrastructure and public transportation presented challenges in the fight against Ebola, so did the disbelief, religious and cultural practices as well as the spread of misinformation. Initially, there were people in Liberia who did not believe that Ebola existed. They thought it was a plot by the government and non-governmental organizations (NGOs) to steal money. The disbeliefs and misinformation through rumour-mongering were highlighted two weeks before I travelled to the United States. It was rumoured that several individuals in various communities were giving children vaccines for protection against Ebola and, after injecting the vaccines, these children died. The Ministry of Health was still struggling to dispel this misinformation when I left Liberia in July 2014.

The impacts of Ebola on funeral rites

In Kpelle, just as in the rest of the sixteen ethnic groups in Liberia, we believe in reincarnation. For those who have passed from this earthly life to enter the new life, we have to perform rituals. Failure to do so may lead to our own destruction. Thus, we wash the bodies of our deceased loved ones, dress them up with the best attire our culture offers and speak to them directly just before burial. If we believe that the cause of death was with wicked intent through witchcraft or poisoning, we give razor blades to the dead and tell them directly to use the weapon to hunt down those responsible for their deaths. Each immediate family member and relatives are required to make this commitment. We also speak to the dead and ask for blessings. We ask them to speak to the rest of our ancestors who have passed away and to convey our best wishes to them. We ask them for a good harvest and long life. If we are facing difficulties in life we ask for their interventions. We do all of these things at the grave site where we face the body and talk to it directly.

At 104 years and probably the oldest elder in the Kpaquelleh Clan, my father was accustomed to the methods of traditional burial in Kpelle culture. His own death was unusual. Normally a man of his age would be sick prior to death. When the elders notice that an older person is sick and the person is likely to die, the rest of the elders of the community take the sick person to a secluded location. Children and sometimes women are not allowed to enter the sick person's room. The elders stay at the side of their colleague until he takes his last breath. If the deceased is female, the body is kept for three days; if a male, his remains are kept for four days before burial. Normally there is not an embalmment. The best way to preserve the corpse is to sit by it and drive the flies. The elders therefore stay with the body and sometimes change shifts while the funeral is arranged.

I had last seen my father in February 2014, when we interviewed him for our documentary. Shortly after I had returned to Madison to continue school after the spring break, news reached me that our father had passed away. The information was that he had refused to eat for an entire day and had slept with hunger that night. The following morning, he had asked to take a sunbath. He had lain on the mat, facing the rising sun, as one of my sisters was preparing soft rice for him. After cooking, she had taken his food to him, but she realized that his eyes were closed and that he was not breathing. Old Taylor Kpekpeh Yarkpawolo had gone to sleep permanently. We were in the middle of the spring semester, and it proved difficult for me to return to Liberia for the burial. My wife and I, along with other family members, remitted some money to help with the funeral. Since he passed just before the Ebola epidemic overtook the country, my father's burial went through all the usual rituals and he received a dignified burial. Barely five months later funeral rites had become completely alien.

On a cool humid day in August 2014, our cameraman captured an unimaginable scene: a blue Hyundai truck full of dead bodies all wrapped in white plastic body bags. Mark Korvayan, head of the Ebola Burial Team, said:

I'm so downhearted, I'm just seeing Liberians just dying, dying, dying … Let us pray that this virus leaves this country, because some people are still in a denial stage … For example, at PHP [Public Health Pond, a community in Monrovia], the man's wife died and we went there, and I took the body. I gave the health tattoo, do not enter the room, we locked the door and everything, we were to send the team to disinfect the room. The moment we left that same day, he went and burst the door and went inside the room. And his body is in this car. You see the challenges. You tell people, don't do this, they pass behind and do it. They say we are eating free money and the government is lying.

The seventeen dead bodies in the truck would be cremated later that day, in a crematorium. Cremation is a completely repugnant to Liberians' way of life.

As the virus spread, the number of people dying increased drastically. There were dead bodies everywhere, particularly in and around health facilities. The government of Liberia struggled to bury them. People resisted the burying of Ebola victims in their communities. Funeral homes could no longer cope with the number of deaths. Also, the traditional method of burying in Kpelle culture is common to other cultures in Liberia.[22] Those methods of burial, where the body is kept for a certain number of days, or where family members and loved ones touch the body, were no longer feasible. In fact, these practices served as major sources of transmission of the disease. One study found that more than 365 people contracted the EBV by attending a single funeral.[23]

On 31 July 2014, the Indian community in Liberia asked the government of Liberia to initiate cremation as a way of reducing the number of dead bodies in the street and as a method of containing the outbreak.[24] This request was in response to President Ellen Johnson Sirleaf's announcement the previous day that the government and its partners would cremate dead bodies.[25] This

---

[22] On the impacts of traditional and religious practices on the spread of Ebola, see Angellar Manguvo and Benford Mafuvadze, 'The Impact of Traditional and Religious Practices on the Spread of Ebola in West Africa: Time for a Strategic Shift', *Pan African Medical Journal*, 22 (2015): 9.

[23] Chulwoo Park, "Traditional Funeral and Burial Rituals and Ebola Outbreaks in West Africa: A Narrative Review of Causes and Strategy Interventions', *Journal of Health and Social Sciences*, 5 (2020): 73–90.

[24] The only crematorium in Liberia was built by the Indian community to cremate the bodies of Indian nationals who wanted to use cremation as burial method. See *Ebola in Liberia: Cremation of victims begins in Marshall* (n.d.). H5N1. Retrieved 17 December 2021, from https://crofsblogs.typepad.com/h5n1/2014/08/ebola-in-liberia-cremation-of-victims-begins-in-marshall.html.

[25] On 30 July 2014, the Liberian government announced sweeping strategies to contain the disease. Among them were the quarantining of several counties where the EBV was discovered; the declaration of 1 August 2014 as a non-working day to allow for 'disinfection and chlorination of all public facilities'; closure of all schools as well as cremation of the bodies of EBV victims. See Javier Blas, 'Liberia Declares Emergency Measures to Contain Ebola Outbreak', *Financial Times*, 30 July 2014. https://www.ft.com/content/c8e2e1b0-1800-11e4-a6e4-00144feabdc0.

announcement became a source of confusion and contempt. Family members' fear of cremation caused them to keep sick people at home and to make secret burials. Even when people suspected that their loved ones were suffering from Ebola, it was impossible not to take care of them. By July 2014, the majority of health facilities were either closed to the public or were overwhelmed by patients and dead bodies. Since touching sick people and dead bodies were major sources of the spreading of the disease, cremation was the only option available. The government of Liberia and partners like the Red Cross recruited and trained specialized burial teams. The teams were responsible for collecting bodies from the streets and from homes and to take them to the crematorium, located in Boys Town, lower Margibi county, some fifty miles east of Monrovia. Some estimates suggest that at least three thousand people were burned at the crematorium.[26]

Final words

Systemic corruption, civil wars, lack of trust in government, human activities in degrading natural habitats and cultural practices of burial all created the space where the EBV would thrive and contributed to its spread.[27] Four thousand eight hundred eight people died.[28] Researchers found that EBV may have jumped from bats to humans because of forest clearance in Liberia and Guinea, replacing them with monoculture oil palms.[29] Government-enforced quarantine via military intervention and unorthodox methods of cremation, with no adequate public awareness, did not stop but rather contributed to the spread of the disease. What was successful was community involvement. For example, during the heat of the outbreak, the people of Gomue self-imposed quarantine and wrote a letter informing everyone in the city not to visit the village until the outbreak was over. Prior to the Ebola outbreak, I had initiated community farming in Gomue. Rice we produced enabled the villagers to self-quarantine without worrying

---

[26] On the estimated number of dead bodies burned at the crematorium, see Al Varney Rogers and Robyn Dixon, 'Ebola's Lingering Pain: Liberians Rue Use of Cremation', *Los Angeles Times*, 11 March 2015. https://www.latimes.com/world/africa/la-fg-ebola-liberia-cremation-20150311-story.html.

[27] On the impacts of cultural practices on the spread of EBC, see Mohamed F. Jalloh et al., 'Evidence of Behaviour Change during an Ebola Virus Disease Outbreak, Sierra Leone', *Bulletin of the World Health Organization*, 98 (2020): 330–40.

[28] On the number Ebola victims, see Nyenswah et al., 'Ebola'.

[29] On the origin of the West African EBV, see Emmanuel Urey, 'Did Palm Oil Expansion Play a Role in the Ebola Crisis?', *Mongabay Environmental News*, 14 January 2015. https://news.mongabay.com/2015/01/did-palm-oil-expansion-play-a-role-in-the-ebola-crisis/.

about food shortages. Civil society organized and promoted hand washing. A combination of these efforts saw the incidence of EBV declining before the broader involvement of the international community. Ebola entangled itself around cultural memories of war and suffering; Ebola disrupted cultural norms and ritual expectations; Ebola exposed the structural flaws in politics, society and economy. In all these ways and more, Ebola was fear.

Postscript: I was able to get Lloyd, our third son, to the United States in September 2014. Bobby, the eldest, joined us in November 2016. We are once again united as a family, facing the coronavirus pandemic together.

2

Ebola *wahala*: Breaching experiments in a Sierra Leonean border town

Luisa Enria and Angus Fayia Tengbeh

On the eve of the Ebola outbreak that was to spread through Sierra Leone between 2014 and 2016, Kambia, a small town on the country's north-western border with Guinea, looked towards the future with anticipation. In 2012, works had been completed on a newly paved highway that finally connected Kambia District to the capital, Freetown. The road had long been a point of contention for Kambians. Frequent stories of day-long journeys, on uneven and dusty roads that would require passengers to bring a change of clothes for when they arrived in the city, were often recounted across town. The road had become a symbol of the District's perceived exclusion from the centres of power. The new highway was widely seen as recognition for the District's support of the government in the 2007 elections, and its re-election in 2012 brought hope of even more change to come.

Two years later, however, change arrived through very different means, first as rumour as the news of a new virus spreading across neighbouring Guinea and then as reality as Ebola made its way from the Eastern District of Kailahun across Sierra Leone. After the country reported its first official case in May 2014, the outbreak rapidly escalated, reaching hundreds of cases a week by the summer. A disease of 'love', as many described it at the time, Ebola spread rapidly through social networks, through acts of care for the sick or burial rites to show respect for

Luisa Enria acknowledges the support of a fellowship from the Economic and Social Research Council (Ref: ES/N01717X/1), which made this research possible, and the assistance and advice of Umarr Kamara, the EBOVAC-Salone team and all research participants. Angus F. Tengbeh acknowledges the support of a MasterCard Foundation Scholarship, Edinburgh, for his research and the Student Development Office, the University of Edinburgh, which partially funded this project through the placement-based dissertation funding opportunity. He would also like to acknowledge the support of Dr Mark Hellowell, dissertation supervisor; advice from Dr Shona Lee and Dr David Ishola; and the management of the EBOVAC-Salone project for serving as the host institution for data collection. Both authors are grateful to Myfanwy James and the editors for insightful comments on earlier drafts.

the dead. In July 2014, following the death of the only haemorrhagic fever expert in the country, Dr Umarr Khan, the President announced a state of emergency. New regulations were imposed, including curfews, checkpoints, fines and jail sentences, for failure to report the illness or death of family members or for secret burials that did not follow infection prevention protocols. In a two-year-long fight against the virus, Kambia became one of the last 'battlegrounds', the centre of the military-led 'Operation Northern Push' to stamp out final clusters of transmission and the site of a large vaccine trial.[1] Ebola, in other words, upended daily life in Kambia, claiming lives and disrupting social practices and relations. The town's very landscape morphed, as derelict buildings turned into emergency operation hubs and new homes sprang up thanks to the 'Ebola money' that benefitted only a few working for the response.

Ebola was undoubtedly a moment of rupture, not simply in terms of illness and death but because of profound upheavals in social practices and relations. The declaration of a state of emergency, or, as Janet Roitman puts it, the epistemological claim that 'this is crisis', has significant consequences in redrawing social and political landscapes.[2] The official denomination of an event, or a moment, as crisis makes certain types of interventions possible, while foreclosing other avenues. During the Ebola outbreak in Sierra Leone, for example, the 'epistemic shift' that followed the declaration of a Public Health Emergency of International Concern (PHEIC) facilitated the mobilization of funding, the rapid development and testing of therapeutics and vaccines and the mobilization of the 'martial global imagination for response to epidemics', as both British and Sierra Leonean armed forces were called in to support the logistical organization of the Ebola response.[3] These configurations of national crisis undoubtedly impacted everyday life even for those not directly affected by the disease, not least through normative distinctions between 'good citizens' complying to new regulations and the 'dangerous bodies' needing to be policed and contained.[4] New regulations and political identities also became intertwined

---

[1] L. Enria, 'The Ebola Crisis in Sierra Leone: Mediating Containment and Engagement in Humanitarian Emergencies', *Development and Change*, 50 (2019): 1602–23; A. F. Tengbeh et al., '"We Are the Heroes Because We Are Ready to Die for This Country": Participants' Decision-Making and Grounded Ethics in an Ebola Vaccine Clinical Trial', *Social Science and Medicine*, 203 (2018): 35–42.
[2] J. Roitman, *Anti-Crisis* (Durham, NC: Duke University Press, 2013).
[3] A. H. Kelly, 'Ebola Vaccines, Evidentiary Charisma and the Rise of Global Health Emergency Research', *Economy and Society*, 47 (2018): 135–61, at 137; A. Desclaux, M. Diop and S. Doyon, 'Fear and Containment', *The Politics of Fear: Médecins Sans Frontières and the West African Ebola Epidemic*, ed. M. Hofman and S. Au (Oxford: Oxford University Press, 2017), 212; A. Benton, 'Whose Security? Militarization and Securitization during West Africa's Ebola Outbreak', *The Politics of Fear*, ed. Hofman and Au.
[4] Enria, 'Ebola Crisis in Sierra Leone'.

with individual experiences of other, often more personal kinds of crisis, as citizens continued to confront the insecure livelihoods that denote the lives of many Sierra Leoneans also in times of 'normality'.

The relationship between crisis and the everyday has been the focus of anthropological enquiries, which have not only highlighted the lived experience of those living in states of emergency but also questioned the very concept of crisis in contexts where it may be seen as chronic. Henrik Vigh, for example, proposes a consideration not of crisis *in context* but rather crisis *as context*. Instead of seeing crisis as an event, a tangible moment of rupture, light is shed on how individuals navigate precarious and uncertain landscapes marked by poverty and violence.[5] Conversely, Veena Das disrupts conceptualizations of the everyday, to focus not only on how it is 'actualized in routine and repetition, but also how it contains the possibilities of innovation and moral striving'.[6] In this chapter, we take these reflections as points of departure to look at the relationship between crisis and the everyday by considering how the disruptions caused by 'crisis as event' afford access to 'crisis as context' – that is, how declarations of crisis and their material consequences make what was once taken for granted in the everyday suddenly and jarringly visible. To do this, we borrow from the work of sociologist Harold Garfinkel whose 'breaching experiments' sought to suspend unspoken rules of social interactions to reveal implicit background knowledge about how societies work.[7] In particular, Garfinkel's work intended to highlight the moral claims people make on each other on a daily basis as they make meaning of the world together. An awareness of the impact of the everyday on broader societal phenomena emerges through a process of being forced to become aware of underlying rules, claims and realities that are embedded in the social fabric and seem to be obvious. In turn, the moral underpinnings of the everyday come into question. More recently, Graham Scambler has invited the study of the Covid-19 pandemic as a breaching experiment, to see how it is 'putting a gigantic spanner in the works of neoliberal governance, in the process exposing the widening cracks and fissures of what [he has] called the

---

[5] H. Vigh, 'Crisis and Chronicity: Anthropological Perspectives on Continuous Conflict and Decline', *Ethnos*, 73 (2008): 5–24.
[6] V. Das, 'On Singularity and the Event: Further Reflections on the Ordinary', *Recovering the Human Subject: Freedom, Creativity and Decision* (Cambridge: Cambridge University Press, 2018), 53–73, at 58.
[7] J. Heritage, 'Harold Garfinkel', *Key Sociological Thinkers* (Houndmills: Palgrave Macmillan, 1998), 175–88.

"fractured society"' in the UK.[8] As a 'natural experiment', he argues, 'COVID has shone a bright light onto UK society, exposing, and then amplifying, its fractures'.[9]

We propose to apply this perspective to explore how the Ebola crisis – or *wahala*, meaning trouble – may have acted as a breaching experiment, highlighting longer-standing fractures in Sierra Leonean society and giving voice to older narratives of social suffering. At the same time, we consider the broader utility of this concept for making sense of crisis, and epidemics more specifically, in relation to ethnographic reflections on the everyday. We draw, therefore, on ethnographic accounts and narratives of individuals directly affected by the outbreak. We explore how Ebola reconfigured lifeworlds and built environments as well as social and political relations. Inspired by Mbembe and Roitman, we start with a focus on the 'physicality' of crisis, taking a tour of Kambia's buildings on which Ebola left a mark, to highlight how 'the crisis is inscribed in the everyday ... landscape, in its material structures such as roads, residences and office buildings and in social interactions and relations of power, profit and subsistence'.[10] Paying particular attention to the affective entanglements generated by the disease and its response, the intersections of fears and hopes, disappointments and anticipation, we consider the role of epidemics like Ebola as 'breaching experiments', where social order is at once revealed and upended.

The data presented in this chapter was collected primarily through two qualitative research projects. The first (led by LE) focused on the effects of the Ebola outbreak on state–society relations in Freetown and Kambia District and entailed five months of ethnographic research, reviews of grey literature and official documents (including those obtained from key agencies involved in the Ebola response), participant observation and in-depth interviews in January 2017, August–November 2017 and May 2017. The second project (led by AFT) focused on the experience of Maternal and Child Health Aide nurses (MCH Aides) during and after the Ebola outbreak, conducted in May 2019. Data was collected through interactive in-depth interviews with MCH Aides in Peripheral Health Units in the Kambia District and senior members of the Kambia District Health Management Team. The data and analysis are contextualized in both authors' experiences conducting ethnographic research during and after the

---

[8] G. Scambler, 'Covid-19 as a "Breaching Experiment": Exposing the Fractured Society', *Health Sociology Review*, 29 (2020): 140–8, at 140.
[9] Scambler, 'Covid-19', 147.
[10] A. Mbembe and J. Roitman, 'Figures of the Subject in Times of Crisis', *Public Culture*, 7 (1995): 323–52, at 327.

Ebola outbreak, over fourteen months of collaboration in the Ebola vaccine trials in Kambia District between 2015 and 2016.[11]

Ebola in Kambia

In the summer of 2015, a year after the first cases of Ebola had been identified in Kailahun, Kambia was targeted as one of two final 'hot spot' districts to end the epidemic. The strict curfews, checkpoints and military patrols of Operation Northern Push reminded Kambians of the eleven-year civil war that ended in 2002. The war had started with a group of rebels entering Eastern Sierra Leone from Liberia and saw some of its final battles in Kambia. People argued that Ebola followed the same trajectory. After many months of hearing about how the virus was taking the lives of healthcare workers (HCWs) and community members in other parts of the country, stories of how Ebola entered the District were varied. Many who worked for the response remembered a truck driver who had arrived from the South and had died, or an older woman who escaped quarantine in a neighbouring District, for example, as the cases that made them realize this was going to become 'a weapon in the lives of our people', as a senior response official put it. Specific transmission chains remained etched in collective memory and were referred to in conversation well beyond the end of the epidemic, to remember how bad things became: a whole family wiped out in the village in Mambolo chiefdom; or a case that sparked a confrontation between a whole village in quarantine and military officials posted from Freetown in Tonko Limba chiefdom.

Ebola's mark on the history of the district was also visible in how it changed Kambia town's built environment, adding onto the visible scars of previous crises. Across the old town, burnt-down buildings, remnants of columns and blackened walls with grass growing between them are permanent reminders of the conflict, as families either refused or were unable to rebuild or demolish the structures after they were torched by the Revolutionary United Front during their attack and siege of the town in 1995. These abandoned buildings posed a silent accusation, evidence that post-war peace dividends had been slow to come to this border town. As cases of Ebola tallied up, and the government realized

---

[11] Tengbeh, 'We Are the Heroes'; L. Enria et al., 'Power, Fairness and Trust: Understanding and Engaging with Vaccine Trial Participants and Communities in the Setting up the EBOVAC-Salone Vaccine Trial in Sierra Leone', *BMC Public Health*, 16 (2016): 1–10.

the need for a decentralized response, old unused buildings like the former Resource Centre were brought back to life to be transformed into a makeshift District Ebola Response Centre. In what used to be meeting halls for the District Council, the Republic of Sierra Leone Armed Forces (RSLAF) presided over evening briefings, reporting the names and circumstances of individual cases and planning the activities of different pillars of the response. These transformations did not go uncontested. Discussions over where a holding (and later treatment) centre for suspected and confirmed Ebola cases would be located generated much debate. An RSLAF Report from 19th August notes these challenges as well as the intertwining of histories of crisis in these deliberations:

> The District Health Medical Team and the Task Force on Ebola are currently engaging the Catholic Mission in Kambia for the use of a building back of the Kolenten Senior Secondary School which was used as a transit centre for refugees. Nonetheless, there is stiff resistance from the community on the establishment of the Holding Centre in the said facility.[12]

Much has been written to critique narratives of 'resistance' that dominated portrayals of communities, especially in the early parts of the epidemic.[13] Social scientists highlighted that portrayals centring on 'resistant communities' and cultural practices to explain challenges in containing transmission misrepresented the role of 'culture', ignored community-level adaptability and failed to engage with the priorities of affected communities when caring for loved ones.[14] Furthermore, these narratives about communities had direct consequences, in terms of creating dividing practices between 'good' and 'bad' citizens, shifting power relations within affected communities and in some areas eroding much-needed trust in the response.[15] These portrayals were at once unique to the Ebola emergency because of the particular connection made between community behaviour and infectious disease dynamics. At the same time, they were firmly rooted in longer-term and much broader narrative

---

[12] Strategic Situation Group (SSG) Report from 19th August, Ministry of Defence, Freetown.
[13] S. A. Abramowitz et al., 'Community-Centered Responses to Ebola in Urban Liberia: The View from Below', *PLoS Neglected Tropical Diseases*, 9 (2015): 1–18; F. Le Marcis, L. Enria, S. Abramowitz, A. Marí-Sáez and S. L. B. Faye, 'Three Acts of Resistance during the 2014–16 West Africa Ebola Epidemic', *Journal of Humanitarian Affairs*, 2 (2019): 23–31; A. Wilkinson, M. Parker, F. Martineau and M. Leach, 'Engaging "Communities": Anthropological Insights from the West African Ebola Epidemic', *Philosophical Transactions of the Royal Society B*, 372 (2017).
[14] C. Chandler et al., 'Ebola: Limitations of Correcting Misinformation', *Lancet*, 385 (2015): 1275–7; P. Richards, *Ebola: How a People's Science Helped End an Epidemic* (London: Zed Books, 2016).
[15] Enria, 'Ebola Crisis in Sierra Leone'; L. Enria, 'Unsettled Authority and Humanitarian Practice: Reflections on Local Legitimacy from Sierra Leone's Borderlands', *Oxford Development Studies*, 48 (2020): 387–99.

structures: those that imagine communities in places like Sierra Leone as 'other' and in need of intervention common to development paradigms, and specific histories of subjectification and marginalization of rural and poor citizens in the making of modern Sierra Leone.[16]

In telling a localized history of Ebola in Kambia, therefore, we consider how these social dynamics and the relationship between Kambians and those in positions of power were shaped by the realities generated by crisis; and we reveal longer-standing processes of marginalization. Here we particularly highlight how these relations and contestations over crisis management were materialized through buildings such as the holding centre and how these processes were written over the prior histories that these buildings represented.

The Catholic Mission that the RSLAF approached for the holding centre had a long but fraught presence in Kambia. European nuns had only recently started returning after a long time away following a kidnapping incident during the war. Ultimately, another of their buildings, a former centre for polio sufferers that lay empty, was chosen as the site for the Ebola centre. Those living in its surroundings tried to protest the decision, expressing their fears that especially during the rainy season the infection might travel from the nearby centre to their homes. These holding centres, as a senior response official noted, were feared to be 'death chambers', especially in the early parts of the epidemic where patients could not be treated in Kambia and would either be taken to the Eastern District of Kenema or die there. With little visibility as to what happened within the centres and mistrust rife in a general atmosphere of anxiety, rumours circulated that when people entered the holding centre they would never come back – that they were being murdered in occult rituals or that they were asphyxiated with chlorine used for decontamination. Neighbourhood protesters ultimately felt powerless in their demands: 'you can't fight government,' one argued, adding that they did not have anyone to turn to: those who would normally hear complaints, such as the Paramount Chief, were working with the Ebola response to confirm these decisions.

Another contentious transformation of the town's landscape similarly revealed simmering tensions over perceived imbalances of the impacts of Ebola on different Kambians. As the epidemic progressed, and as funding ramped up,

---

[16] T. M. Li, *The Will to Improve: Governmentality, Development and the Practice of Politics* (Durham, NC: Duke University Press, 2007); L. Enria and S. Lees, 'Citizens, Dependents, Sons of the Soil: Defining Political Subjectivities through Encounters with Biomedicine during the Ebola Epidemic in Sierra Leone', *Medicine Anthropology Theory*, 5 (2018): 30–55; D. Harris, *Sierra Leone: A Political History* (London: Hurst, 2013).

especially following the PHEIC announcement, a response that had largely been made up of volunteers was gradually formalized, with opportunities for jobs and incentives across the range of response pillars: members of burial teams, decontamination, social mobilization and swabbers. Initially, these were far from coveted positions, not only because of the significant risk associated with coming into contact with potentially infected patients but also because of the stigma associated with these roles given the widespread mistrust of the Ebola response noted above. However, as the epidemic developed, these unpopular jobs also became one of the main sources of employment in a District that had often been overlooked by development or investment opportunities prior to the crisis. The response, in other words, gave rise to a particular emergency economy that was known in local discussions as 'Ebola money'. Ebola money materialized most visibly in new houses being built across town, as response workers attempted to invest in the future, making the most of what they knew would be a short-term opportunity. Narratives around Ebola money, and specifically those who had been 'eating it' and those who had not, were rife around Kambia and loaded with moral judgement. The new buildings, for some, symbolized an accumulation of wealth, the morality of which was at best ambiguous, as it was seen to rely on the suffering of others. These concerns were expressed, for example, through rumours that new cases of Ebola at the tail end of the epidemic were fabricated to ensure Ebola workers could continue profiting, or that announcements of new infections were met with jubilation in the notorious holding centre. In practice of course, the story was far more complex, including experiences of trauma, burnout and exclusion for response workers, as discussed below. However, the materiality of the Ebola crisis, visible in its changes on Kambia's landscape, sets the stage for a broader discussion of how this moment of rupture cast light on dynamics of inequality and power(lessness), giving new vocabularies for moral and political critiques with much deeper roots than the arrival of Ebola on the scene.

Experiences of the crisis

Ebola's arrival in Kambia, in its many guises, from state-of-emergency regulations, deaths and shifting physical and social landscape, was experienced by its inhabitants through a range of feelings. Retellings of what happened during that time were emotionally charged, reflecting for some the trauma of individual experiences with the disease, as well as the anger, frustration, hopes and expectations roused by a multifaceted crisis and its effects on the town's daily life. Affective engagements with memories of Ebola allow us to consider both the moral upheaval of the state of emergency and how this moment of rupture cast light on much longer-standing realities that may have otherwise been left unspoken. We focus on three examples to highlight this: MCH Aides, Ebola response workers and families placed in quarantine.[17]

The experience of HCWs is an obvious starting point to think about the wide range of emotions imbued in memories of the outbreak. HCWs played a crucial role in controlling the outbreak, while also trying to ensure the continued running of their health facilities and the provision of routine health services. When recounting their experiences at the start of the outbreak, HCWs remembered feeling unprepared, both in terms of their experiences and the available structures, supplies and amenities. The death of the country's only virologist in the early stages of the outbreak had shaken up the whole profession, highlighting a sense of collective inexperience in dealing with this 'new virus'. Health staff were also painfully aware that their colleagues were among the most affected, reporting high rates of infection and deaths among those working on the front lines, often 'with bare hands', as supplies of personal protective equipment (PPE) were often limited.[18] The constant reports exacerbated fear, as HCWs continued to provide services in facilities that were ill-equipped to protect them. This meant also that HCWs increasingly became suspicious of their patients, frightened that they may not disclose their exposure to the disease. As a nurse in one of the health facilities argued:

> Some [patients] would run from quarantine homes, but they would not tell you the health worker about it. At the end of the day, you would treat them and become infected. When we knew about this dishonesty, our bosses told us to treat every patient as a potential case.

Especially in the early days of the epidemic, poor conditions in quarantine homes and widespread anxiety that people in quarantine would become infected or lose their livelihoods meant that there were frequent reports of suspected Ebola cases running away. While community-level mistrust has been the focus

---

[17] The quotes and observations relating to MCH Aides come from ethnographic field notes and transcripts of in-depth interviews with nurses conducted in Kambia District in May 2019 for the project led by AFT, outlined in the introduction. Quotes and observations regarding response workers and families come from ethnographic research and transcripts of in-depth interviews with key informants in Kambia District between August and November 2017.

[18] I. Abdullah and A. B. Kamara, 'Confronting Ebola with Bare Hands: Sierra Leone's Health Sector on the Eve of the Ebola Epidemic', *Understanding West Africa's Ebola Epidemic: Towards a Political Economy*, ed. I. Abdullah and I. O. D. Rashid (Chicago: University of Chicago Press, 2017).

of attention of post-epidemic analyses, the concern generated by these events, and the fear that these cases would show up at other facilities without disclosing where they came from (so as not to be taken to a treatment centre), also eroded HCWs' trust in their patients. This was particularly marked for Maternal and Child Health Aide nurses who, while being among the lowest cadre of staff, were also directly involved in handling childbirth in Kambia's rural areas. This meant that they felt they did not have a choice: 'If a pregnant woman comes in labour, you just have to see her.'

Fears associated with experiences in the workplace were augmented by concerns about infecting close family members and loved ones. To protect those closest to them, some HCWs self-isolated or stopped going home after work at the peak of the outbreak. One nurse who was breastfeeding at the time of Ebola found herself quarantined with her baby and emphasized seeing this as a cost of her sacrifice:

> I took care of one pregnant woman because all our friends were afraid. But I went and looked after her because she was in labour. At the end of the day, she died, and it was later discovered that she was [EVD] positive. They had to put all of us that took care of her under quarantine. For me I was quarantined with my baby. So, you see!

Many described the daily rituals they put in place to try and protect their loved ones and to assuage the common ostracization faced by those associated with the Ebola response, including changing clothes before returning home.

These fears were explicitly not articulated as inevitable side effects of an unfolding crisis. They were in fact accompanied by profound anger and frustration that resonated across all our conversations with HCWs as they recalled the challenges they faced during the epidemic. Feeling unprepared and at risk was a result of insufficient supply of PPE and required training. Experiences of quarantine were also a source of anger as HCWs felt that although they had made a sacrifice and had put their lives on the line, they had not been treated with the respect they deserved by those in charge of the response:

> We were quarantined with no food and water and [when] they finally started bringing food, they would stand there and throw the food at us. But like for me, I never gave up because this is something I signed up for.

This situation was common in Sierra Leone, especially during the early stages of the response. As transmissions increased, there were reports of quarantine homes not receiving supplies of food, water and other sanitary facilities. This was also one of the reasons responsible for people escaping from quarantine homes as they went in search of food and water.

Then again, the evolution of the epidemic response revealed a sharp contrast between the deep challenges for the Sierra Leonean health system and what was possible when provided adequate funding and support through an emergency response. The increase in the number of partners working on the response meant that supplies of PPE and other equipment also increased. In addition, there was a rise in training and supportive supervision for mentorship and support for frontline health workers: 'We hardly ran out of supplies during the [later parts of the] outbreak. We had enough gloves, PPEs, gowns, boots, kits and drugs. All the NGOs used to bring supplies for us in the centre.'

Some facilities also benefited from renovations, in particular to their water and sanitation services and labour wards. The outbreak brought sudden international attention to poor health outcomes and health system fragilities in Sierra Leone, including renovations, capacity building, the arrival of foreign doctors supporting the Kambia government hospital and the allocation of five new ambulances for swift patient referrals. These developments brought hope to Kambian HCWs that the crisis might serve to draw attention to the long-standing under-resourcing of the healthcare system, crippled by structural adjustment programmes, civil war and narrowly focused vertical programming.[19] The extreme examples of what they faced during the outbreak made it possible to question and point to everyday challenges faced by a largely volunteer-based workforce. In practice however, these hopes were as short-lived as the international attention span, which quickly moved to the next crisis, as did a new government, hoping to refocus its attention on education. In 2019, for example, most health facilities we visited had no running water, either because wells had dried up or because there were no or broken connection pipes, with no means for repair.

Similar emotional trajectories, excavating both the ordinary and the extraordinary, could be found in the memories of those involved directly in the Ebola response.[20] Alhassan, who was twenty-five years old at the time Ebola started, heard that the newly established DERC was calling people to work for the response. At first, he said: 'When the work came, none of us had the *mind* [courage] to go and work,' but after some time him and his friends

---

[19] A. Benton and K. Y. Dionne, 'International Political Economy and the 2014 West African Ebola Outbreak', *African Studies Review*, 58 (2015): 223–36.

[20] Names have been changed.

thought they should go and hear what was being offered. In that meeting a team of decontaminators from Nigeria explained the nature of the work, including the fact that in the process of undressing from the PPE it would be possible to become infected. Initially they all refused. After a one-on-one conversation with a member of the team who promised he would be well trained to protect himself, Alhassan tried to put his fears aside and was among the first to join the decontamination team. He began working but recalled: 'my heart was not at rest because people were talking that [they] were going to die [on the job].' His job was particularly contentious because of the widespread rumours circulating around town that Ebola was not real but that the response was killing people by suffocating them with chlorine. Alhassan himself was not really convinced initially about the disease, its origins or whether the epidemic hid nefarious intentions by the government or the international community. Everything changed for him the first time he entered the holding centre:

> I saw blood all over the place. That was the time I said the thing is true because I saw blood all over. ... They also had pans where they were vomiting and all of those; we were the ones who disinfected all of them. So, when I began seeing those things that was the time I believed, because I was also denying. ... That work on that day, I did not feel fine. I didn't know we were to wear the PPE, after using the PPE, when you go back your head would spin.

Within one week he started feeling sick and was concerned he had been infected. He quickly recovered but the fear of contracting Ebola remained. His family had similar concerns and for the duration of his contract he had to rent a room away from his family home. This bad feeling was hard to shake as people started dying around him, from swabbers to ambulance drivers.

The job felt risky in more than one way. Alhassan recalled being sent to a very distant community close to the Guinean border, where he had to negotiate broken trust in order to do his job. The people who needed to be quarantined had crossed over to an island to escape, as they had been told that soldiers were coming to beat them up. This was following a recent confrontation that saw community members beat a soldier, and they now feared retaliation. As he went in, he had no idea what to expect:

> When we went, we dressed [in PPE] and went into the huts. But when I entered, I heard a voice, but I thought it was just something else. Since I talk Temne, so I had to ask in Temne; '*Kaneh yi do-a*' [who is there]? then the person answered saying '*mineŋ*' [is me]. So when I went to him and began to interview him and he told me he is not well. Then I asked him if he is the only one there and he said

no, and that the other woman is in the other corner. She had isolated herself into a corner. So, I had to look for her and I saw her.

Because this was a riverine area there was no way of transporting the two sick people except by getting on a bike with them. Alhassan's memories centred on the fears and uncertainty associated with his job, but he also reflected on the opportunities that became available to him that he would not have had otherwise. From being unemployed and relying on others for his daily living he became, for a short time, a patron for his friends:

> They were surviving from us [who worked in the response], because when they paid us we would give them some hundred thousand or fifty thousand [Leones], because 'Ebola money', when they pay it cannot be hidden. They will just come and pay and everybody will know about it. So those who were not working were the ones who would follow us where they were going to pay us. Some will go and stand in the corner so that when they pay us we could be able to give them their fifty thousand, twenty or ten thousand. They also wanted to begin the work but there was no way again [they were no longer hiring].

This new situation generated significant social pressure for Alhassan but it also, at least temporarily, improved his social standing and allowed him to make changes to his and his family's life. From his time in the response, he was able to build a home for himself and his family, making an addition to the contentious 'Ebola money' buildings. Rejoining the very large rank of unemployed youth in Sierra Leone immediately after the outbreak, Alhassan's reflections on this difficult time mirrored the ambiguous nature of the crisis and its relationship to the underlying political economy of Sierra Leone. Alhassan had also been part of the initial protest at the holding centre site, who dissipated because of a feeling of powerlessness to change the course of the decision. 'You can't fight government', those involved in the protest said.

The same sentiment was often repeated to describe reactions to being quarantined by those who were directly affected. The last case of the Sierra Leonean epidemic, for example, resulted in the need to quarantine several homes in a town in Kambia District. Members of the compound recalled how a relative who had come to visit them over the holidays had later died and a swab of her corpse had proved positive. When they heard the news, some family members had tried to run away. Fatmata, one of the women whose house was quarantined, said it was *fraidness* (fear) that prompted the decision, but that she was found and taken back in a jeep. They stayed in the quarantine for twenty-two days, and in the initial days, the Ebola response had been able to provide them with food and cooking materials to sustain themselves. During the period of their quarantine, however, their town experienced a riot as young people rebelled against a rumour that the local market was to be shut because of Ebola regulations. Over two days tensions escalated, and confrontations between security officers and young town residents resulted in the burning of a police station and the wounding of a young man by a police firearm. At night, town residents put up a checkpoint and rumours circulated that jeeps associated with the response or carrying local leaders responsible for implementing regulations would be attacked. Fatmata and her family had not seen the protests – they had remained in quarantine – but they had heard the *hala hala* (commotion). Their supplies stopped over those days, but they had understood and at least partly shared the frustrations that led to the riot. Fatmata noted: 'We had no chance to protest but we were not happy, we were surrounded by soldiers, we took it like, if we tried to do anything, they'd shoot at us.'

Discussions with Fatmata and others who had been quarantined over this period highlighted the tensions inherent in a wide range of emotions, from frustrations with the Ebola response and fears associated with a militarized response to a level of acceptance of a power that was beyond their control and expectations that the powerful might provide for the poor in times of crisis. For example, provisions of rice and other supplies for those in quarantine had made clear that it was possible for government to take care of its people, but expectations of care tended to be fulfilled solely in moments of crisis. A year after the outbreak had ended, the family continued to struggle to make ends meet, as the head of household had left them on their own, finding better opportunities in the town to which he had escaped during quarantine. In addition, expectations of provision and care were outweighed by anxieties associated with being 'surrounded by soldiers' during quarantine, as well as apprehension as to what happened to those who tried to 'fight government'. Instead, our discussions were punctuated by repetitions that, ultimately, you just had to *biyah* (bear it or endure it). These tensions gave voice to citizens' assumptions about their relationship to government, as expectations of services gave way to deeper convictions that power is something to be endured and that there are limited possibilities for change through confrontation. Compliance with Ebola regulations, then, while often interpreted as a sign of trust and contrasted with forms of resistance, may have been instead a result of fear and concerns about what might happen if they did not comply, at least in some cases. Rumours about the epidemic or defiance of regulations were not the only symptoms of a fragile social contract that came apart at the seams under the spotlight of the emergency.

Ebola as a breaching experiment

We started this chapter considering how the Kambia-Freetown road generated feelings of hope and expectations that were swiftly replaced by fear, anxiety and disillusionment ushered in by the *wahala* caused by the 2014–16 Ebola epidemic. By recounting the history of Ebola in a border town, through the personal experiences of some of its inhabitants, we have proposed to see this period of considerable social change as a 'breaching experiment'. Framing Ebola as a breaching experiment allows us to explore the relationship between crisis and the everyday by noting how a temporary state of emergency rendered visible the pre-existing, chronic crises that lay underneath. The Ebola crisis breached social conventions of 'normality', altering practices of life and death, fuelling mistrust within communities and introducing a militarized state of exception. In so doing, it simultaneously revealed existing fractures and gave voice to contestations that predated the emergency but only found expression in this moment of disjuncture. We agree therefore with Vigh's argument that notions of crisis as a singular event are unsatisfactory in helping us understand how people navigate terrains marked by chronic crisis, and that we are better served by a focus on crisis *as context*.[21] We add to this discussion by reflecting on how singular events that come to be collectively understood as 'crisis' not only produce specific crisis terrains that become intertwined with personal efforts to navigate already uncertain waters but also bring into relief the cracks in what was considered to be 'normal'.

Following Mbembe and Roitman's suggestion, we traced a 'geography of the crisis' to explore 'the forms of inscription of the crisis in public space, the body and material life, in brief, its physicality'.[22] In Kambia, different histories of crises became superimposed, as memories of the war and failed post-conflict development ambitions were brought back to life as the town's built environment was transformed by the arrival of the Ebola response. Tracing the emotions roused by efforts to convert old buildings to house disease-control operations, the fears surrounding rumoured 'death chambers' and unscrupulous response workers, and the erection of new homes built on 'Ebola money', pointed us to simmering tensions and contestations. As has been argued elsewhere, rumours, far from being a sign of misinformation, are rather better understood as

---

[21] Vigh, 'Crisis and Chronicity'.
[22] Mbembe and Roitman, 'Figures of the Subject'.

indicators of deeper anxieties and mistrust.[23] Perceptions of the Ebola response's possibly murderous or occult intentions, for example, cannot be extricated from longer-term histories of extraction and violence that have characterized Sierra Leone's colonial and postcolonial engagement with external interventions.[24] Similarly, the individual stories and affective engagements with the crisis of the nurses, response workers and families shared in this chapter highlight both the extreme challenges and often traumatic lived experiences of the Ebola crisis and at the same time how they brought to the surface individual and collective navigations of other kinds of crises that unfold in the everyday.

Reflections from maternal and child health nurses, for example, highlighted the anxieties and frustrations associated with carrying out their duties in the midst of an epidemic, where trust in their patients and in each other felt at breaking point. These feelings were connected to the perception of neglect, of nurses having been left to sacrifice themselves to fight against the virus without supplies. Their hopes, later turned to disillusionment, were that the crisis would bring attention to the much deeper problems facing the health system. Ebola, in other words, created an opportunity, however temporary, for everyone to see what the nurses had known all along: beyond the pressures of the crisis, health centres had been operating with limited supplies of water and electricity, often reliant on volunteer labour. Just as social scientists writing on the response emphasized the structural causes of the Ebola outbreak, nurses' affective engagements with Ebola and its aftermath highlighted that while the crisis heightened their fears, the waters they had been navigating prior to the crisis were already turbulent.

Similarly, contestations around 'Ebola money' and the experiences of young men like Alhassan highlighted the underpinnings of an economic crisis as well as a crisis of moral economy. Youth unemployment had been at the centre of policy debates since the end of the war, identified as a root cause of conflict and as such a key peacebuilding priority.[25] More than a decade after the end of the civil war, it had remained difficult to create opportunities for young people like Alhassan. The Ebola outbreak exacerbated this situation as investment withdrew (not least as it coincided with a drop in the price of iron ore, Sierra Leone's primary export) and state-of-emergency regulations decimated livelihoods. Yet Alhassan's reflections on whether to join the Ebola response and what this meant

---

[23] L. White, *Speaking with Vampires: Rumor and History in Colonial Africa* (Berkeley: University of California Press, 2000).

[24] Tengbeh et al., 'We Are the Heroes'; Enria et al., 'Power, Fairness and Trust'.

[25] K. Mitton, 'Where Is the War? Explaining Peace in Sierra Leone', *International Peacekeeping*, 20 (2013): 321–37.

for his life trajectory shed light on a particular political economy of crisis with roots predating the epidemic, whereby an emergency response in extremely risky conditions became the only opportunity for someone like him to make a living and provide for his family. The queues of friends waiting for 'Ebola money' to be redistributed to those who were not employed, and critiques of individual accumulation off the back of the suffering of others (expressed in the rumours of a jubilant response of workers when new cases were announced), point to the complex moral deliberations surrounding this political economy of crisis. The grammar of critique underpinning 'Ebola money' accusations applies more broadly to a pointed questioning of the 'background knowledge', or unspoken rules, of an exclusionary economy where individual accumulation in the face of widespread unemployment could be interpreted as moral failure or even greed.[26] The intensity of emotion sparked by the crisis and the extreme distance between those seemingly profiting and those whose lives and livelihoods had been cut short gave voice to new, more urgent articulations of the unjust underpinnings of the post-war economy.

Finally, the stories of those who tried to protest the holding centre and the family who was quarantined at the tail end of the epidemic point to a simmering political crisis. The Ebola outbreak and its associated response measures undoubtedly generated fear and mistrust. Deeper analysis of the crisis pointed to the historical foundations of mistrust, tracing a genealogy of exclusion, state erosion and violence that contributed to diffidence about and in some cases resistance to the Ebola response. The crisis, in other words, generated feelings of insecurity with deeper roots. But our conversations in Kambia also show the converse to be true: experiences of the crisis and reactions to the extreme realities of the state of emergency tell us something about citizens' perceptions of their standing in relation to state forces in the everyday. Feelings of 'powerlessness' in questioning the regulations and their impact, or the fear associated with quarantines manned by military officers, raise questions about the nature of the social contract.

The Ebola crisis, as a moment of rupture, brought into sharp relief a range of fractures in the social fabric. The moral, political and economic underpinnings of the 'normal' were questioned and made more urgent through the intense manifestation of crisis. A burgeoning social science of epidemics urges us to see these phenomena not simply as biological but profoundly social events.[27] Seeing

---

[26] L. Enria, *The Politics of Work in a Post-Conflict State: Youth, Labour & Violence in Sierra Leone* (Oxford: James Currey, 2018).

[27] A. H. Kelly, F. Keck and C. Lynteris, *The Anthropology of Epidemics* (London: Routledge, 2019).

Ebola as a breaching experiment in Kambia, we have proposed that epidemics are not simply social in the conditions of their production or in the social impact they have but in what they make visible. The intensity of Kambians' emotions and affective engagement with a moment of crisis made it possible to question the underpinnings of the everyday, challenging crisis 'as context'.

3

History before corona: Memory, experience and emotions

Bettina Hitzer

Shortly after everything had unexpectedly gone silent on the streets of Germany in the spring of 2020 – when strict preventive measures suddenly shut down most businesses and venues of social life – experts working from home began trying to make sense of it all. Perhaps unsurprisingly, not a few proclaimed that the lockdown occasioned by the virus represented a caesura, and even a 'world-historical caesura', as Kassel-based sociologist Heinz Bude put it in a much-quoted interview with the Berlin daily *Tagesspiegel*.[1] Historian Martin Sabrow also described the immediate reaction to the virus's spread as the 'shock of the unprecedented', a shock that temporarily blinded many to the numerous historical continuities.[2] But most historians of medicine insistently sought to draw attention to such precedents. Published in the year *before* the coronavirus, historian Mark Honigsbaum's book *The Pandemic Century* detailed the series of pandemics that came before this moment. In 2020, he added a new chapter that contextualized the 'corona crisis' within this broader historical trajectory.[3]

At the beginning of the pandemic, a similarly large gap could be witnessed in the divergence between the reactions of virologists, epidemiologists and

---

This is the revised and translated version of Bettina Hitzer, 'Die Geschichte vor Corona: Erinnerung, Erfahrung und Emotion', *Leviathan*, 49 (2021): 111–32 (doi: 10.5771/0340-0425-2021-1-86). Used with permission. Translated by Adam Bresnahan.

[1] Christian Schröder, 'Verwundbarkeit macht solidarisch', interview with Heinz Bude, *Der Tagesspiegel*, 20 April 2020, https://www.tagesspiegel.de/kultur/soziologe-bude-ueber-corona-folgen-fuer-die-gesellschaft-verwundbarkeit-macht-solidarisch/25757924.html.

[2] Martin Sabrow, 'Geschichte im Ausnahmezustand: Vier Thesen über Corona und die gesellschaftlichen Folgen', *Deutschland-Archiv*, 1 May 2020, https://www.bpb.de/308316.

[3] Mark Honigsbaum, *The Pandemic Century: One Hundred Years of Panic, Hysteria, and Hubris* (New York: W. W. Norton, 2020); Mark Honigsbaum, 'The Art of Medicine: Revisiting the 1957 and 1968 Influenza Pandemics', *Lancet*, 395 (2020): 1824–6.

the World Health Organization (WHO), on the one hand, and the general public, on the other. The former had long expected a serious pandemic, while the latter realized for the first time that pandemics were part of national and international emergency planning. At the time this chapter was written, Germany had escaped the most catastrophic effects of the pandemic, though it remains to be seen how it will fare in the future. Nevertheless, many predict that the 'world after corona' will be quite different.[4] It is uncertain, though, whether this world will evidence greater solidarity and consideration of others, whether social inequities will be exacerbated and the shape of globalization will change and whether grave public health emergencies like the fight against malaria in the Global South will, over the long term, be pushed aside by the focus on so-called newly emerging infectious diseases. One primary reason for this uncertainty is that this future is still being shaped by the decisions of the present. The end result will to a large extent depend on the assessment of the origins of the 'corona crisis' and the measures taken to combat it. But developing an accurate understanding of the crisis demands identifying why the realization of being seriously threatened by a novel infectious disease came as a shock for so many people in Europe and why their reactions ranged from fear to uncertainty to denial. Similarly important is explaining why public health officials of the WHO and the governments of the Global North took, after some hesitation, such far-reaching measures, especially in comparison to their reactions to other pandemics over the past seventy-five years.

Two historical perspectives play an important role here: first, the interactions between memory, future expectations and available instruments of scientific observation, and second, the history of disease in the second half of the twentieth century, the history of the experience of it and the history of the emotions felt about it. While the first point primarily concerns the reactions of governments and scientists, the latter has more to do with everyday life. This article focuses on Germany. However, its history with these issues cannot be adequately understood without looking at the history of international health organizations. The article compares Germany's experiences with trends in other European countries and in the United States to underscore the extent to which Germany's history is part of a broader context.

---

[4] Such as German President Frank-Walter Steinmeier in his televised Easter address from 11 April 2020.

Memory, observation, and expectation: The coordinates of combatting epidemics

Whether governments, health officials and societies decide to view a disease as a threat does not necessarily have any direct correlation with the number of cases or deaths. Neither does their reaction to it. For instance, cholera is considered to have been *the* disease of nineteenth-century Europe, because it terrified and unsettled society like no other, dominated newspaper headlines, occasioned municipal and national governments to take drastic measures and for years divided the field of medicine into two groups, the miasmists and the contagionists.[5] However, it was not the leading cause of death in contemporaneous statistics, and in retrospect, the number of people it claimed as its victims did not come anywhere close to those of 'common diarrhoea', which in some places killed one in two children before their first birthday.[6] Alfons Labisch coined the term 'scandalized illnesses' to describe this discrepancy between public perception and statistical danger, thus shining a light on the non-epidemiological factors that can move an illness to the centre of public attention.[7] They include the way in which the disease affects the body and causes death, or how well it lends itself to being blamed on already marginalized groups inside or outside a nation. The 'scandalizing' of an illness exerts pressure on the health system and can influence political and administrative decision-making. Moreover, as the concept of 'emotional epidemiology' underscores, the 'scandalizing' of illness can itself lead to health problems like anxiety disorders that have no direct biological connection to the disease.[8]

But the current coronavirus pandemic and its historical context seem to pose questions of another sort: Why did most Europeans pay relatively little heed to the pandemics of the twentieth century? Conversely, why have pandemics been a central topic of scholarly discourse for the past thirty years – thus, before

---

[5] Adherents of the miasma theory were convinced that infectious diseases were transmitted through bad air and smells from the earth and water ('miasmas'). In contrast, contagionists believed that people were infected by germs. During the cholera epidemic in Hamburg in 1892, Max Pettenkofer represented the miasmists and Robert Koch the contagionists.

[6] This point was recently made again in a discussion on the coronavirus pandemic: Alfons Labisch and Heiner Fangerau, *Pest und Corona: Pandemien in Geschichte, Gegenwart und Zukunft* (Frankfurt am Main: Herder, 2020), 38–41.

[7] Alfons Labisch, '"Skandalisierte Krankheiten" und "echte Killer" – zur Wahrnehmung von Krankheiten in Presse und Öffentlichkeit', *Propaganda, (Selbst-)Zensur, Sensation: Grenzen von Presse- und Wirtschaftsfreiheit in Deutschland und Tschechien seit 1871*, ed. Michael Andel, Detlef Brandes, Alfons Labisch, Jiri Presek and Thomas Ruzicka (Essen: Klartext, 2005), 273–89.

[8] Danielle Ofri, 'The Emotional Epidemiology of H1N1 Influenza Vaccination', *New England Journal of Medicine*, 361 (2009): 2594–5.

the coronavirus pandemic? And to what extent did these two historical factors influence reactions in spring 2020?

Why forget? The 'mother of all pandemics' between 1918 and 1920

Reflecting on the twentieth century, virologists and epidemiologists called the so-called Spanish flu pandemic of 1918–20 the 'mother of all pandemics'.[9] It was notorious for two reasons. First, in just two years, it claimed the lives of between fifty and one hundred million people around the world – more than any other pandemic before or after in such a short span of time. Second, it was caused by a virus that developed out of a recombination of viruses from animal and human hosts. The flu of 1918–20 thus posed a threat that, since the early 1990s, has been discussed under the heading of (re)emerging infectious diseases.[10] But both the pandemic's death count and its zoonotic origins were late discoveries. For most of the twentieth century, only a few people in Europe and the United States remembered what Alfred W. Crosby assessed as a 'national catastrophe' in his book *America's Forgotten Pandemic*, originally written in 1976 and released under this new title in 1989.[11]

This sweeping forgetfulness had many causes, some of which reached back to the time of the events themselves. Like many other belligerent states in Europe, Germany's wartime censorship authorities prevented the press from reporting on the increasing case numbers. But even as newspapers began writing about the flu towards the end of June 1918, their tone was one of reassurance. Even at the crest of the second wave in October and November 1918, articles about the flu did not make it onto the front pages of large German newspapers.[12] On the one hand, this was an expression of the press conforming to the government's appeal to not frighten and panic the populace during a period of military and, later, political instability. After all, in the assessment of Germany's public health authority, the Imperial Health Council, there were neither effective medicines

---

[9] Jeffery K. Taubenberger and David Morens, '1918 Influenza: The Mother of All Pandemics', *Emerging Infectious Diseases*, 12, no. 1 (2005): 15–22.

[10] Mark Harrison, 'Pandemics', *The Routledge History of Disease*, ed. Mark Jackson (London: Routledge, 2017), 137.

[11] Quoted in David Rengeling, *Vom geduldigen Ausharren zur allumfassenden Prävention: Grippe-Pandemien im Spiegel von Wissenschaft, Politik und Öffentlichkeit* (Baden-Baden: Nomos, 2017), 411. See also Alfred W. Crosby, *Epidemic and Peace, 1918* (Westport, CT: Greenwood Press, 1976); Alfred W. Crosby, *America's Forgotten Pandemic: The Influenza of 1918* (Cambridge: Cambridge University Press, 1989).

[12] Eckard Michels, 'Die "Spanische Grippe" 1918/19. Verlauf, Folgen und Deutungen im Kontext des Ersten Weltkriegs', *Vierteljahrshefte für Zeitgeschichte*, 58, no. 1 (2010): 10–11, 22.

against this disease nor any adequate preventive measures.[13] On the other, this type of reporting seems to have reflected the widespread assumption that the flu represented just one danger among many at the time, one that simply had to be accepted because there was nothing anybody could do about it anyway.[14]

Moreover, the case numbers showed stark regional variations and, amidst the complex situation of an ending war, a revolution and the conflict-laden founding of the Weimar Republic, public health authorities had a difficult time getting an overview of the flu's death toll.[15] Thus, the 1918–20 flu pandemic never really had an opportunity to enter into German collective memory[16] and has been and continues to be passed over in almost all well-known surveys of German history.[17] The same holds for many other Western countries.[18]

Things looked quite different in the United States – and particularly in the American military – as well as at international organizations. Preventing pandemics was a primary objective of the Health Organization of the League of Nations. The Surgeon General of the US army built up a system of medical information and surveillance and, in 1941, shortly before the United States entered the Second World War, it established the Commission on Influenza and Vaccine Development. These initiatives treated the memory of the Spanish flu as a warning.[19] Indeed, while it was ongoing in 1918–20, the pandemic had drawn much more media attention in the United States than was the case in Germany. One reason was that the First World War was not fought on US territory, thus making flu deaths and severe cases more 'visible'. Additionally, in contrast to Germany's largest metropolises, some American cities enforced considerable restrictions on public life in order to stop the spread of the virus.[20] The military was sensitive to the virus early on because the first cases appeared

---

[13] Michels, 'Die "Spanische Grippe"', 11–12.
[14] Michels, 'Die "Spanische Grippe"', 22–4. On France, see Marc Hieronimus, *Krankheit und Tod 1918: Zum Umgang mit der Spanischen Grippe in Frankreich, England und dem Deutschen Reich* (Münster: LIT Verlag, 2006), 86–9.
[15] Wilfried Witte, *Erklärungsnotstand: Die Grippe-Epidemie 1918-1920 in Deutschland unter besonderer Berücksichtigung Badens* (Herbolzheim: Cerbaurus, 2006), 317–34.
[16] This term denotes both communicative memory (memories shared orally within a group) and cultural memory (memories shared through cultural artefacts), two concepts defined in Jan Assmann, 'Kollektives Gedächtnis und kulturelle Identität', in *Kultur und Gedächtnis*, ed. Jan Assmann and Tonio Hölscher (Frankfurt am Main: Suhrkamp, 1988), 9–19. Aleida Assmann notes that forgetting plays a central role in cultural memory. The acts of concealing, staying silent and ignoring are primarily responsible for the type of forgetting discussed in this article. See Aleida Assmann, *Formen des Gedächtnisses* (2nd edition, Göttingen: Wallstein, 2016), 22–5.
[17] Rengeling, *Vom geduldigen Ausharren*, 20.
[18] Wilfried Witte, *Tollkirschen und Quarantäne: Die Geschichte der Spanischen Grippe* (Berlin: Wagenbach, 2008), 95–6.
[19] Harrison, 'Pandemics', 135.
[20] Honigsbaum, *Pandemic Century*, 48–51.

at domestic bases and spread rapidly due to the barracks' close quarters.[21] While most German medical scientists assumed that the disease was caused by *Bacillus influenzae*, American military doctors' ability to extensively study the flu and its devastating effects on the lungs of healthy young men away from the battlefields of the First World War led them to conclude that it must have been caused by a yet unknown germ – a virus – invisible to microscopes of the era.[22]

Thus, the memory of the 1918 influenza epidemic remained particularly alive within the US military, despite what the 1989 title of Crosby's book – *America's Forgotten Pandemic* – might suggest. This was particularly apparent in the year 1976 – when the book was first published under the title *Epidemic and Peace* – as a flu outbreak again struck an American military base. The flu virus had been discovered in the intervening years (in 1933 to be exact), and scientists were then speculating that the reason the 1918–20 pandemic was so deadly was because it was caused by a virus endemic to an animal host. As the 1976 outbreak that started at Fort Dix was caused by a swine flu of the influenza A virus subtype H1N1, the Ford Administration quickly decided to activate a national vaccination drive of unprecedented scale. Forty million Americans were vaccinated. But in the end, the flu turned out to be relatively harmless, and the vaccination program was heavily criticized not only because the virus turned out to be a mild threat but also because the vaccine was developed hastily and triggered numerous side effects. It remains a subject of debate whether it was actually the cause of an increase in cases of Guillain–Barré syndrome.[23]

Flu management 1957–8 and 1968–70

This failure was publicly discussed in West Germany and other West European countries. It bolstered the scepticism of those who did not believe the flu posed a special threat and thus did not think that the state should take any measures against it.[24] As historian David Rengeling has analysed in detail, this kind of 'patient perseverance' defined the West German federal government's approach to the flu pandemics of 1957–8 and 1968–70.[25] The choice of strategy illustrates

---

[21] Honigsbaum, *Pandemic Century*, 24–35.
[22] Honigsbaum, *Pandemic Century*, 35–46.
[23] Harrison, 'Pandemics', 135–6; Witte, *Tollkirschen und Quarantäne*, 81–92. Guillain–Barré syndrome is a neurological condition that causes muscle weakness that can inhibit a person's movement. The weakness usually begins in the legs and then moves up over the back to the arms and head. It can affect the breathing muscles and cause potentially fatal respiratory failure. The weakness gradually subsides after four weeks, though sometimes some effects endure.
[24] Rengeling, *Vom geduldigen Ausharren*, 275–6.
[25] Rengeling, *Vom geduldigen Ausharren*, 134–62, 185–235.

with particular clarity how memory, expectations about the future and the capabilities of epidemiological observation interact with emotional and social-historical factors and how this interaction can influence political and media responses. Because although contemporary statistics demonstrate that both pandemics each led to between 30,000 and 40,000 deaths, neither occasioned any serious public health measures when they were ongoing. The media reported little on flu cases, and when they did, it was generally with a conciliatory tone.[26] The situation in France and Great Britain was similar.[27]

One explanation is that health officials simply lacked a comprehensive sense of the actual extent of these flu pandemics. This was particularly true of West Germany, where the federalist system of government posed an extra hurdle to data collection. After the WHO's Director-General warned the Federal Ministry of the Interior by telegraph and recommended that it procure vaccines, it took two months for the ministry to order the health departments of West Germany's ten states to submit case numbers twice a month. But the health departments did not regularly comply.[28] Moreover, West Germany's Federal Health Agency only counted deaths as having been caused by the flu if the person had tested positive. But because test rates were low, the federal health authority counted only a total of about two hundred deaths for both the 1957–8 and 1968–70 pandemics together.[29] The Federal Health Agency insisted on this method, even though doctors, particularly during the 1968–70 epidemic, heavily criticized it and demanded that excess deaths be integrated into the numbers.[30] The Federal Health Agency's counting allowed the federal government to assert that there was no pandemic in West Germany, despite the fact that around New Year 1969/70, hospitals sounded the alarm that they were confronting an 'unprecedented situation'.[31]

The hesitancy to rethink epidemiological data collection methods was informed by the conviction that the flu was generally harmless. The memory of

---

[26] During the 1968–70 epidemic, the media did depict the risk more seriously, while at the same time promoting vaccinations as a promising form of protection. See Rengeling, *Vom geduldigen Ausharren zur allumfassenden Prävention*, 173–8, 244–9; Bettina Hitzer, 'Angst, Panik?! Eine vergleichende Gefühlsgeschichte von Grippe und Krebs in der Bundesrepublik', *Infiziertes Europa. Seuchen im langen 20. Jahrhundert*, ed. Malte Thießen (Frankfurt am Main: Beihefte der Historischen Zeitschrift, 2014), 143–5.

[27] 'Grippe des Hongkong: pourquoi on l'a tous oubliée', *Podcast Le Monde*, https://www.lemonde.fr/podcasts/article/2020/05/09/grippe-de-hongkong-en-1968-pourquoi-on-l-a-tous-oubliee_6039185_5463015.html; Honigsbaum, 'Art of Medicine'.

[28] Rengeling, *Vom geduldigen Ausharren*, 146, 148.

[29] Rengeling, *Vom geduldigen Ausharren*, 417.

[30] Rengeling, *Vom geduldigen Ausharren*, 417.

[31] Quoted in Rengeling, *Vom geduldigen Ausharren*, 211.

the Spanish flu played a role here. By no means had it been completely forgotten, and indeed, some newspapers and magazines used it as a point of comparison. However, the memory was stripped of all sense of urgency.[32] Articles that did reference the 1918 influenza pandemic featured neither images nor concrete accounts, but simply worldwide death numbers. For their part, these numbers were also far below contemporary estimates, because they did not contain any data on colonized territories like India, which were some of the hardest hit regions in 1918–20.[33] Moreover, the memory of the Spanish flu was coloured by the assumption that the pandemic had only been so severe because of the catastrophic conditions unleashed by the ending war. Thus, it was pigeonholed as an exception in the history of pandemics, an assessment that implied that there was no reason to fear that future pandemics of such intensity would come about. Indeed, comparisons with 1918–20 generally had a reassuring effect, because many medical scientists hypothesized that older generations who had lived through the Spanish flu would be immune to other flu pandemics.[34] Accordingly, the field of virology and medical research on the flu only slowly gained more attention and funding in the Federal Republic of Germany.[35]

Health authorities' and many doctors' doubts about the efficacy of the available treatments compounded these issues. Intensive care units had much fewer options than they do today, and respirator technology was at a rudimentary stage. Thus, to many, it seemed pointless to require quarantine to avoid overfilling hospitals, since, with a lack of alternatives, flu patients were already being advised just to call their house doctors and receive care at home.[36] Flu vaccines, in contrast, were a subject of contested debate. In Western countries, and particularly in the United States, they were seeing use as early as 1957.[37] In West Germany, on the other hand, scepticism towards the effectiveness and safety of flu vaccines was widespread.[38] Alongside insufficient production capacity and the low estimation of the threat posed by the flu, West Germany's government decided against advising everyone to get vaccinated during the 1968–70 pandemic, because the government did not want to accept legal liability for potential harms caused by the vaccine.[39] On the issue of vaccines, almost all media outlets took a different

[32] See, for example, 'Viren aus Singapur', *Der Spiegel*, 27, 3 July 1957, 46–7.
[33] The numbers were first officially recognized in the 1990s. See Rengeling, *Vom geduldigen Ausharren*, 305.
[34] Rengeling, *Vom geduldigen Ausharren*, 411.
[35] Rengeling, *Vom geduldigen Ausharren*, 137–41.
[36] Honigsbaum, 'Art of Medicine', 1826.
[37] See Honigsbaum, 'Art of Medicine', 1826.
[38] On scepticism towards vaccines see Malte Thießen, *Immunisierte Gesellschaft: Impfen in Deutschland im 19. und 20. Jahrhundert* (Göttingen: Vandenhoeck & Ruprecht, 2017), 215–27.
[39] Rengeling, *Vom geduldigen Ausharren*, 152–3, 217.

position, without, however, formulating it as a critique of the government's strategy. Already in 1957, many newspapers described vaccines as providing good protection.[40] And by 1968–70, editorials assertively promoted vaccination.[41] Still, with their generally reserved reporting style, German newspapers adhered to the government and the Federal Health Agency's strategy of trying to reassure the populace, of avoiding anything that might provoke fears and of not reporting on already existing anxieties. There certainly were some people concerned about reports on the flu spreading throughout Asia and other European countries who turned to health authorities for help. But in the cases when they received any reply at all, it was usually just to flatly deny that there was a flu pandemic.[42]

Government responses and journalistic reporting were informed by an emotional regime that extended far beyond the realm of public health. This was a regime in which speaking about fears, risks and the limits of knowledge was supposed to have no place in public discourse, and particularly not when it concerned domestic policy or the health and safety of citizens.[43] Different rules applied to foreign policy issues, such as the Sputnik shock that dominated West German media in the autumn of 1957, in which fear played a key role in a nuanced strategy of political emotional management.[44]

Thus, the emotional regime around fear differed from today's. But so too did emotional attitudes towards (early) death from illness. Infectious diseases like typhus and diphtheria caused many deaths in the first years after the Second World War. The year 1952 marked the worst year of a lengthy polio epidemic in West Germany that afflicted more than nine thousand people, many of whom were permanently paralysed, and killed over seven hundred people, many of whom were children.[45] The main difference to today did not consist in people

---

[40] See, for example, 'Viren aus Singapur'.
[41] See, for instance, 'Schuß mit atü', *Der Spiegel*, 7, 12 February 1968, 116–18; 'Herr Meier kommt nicht. Er hat Grippe', *Stern*, 46, 17 November 1968, 193. See also Rengeling, *Vom geduldigen Ausharren*, 244–6.
[42] Rengeling, *Vom geduldigen Ausharren*, 144, 194–5.
[43] Frank Biess, 'Corona-Angst und die Geschichte der Bundesrepublik', *Aus Politik und Zeitgeschichte*, 35–7 (2020): 5, https://www.bpb.de/apuz/314351/corona-angst-und-die-geschichte-der-bundesr epublik. A certain parallel can be found in media and political treatment of corruption during West Germany's early years, as it was generally only reported on with reserve and in very 'matter-of-fact' terms. See Jens-Ivo Engels, *Alles nur gekauft? Korruption in der Bundesrepublik seit 1949* (Darmstadt: Wissenschaftliche Buchgesellschaft, 2019), 25–43.
[44] Honigsbaum, 'Art of Medicine', 1826. Frank Biess refers to a 'carefully calibrated emotional balance' during the Cold War, writing that West German chancellor Konrad Adenauer's government sought to mobilize fear of communism while seeking to contain fears of nuclear war by making grand promises about security in civil defence campaigns. Frank Biess, *German Angst: Fear and Democracy in the Federal Republic of Germany* (Oxford: Oxford University Press, 2020), 107, 95–129.
[45] Ulrike Lindner, *Gesundheitspolitik in der Nachkriegszeit: Großbritannien und die Bundesrepublik Deutschland im Vergleich* (Munich: Oldenbourg, 2004), 221–82.

mourning the dead with less intensity, but rather that their deaths were more or less accepted as being unavoidable.

This difference in perception has a close relation with the history of prevention and security, a point that can be illustrated by a comparative look at East Germany, where prophylaxis was considered the primary purpose of public health. Early in the flu pandemic of 1968–70, the East German government sought to acquire vaccines and took the fears of its citizenry more seriously than did its West German counterpart.[46] The West German government's approach to other potentially fatal risks underscores this difference. Whether it was traffic fatalities or the health risks of smoking, the population of the Federal Republic of Germany in the 1950s and 1960s generally accepted such dangers without demanding that the government act to mitigate them and without showing a particularly widespread willingness to change their own behaviours.[47] Even though the end of the 1960s saw the Federal Centre for Health Education produce some informational films about preventing smoking, it took until the 1970s for the definition of these risks as avoidable to slowly become established, and then only in the context of a more generally increased focus on security in many spheres of society. During this period, many people came to expect the state to function as the guarantor of a notion of security that became ever more all-encompassing.[48] In the field of medicine, disease prevention was prioritized, and, beginning in the 1980s, so was healthy living. In this context, the governmental strategy of 'patient perseverance' no longer seemed adequate.

'Newly emerging infectious diseases' and the rise of 'preparedness'

Since the 1990s, these developments have opened up new expectations about governmental strategies against pandemics. In the 1950s and 1960s, the WHO focused on fighting certain infectious diseases that had been widespread for a long time. Among its most ambitious projects was the campaign started in 1955

---

[46] Rengeling, *Vom geduldigen Ausharren*, 220–2, 226.
[47] On the treatment of traffic fatalities see Thomas Zeller, 'Loving the Automobile to Death? Injuries, Mortality, Fear, and Automobility in West Germany and the United States, 1950–1980', *Technikgeschichte*, 86, no. 3, special issue 'Tech-Fear: Histories of a Multifaceted Relationship', ed. Alexander Gall, Martina Heßler, Bettina Hitzer, Karena Kalmbach, Anne Schmidt and Andreas Spahn (2019): 201–25.
[48] See Nicolai Hannig, 'Erforschungen des Gefährlichen. Zur Versicherheitlichung der Natur in den 1970er Jahren', *Jenseits der Moderne? Die Siebziger Jahre als Gegenstand der deutschen und der italienischen Geschichtswissenschaft*, ed. Thomas Großbölting, Massimiliano Livi and Carlo Spagnolo (Berlin: Duncker & Humblot, 2014), 175–93.

to eradicate malaria and the successful campaign to eradicate smallpox, which ran from 1967 to 1980.[49] Both occasioned optimism that infectious diseases could, over the long term, be beaten. During this period, pandemics were not considered a particular security risk, nor did anyone seriously anticipate that new infectious diseases would come about.[50]

This began to change with the first cases of HIV/AIDS in the early 1980s. But not from the WHO's perspective, which categorized AIDS as an exclusively Western problem and thus as outside of the WHO's sphere of responsibility.[51] The then relatively new discipline of virology viewed things differently. The emergence of HIV led virologists to the realization that the globalized world would consistently be confronted with new infectious diseases that had the potential to explode into pandemics. By 1989, the US National Institute of Allergy and Infectious Diseases and other research institutes convened a large conference on 'newly emerging viruses'. After the conference, a research group led by molecular biologist Joshua Lederberg from the Institute of Medicine (now called the National Academy of Medicine) was formed to develop a comprehensive overview of the extent of this newly identified danger. In 1992, the committee published their study, *Emerging Infections: Microbial Threats to Health in the United States*.[52] In 1996, the WHO came to adopt the position that newly emerging infectious diseases posed a considerable threat to the world's health and security. Hiroshi Nokojima, then Director-General of the WHO, began the organization's annual report that year with the message that the world stood 'on the brink of a global crisis in infectious diseases', a threat that no state would be spared.[53]

In the same year, a research group led by American virologist Jeffery K. Taubenberger succeeded in sequencing the genome of the virus that caused the Spanish flu.[54] The findings confirmed previous assumptions that the virus was, like HIV, zoonotic. The discovery permanently altered the memory of the

---

[49] Thomas Zimmer, 'Weltgesundheitspolitik zwischen Panik und Verdrängung', *Geschichte der Gegenwart*, 2020, https://geschichtedergegenwart.ch/weltgesundheitspolitik-zwischen-panik-und-verdraengung/.
[50] Harrison, 'Pandemics', 136.
[51] Thomas Zimmer, *Welt ohne Krankheit: Geschichte der internationalen Gesundheitspolitik 1940–1970* (Göttingen: Wallstein, 2017), 369.
[52] Joshua Lederberg, Stanley C. Oaks and Robert E. Shopes, eds, *Emerging Infections: Microbial Threats to Health in the United States* (Washington, DC: National Academics, 1992). On the 1989 conference, see page 1.
[53] See Hiroshi Nokojima, 'Message from the Director-General', *The World Health Report 1996: Fighting Disease, Fostering Development*, ed. World Health Organization (Geneva: WHO, 1996), v–vi.
[54] Jeffery K. Taubenberger, Ann H. Reid, Amy E. Krafft, Karen E. Bijwaard and Thomas G. Fanning, 'Initial Genetic Characterization of the 1918 "Spanish" Influenza Virus', *Science*, 257 (1997): 1793–6.

1918–20 pandemic. No longer considered an exceptional event, it was now seen as a harbinger of a future defined by pandemics. Its extraordinary lethality could no longer be adequately explained by the conditions created by the ending war. Rather, its lethality was a factor of its zoonotic origins. And both virologists and epidemiologists were convinced that the probability that new, previously unknown zoonotic diseases would appear and bloom into pandemics would only increase with accelerating globalization and the environmental destruction that goes along with it.[55] In 1997, just one year later, their worst fears seemed verified. In Hong Kong, people became infected with the novel avian influenza A virus subtype H5N1, which had a high mortality rate: 50 per cent of those infected died.[56] However, because the virus could only be transmitted from animals to humans and not from humans to humans (which remains true today), the total number of cases was low. The anticipated catastrophe had not yet arrived.

Newly emerging infectious diseases would never again disappear from the agenda of both international and national health organizations and authorities. The influenza pandemic of 1918–20 now served as a model of modern global pandemics that could spread throughout the world over the span of just a few weeks. This insight slowly altered understandings of global health security. Prevention was now joined by the principle of preparedness. In contrast to prevention, which seeks to keep negative events from taking place, preparedness is rooted in the assumption that certain emergencies or catastrophes cannot be prevented, even if it is difficult or impossible to predict if and when they will occur. Minimizing the negative effects of these potential events necessitates preparation through means like bolstering the resiliency of existing structures, developing countermeasures and implementing constant surveillance to identify signs of an impending catastrophe as early as possible.[57]

The WHO therefore released an influenza pandemic preparedness plan in 1999 that has been regularly updated since. It provides guidelines for how member states should shape their national pandemic preparation measures.

---

[55] Nokojima, 'Message from the Director-General'.
[56] However, there are doubts that the mortality rate was really so high or whether this might have partially been an effect of insufficient testing. See Martin Enserink, 'Controversial Studies Give a Deadly Flu Virus Wings', *Science*, 334, no. 6060 (2011): 1192–3.
[57] See Andrew Lakoff, *Unprepared: Global Health in a Time of Emergency* (Oakland: University of California Press, 2017), which details how the logic of preparedness was developed by civil engineering and emergency management and then adopted by global health in the 1990s. On this topic from the perspective of the coronavirus pandemic, see Ulrich Bröckling, 'Optimierung, Preparedness, Priorisierung. Soziologische Bemerkungen zu drei Schlüsselbegriffen der Gegenwart', *Soziopolis*, 13 April 2020, https://www.soziopolis.de/beobachten/gesellschaft/artikel/optimierung-preparedness-priorisierung/; Carolin Mezes and Sven Opitz, 'Die (un)vorbereitete Pandemie und die Grenzen der Preparedness', *Leviathan*, 48, no. 3 (2020): 381–406.

The plan helped usher in a global observation system that is coordinated by the WHO's Pandemic Task Force with assistance from select National Influenza Laboratories, which continuously collect and report on samples of new influenza strains.[58] On the basis of this plan, the WHO defined different threat levels intended to trigger the execution of certain preparatory measures, which, for their part, were to be defined by the national plans developed on the basis of the WHO's guidelines. In Germany, the first such plan was formed by the Robert Koch Institute – the country's governmental disease control agency – in 2005.[59]

Also in 2005, the WHO revised its International Health Regulations (IHR) for the first time since 1969.[60] Entering into effect in 2007, the revised IHR implemented three fundamental innovations in global public health security. First, it introduced the new, expansive concept of a 'public health emergency of international concern'. Second, it enabled the WHO to use information from non-governmental actors to diagnose such 'public health emergencies'. Third, it required that all member states set up public health institutions by the year 2016. These resolutions, binding under international law, substantially expanded the global network of health surveillance. The revision of the IHR thus represents one of the most fundamental shifts in international public health law since the nineteenth century.[61] Moreover, it codified an understanding of newly emerging infectious diseases as primarily resulting out of the increasing worldwide mobility of people, goods and services.

Meanwhile, the concept of excess deaths had become established in Germany for calculating mortality rates.[62] German health authorities laid out the measures to be taken in continuously revised pandemic plans, which culminated in the crisis management test (LÜKEX) of 2007. Spanning all of Germany's sixteen federal states and multiple state and federal ministries, the test used three thousand participants to simulate a 'medium serious pandemic', defined as involving about twenty-seven million cases, of which 370,000 would have to be treated in hospitals and 102,000 would die.[63] Such calculations were derived

---

[58] World Health Organization (WHO), *Influenza Pandemic Plan: The Role of WHO and Guidelines for National and Regional Planning 1999* (Geneva: WHO, Department of Communicable Disease Surveillance and Response, 1999), 9.

[59] Robert Koch Institute (RKI), *Nationaler Pandemieplan. Teil I: Strukturen und Massnahmen*, 2017, 5–6, https://edoc.rki.de/bitstream/handle/176904/187/28Zz7BQWW2582iZMQ.pdf?sequence=1&isAllowed=y.

[60] World Health Organization (WHO), *International Health Regulations (2005)* (3rd edition, Geneva: WHO, 2016).

[61] David P. Fidler, 'From International Sanitary Conventions to Global Health Security: The New International Health Regulations', *Chinese Journal of International Law*, 4, no. 2 (2005): 326.

[62] Rengeling, *Vom geduldigen Ausharren*, 420.

[63] Bundesministerium des Innern (BMI) and Bundesministerium für Gesundheit (BMG), *Kurzfassung des Auswertungsberichtes der dritten länderübergreifenden Krisenmanagementübung 'Lükex 2007',*

from epidemiological models generated by computer programs like FluAid 2.0 (one of the first such programs, it was developed in the year 2000 by the American Centers for Disease Control and Prevention).[64]

The revised memory of the Spanish flu thus created a new horizon of expectations, which, for its part, completely transformed instruments of epidemiological observation and data collection. The system of preparedness forged around the turn of the millennium rested and continues to rest on the certain expectation that a global pandemic *will* come in the near future. According to anthropologist Carlo Caduff, this gave rise to a culture of anticipated danger that was constantly being updated by virologists in the labs and by national and international organizations tasked with combatting pandemics.[65] This awareness of imminent danger was reflected in and shaped by an altered political culture and a new media landscape in which open discussion of fears and concerns came to be seen as indicative of a critical perspective.[66] Works of non-fiction, novels and films produced after the mid-1990s have all thematized the possibility of a 'coming plague'.[67] Indeed, it seemed to have arrived in November 2002, when the first cases of the atypical lung infection SARS were diagnosed. During some stretches, German media reported almost daily on the disease that was spreading throughout Asia and, later, Canada, as well as on the few cases in Germany that were quickly placed under quarantine.[68] Nevertheless, SARS did not end up being the feared pandemic for Europe.

The WHO declared a pandemic again in 2009. A strain of influenza A subtype H1N1 spread from Mexico throughout the rest of the world. A recombination of multiple swine flu viruses, it was, like the Spanish flu, a zoonotic disease and could be spread from human to human. The 'swine flu' thus showed some of the primary attributes of the long-expected pandemic; however, at the time, there was no evidence that the illness it caused was particularly severe. Still, the German government rushed to order fifty million doses of vaccine and large quantities of antiviral drugs. But the unexpectedly mild symptoms of what was officially being called the 'new influenza' ultimately made these measures

---

2007, 4, https://www.bbk.bund.de/SharedDocs/Downloads/BBK/DE/Downloads/Luekex/LUEKEX07_Auswertungsbericht.html.

[64] Labisch and Fangerau, *Pest und Corona*, 144.
[65] Carlo Caduff, *The Pandemic Perhaps: Dramatic Events in a Public Culture of Danger* (Oakland: University of California Press, 2015). See also Lakoff, *Unprepared*, 167.
[66] See Biess, *German Angst*, 251–71, 290–330.
[67] This is the title of a bestseller by science journalist Laurie Garrett, *The Coming Plague: Newly Emerging Diseases in a World Out of Balance* (New York: Farrar, Straus and Giroux, 2014). See also Hitzer, 'Angst, Panik?!', 146–7.
[68] A search of www.stern.de for the period between March 2002 and October 2003 returns 140 hits.

superfluous. At the end of 2011, most of the vaccine doses expired and had to be destroyed, representing a loss of 239 million euros.[69] This costly false alarm illustrates well how the combination of memory, future expectations and epidemiological observation can develop its own momentum within a political and media culture defined by fears and demands that the state provide security.[70]

Reacting to criticism of how it handled the 'swine flu', the WHO published a revised pandemic plan in 2013. The Robert Koch Institute, too, issued a revised national pandemic plan in 2014. The WHO reworked its definition of what constitutes a pandemic by giving more weight to the disease's lethality, while the Robert Koch Institute advised that Germany's own health authorities should play a greater role in determining whether a given disease rose to the level of a pandemic.[71] However, the fundamental logic of preparedness and the extant instruments of combatting pandemics remained untouched. When Tedros Adhanom Ghebreyesus, the Director-General of the WHO, officially declared on 11 March 2020 that Covid-19 was a pandemic, the measures long prepared in various national and international pandemic plans were set in motion, with one significant addition: 'Lockdowns' were not originally part of these plans, but public pressure led to their quick integration into the arsenal of pandemic crisis management strategies.[72] Despite these plans, there was a lack of sufficient personal protective equipment like gowns and masks, which might be explained by the fact that European and North American pandemic plans were primarily focused on influenzas and thus on stockpiling antiviral medicines and the quick development and production of a flu vaccine. Another explanatory factor might be that the false alarm of 2009 had altered European and American governments' and health authorities' threat assessments.

The notion that the Covid-19 pandemic blindsided these governments and health authorities is incorrect. However, the same cannot be said for the majority of these countries' populations. Certainly, neither pandemic plans nor

---

[69] Jörg Vögele (with Ulrich Koppitz and Hideharu Umehara), 'Epidemien und Pandemien in historischer Perspektive', *Epidemien und Pandemien in historischer Perspektive: Epidemics and Pandemics in Historical Perspective*, ed. Jörg Vögele, Stefanie Knöll and Thorsten Noack (Wiesbaden: Springer, 2016), 11.

[70] See also Andrew Lakoff, 'Global Health Security and the Pathogenic Imaginary', *Dreamscapes of Modernity: Sociotechnical Imaginaries and the Fabrication of Power*, ed. Sheila Jasanoff and Sang-Hyun Kim (Chicago: University of Chicago Press, 2015), 315–16. No evidence has been found to substantiate some critics' claims that this was in part the result of impermissibly close relations between the WHO and the pharmaceutical industry. For an example of such criticisms see Fiona Godlee, 'Conflicts of Interest and Pandemic Flu', *British Medical Journal*, 340 (2010): c2947.

[71] Rengeling, *Vom geduldigen Ausharren*, 358–61.

[72] Pascal Berger, 'Zwei Wochen im März: zum Zusammenspiel von Medien, Wissenschaft und Politik während der SARS-CoV-2 Pandemie', *Zeitschrift für theoretische Soziologie*, 1 (2021): 34–47.

the laws undergirding them were created in secret – all documents were and are publicly available. But clearly, only a handful of people in Europe and the United States seriously believed in early 2020, when the first reports from China about the new coronavirus were broadcast, that a serious pandemic could affect their countries too. The reasons for this lie primarily in the history of emotions and experiences related to disease in the second half of the twentieth century.

Who's afraid of which disease? Perspectives from the history of emotions and history of experience

Historian of medicine Fritz Dross recently noted that most people in the premodern era were 'survivors of epidemics', because 'every forty-year-old person … had survived at least two serious plagues'.[73] But in modernity, too, pandemics and potentially fatal endemic infectious diseases long remained part of everyday life. Still, since the second half of the nineteenth century – and in some places even earlier – large-scale epidemics have become less common.[74] Even before 1850, many infectious diseases like smallpox, measles and scarlet fever had transformed from non-age-specific illnesses into childhood illnesses. Life expectancy rose continuously. In the 1970s, epidemiologist Abdel R. Omran summarized these findings in his model of epidemiological transition. According to this theory, the history of disease can be divided into three phases: the phase of pestilence and famine is followed by a transitional period in which epidemics lose significance and death rates gradually decline. In the third and final phase, infectious diseases are relegated to a secondary role and are supplanted by lifestyle and chronic diseases. Mortality rates nevertheless remain low and life expectancy high, because chronic diseases often first appear when a person has reached an advanced age.[75]

Most researchers date the beginning of the third phase in Europe and North America at around the middle of the twentieth century. Omran's model, though often criticized in its details and modified by others, defined research on the history of medicine and demographics for decades.[76] The claim that infectious diseases no longer posed a serious threat and would, over the long term, fade into the past around the world is reflective of the overarching optimism of

---

[73] Fritz Dross, 'Vergesellschaftung unter Ansteckenden – für eine Körpergeschichte der Seuche', *NTM – Zeitschrift für Geschichte der Wissenschaften, Technik und Medizin*, 28, no. 2 (2020): 198.
[74] On the following see Vögele, 'Epidemien und Pandemien', 5–6.
[75] See Abdel R. Omran, 'The Epidemiological Transition: A Theory of Epidemiology of Population Change', *Milbank Memorial Fund Quarterly*, 49, no. 1 (1971): 509–38.
[76] For instance, Omran completely omitted data from Africa, thus failing to consider a majority of cases of malaria. See Vögele, 'Epidemien und Pandemien', 6.

the 1970s. Medical scientists' optimistic belief in progress made itself felt in the everyday lives of people in Europe and North America. While diphtheria, typhus and polio raged in the early post-war period, they were almost entirely stamped out by antibiotics, vaccines and improved hygienic measures. These successes convinced many that infectious diseases of all types could in principle be defeated by modern medicine. The influenza pandemics of 1957–8 and 1968–70, which received little attention from politicians and the media, seemed to have negligible impact on this optimism.

But the model of epidemiological transition was in no way just a bet about the future. In Europe and North America, infectious diseases were indeed waning in significance as causes of death. As a consequence, fewer and fewer people experienced how severe infectious diseases could be. By downplaying the risks, the West German government left its citizens in the dark as to the actual extent of the influenza pandemics of 1957–8 and 1968–70, which never entered into German collective memory despite many – above all doctors – having had to grapple with their detrimental effects. These factors changed part of the population's assessment of risks. Although the Robert Koch Institute established a Standing Committee on Vaccination in 1972 that recommended all children receive certain vaccinations, many parents did not vaccinate their children, not necessarily because they rejected vaccinations as such, but simply because they forgot, so little were the risks of infectious diseases part of their everyday thinking. 'Impfmüdigkeit', or 'vaccine fatigue', was a recurring topic of discussion in West German health policy after the late 1960s, which, in contrast to East Germany, for the most part did not mandate vaccinations.[77]

Fears of infectious disease popped up only sporadically when viruses were 'imported' from abroad. Up into the 1970s, West Germany experienced a few isolated smallpox outbreaks; the virus was first transmitted in these instances by travellers or migrants.[78] In 1967, employees of a laboratory in Marburg fell ill with a haemorrhagic fever caused by a previously unknown virus that was surmised to have been transmitted by lab monkeys from Uganda.[79] These 'incidents' stuck out in a country that otherwise did not have to contend much with infectious diseases, and (sometimes sensationalized) media reporting on them drew peoples' attention to the danger they could pose. But in the end, they mostly served to bolster the feeling that the territory of West Germany was a safe

---

[77] Thießen, *Immunisierte Gesellschaft*, 294–5.
[78] Thießen, *Immunisierte Gesellschaft*, 241–6.
[79] The virus was named the 'Marburg Virus' after the city where the first documented infection occurred.

zone, because the outbreaks were quickly contained and affected only a small number of people. They thus intensified the general impression that infectious diseases were a problem of other parts of the world – in these cases, above all Africa and Asia – and not of West Germany or Europe more generally.

Instead, Europeans and North Americans were gradually training their focus on chronic illnesses. Long-term epidemiological studies like the Framingham Heart Study, which has been ongoing since it started in 1948, sought to identify the factors that could increase risks of heart disease and other chronic conditions.[80] In the 1970s, doctors and health officials began studying protective factors. The goal of avoiding illness was now being rounded out by the principles of health maintenance and healthy living, which were consecrated in the Ottawa Charter for Health Promotion, adopted by the WHO in 1986.[81] Analyses of risk factors and protective factors modelled the relation between an individual's lifestyle and their chance of being affected by certain chronic health conditions. Stress and a general feeling of coherence in one's life could be influenced by individual behaviour; people could quit smoking, choose a healthier diet and get more exercise. Minimizing risk and improving one's health, the hypothesis went, were thus matters of individual behaviour. Models of risk factors and protective factors go hand in hand with the concept of prevention, which, while centred on individual behaviour, has been assisted by measures to minimize unhealthy environmental factors and cultivate communities that promote health.[82]

A different approach has been taken towards diseases like cancer. Until recently, early detection, and not prevention in the strict sense, was the dominant strategy. But here, too, personal responsibility was and remains a significant component of mitigation, as early detection campaigns since the early twentieth century have often centred on the notion that the mindful patient who regularly monitors their own body will always detect irregularities early on and will thus be able to be quickly cured.[83] These ideas exerted an

---

[80] See Carsten Timmermann, 'Risikofaktoren: Der scheinbar unaufhaltsame Erfolg eines Ansatzes aus der amerikanischen Epidemiologie in der deutschen Nachkriegsmedizin', *Das präventive Selbst: Eine Kulturgeschichte moderner Gesundheitspolitik*, ed. Martin Lengwiler and Jeannette Madarász (Bielefeld: transcript, 2009), 251–77; Robert A. Aronowitz, 'The Social Construction of Coronary Heart Disease Risk', *Making Sense of Illness*, ed. Robert A. Aronowitz (Cambridge: Cambridge University Press, 1998), 111–44.

[81] Aaron Antonovsky's concept of salutogenesis played an important role here. See Aaron Antonovsky, *Unraveling the Mystery of Health: How People Manage Stress and Stay Well* (San Francisco, CA: Jossey-Bass, 1987).

[82] Matthias Leanza, *Zeit der Prävention: Eine Genealogie* (Weilerswist: Velbrück Wissenschaft, 2017), 221–43.

[83] Bettina Hitzer, *Krebs fühlen: Eine Emotionsgeschichte des 20. Jahrhunderts* (Stuttgart: Klett-Cotta, 2020), 103–77.

enormous influence on experiences and feelings of health and sickness in the West, because they were communicated to people through the most multifarious media. Exhibitions, posters, pamphlets, films and television shows funded by the state or public health insurers delivered this message to homes and schools. Health advice books written by experts, newspaper and magazine articles and podcasts also engaged with the subject, while early detection programs and bonuses from statutory health insurers nudged people to make these practices into habits.

Early detection measures continued (and continue) to be wrapped up in a delicate balance between promises of security and feelings of fear. While they claim to offer people a certain degree of control over their own health risks, they also unremittingly direct people's attention towards the possibility of falling ill with one of the diseases that stands in the focus of early detection and prevention. The primary ones are heart disease and cancer, which is to say, noncommunicable diseases.[84] Both are among the most feared illnesses, along with Alzheimer's, against which there are still no known preventive measures.[85] In contrast, up until 2019, few people feared catching an infectious disease, and when they did, it was generally only sexually transmitted diseases.[86]

This might sound surprising, since, as discussed above, virologists and epidemiologists took HIV/AIDS as a warning that could not be ignored, which helped turn newly emerging infectious diseases into a priority of medical research. In the 1980s, HIV/AIDS did spark fears and for a time was widely discussed in newspapers and television. However, in the media – and, in the early years of the epidemic, in science – it was quickly identified with marginalized 'risk groups', directing fears of the disease towards homosexuals and intravenous

---

[84] Only since the discovery of an HPV vaccine for girls in 2006 have large swathes of the population been aware of the fact that viruses, and thus infection, can play a role in some types of cancer. However, this has not changed the general perception of cancer, because viral infections have been demonstrably identified as significant factors for only a very small number of cancers, and even in these cases, viral infections only increase one's disposition to get cancer and do not themselves cause cancer.

[85] As demonstrated, for instance, by a Forsa Institute survey of about 2,800 German citizens conducted annually since 2010. Commissioned by the public health insurer DAK, it shows that between 65 per cent (2017) and 73 per cent (2010–11) of respondents listed cancer as their most feared disease. There is a large gap between it and the next on the list: Alzheimer's/dementia (39–54 per cent), stroke (40–54 per cent) and heart attack (33–45 per cent). Fear of an accident resulting in serious injuries (37–57 per cent) is roughly on the same level as these health problems. 'Junge Leute haben Angst vor psychischen Erkrankungen', DAK Gesundheit, https://www.dak.de/dak/bundesthemen/angst-vor-krankheiten-2179528.html#/.

[86] In the Forsa survey, the numbers fluctuate between 19 per cent (2011) and 9 per cent (2017). In 2019, 11 per cent of respondents said they most feared venereal disease; among those aged fourteen to twenty-nine it was 28 per cent, while 74 per cent in this age group most feared cancer (multiple responses were allowed).

drug users.[87] Othering the danger made the fear seem manageable – but only at the high price of wide-scale discrimination against those identified with the 'risk groups'.[88] By the late 1980s, when most people had learned that anyone could get infected, some simple and efficacious methods of preventing transmission, such as condom use, had become known, and the discovery of AZT represented the first effective antiretroviral drug, even if the dosage prescribed at the time caused numerous side effects. Infection rates in Europe remained well below the numbers feared.[89] Thus, in the long run, HIV/AIDS did little to change the perception of many people in Europe that infectious diseases do not pose a serious danger to the population as a whole.

In some respects, the 2002–3 SARS pandemic presented a similar scenario. Extensive media coverage quickly engaged in othering, albeit of a different sort. A 'virus from the witch's cauldron', namely Southeast China, was raging in Asia, while papers reassured people that 'fears of a SARS epidemic' in Germany were baseless.[90] In the early summer of 2003, there was a brief period when German media speculated about whether SARS might reach Europe and develop into one of the 'first global epidemics of the twenty-first century', but the general consensus that its spread was 'manageable' did not take long to return.[91] In short, the media reported with a feeling of safe distance. And they pointed to the perception that Asian countries had insufficient hygienic standards and allowed people and animals to live too close together in order to justify their claim that the continent was particularly ripe ground for the emergence of new zoonotic diseases like SARS.[92]

At the same time, the search for the SARS virus was depicted as a kind of real-life crime drama with global 'virus hunters'. This framing clearly drew on narrative techniques from non-fiction books as well as films from the 1990s about the search for the virus that caused the Spanish flu or the viruses responsible for fictional pandemics, as in the movie *Outbreak*

---

[87] Henning Tümmers, 'AIDS und die Mauer: Deutsch-deutsche Reaktionen auf eine komplexe Bedrohung', in Thießen, *Infiziertes Europa*, 158.
[88] Susan Sontag, *AIDS and Its Metaphors* (New York: Farrar, Straus and Giroux, 1989), 25.
[89] Tümmers, 'AIDS und die Mauer', 163, 170.
[90] Jörg Blech and Andreas Lorenz, 'Erreger aus dem Hexenkessel', *Der Spiegel*, 24 March 2003, 184–6; 'Experten: Angst vor SARS-Epidemie in Deutschland unbegründet', *Stern*, 3 April 2003, https://www.stern.de/gesundheit/epidemie-experten--angst-vor-sars-epidemie-in-deutschland-unbegruendet-3349102.html.
[91] 'SARS. Wissenschaftler im Wettlauf gegen die erste globale Seuche des 21. Jahrhunderts', *Der Spiegel*, 5 May 2003; 'Seuche bedroht auch Europa', *Stern*, 27 April 2003, https://www.stern.de/gesundheit/sars-seuche-bedroht-auch-europa-3350286.html; 'Die Gefahr ist überschaubar', *Stern*, 29 April 2003, https://www.stern.de/gesundheit/deutschland--die-gefahr-ist-ueberschaubar--3351954.html.
[92] Blech and Lorenz, 'Erreger aus dem Hexenkessel'. Similar comparisons were drawn during the flu pandemics in 1957–8 und 1968–70. See Hitzer, 'Angst, Panik?!', 145–9.

(1995).⁹³ Thus, in 2002–3, the observer position opened up by newspapers and television was supplemented with an element of fiction. The next pandemic – the 'swine flu' of 2009 – did come to Europe and, like SARS, created a lot of noise, but its lack of severity only bolstered the feeling of many that Europe was safe from pandemics. Accordingly, neither the West African Ebola epidemic in 2014–16 nor the Ebola outbreak in the Democratic Republic of Congo and Uganda generated much fear in Europe.

Conclusion

In the spring of 2020, people in Europe and the United States were quickly and painfully shaken out of their position as mere observers. After the model of the first SARS pandemic, many in the West tried to channel fears through othering, as emblematized by Donald Trump calling SARS-CoV-2 the 'China Virus' or 'Wuhan Virus'. But these attempts failed in the face of rising case numbers.

In most of Europe, however, far-reaching measures to fight the pandemic were implemented, even if with a bit of delay in some places. In comparison with the strategies against pandemics in the twentieth century, the restrictions they placed on everyday life were unprecedented. Looking back, neither the Spanish flu nor the later flu pandemics of 1957–8 and 1968–70 were countered with such intense reactions. Three factors were responsible for this. First, the death rate was underestimated in all three earlier pandemics, because proper epidemiological observational techniques were lacking or were not adequately applied and because the mortality rates were calculated differently. Second, unlike the coronavirus, they were not predated by expectations about a coming, potentially catastrophic pandemic. Thus, their prospective course was assessed differently from the very beginning. Third, government responses, and, to an extent, those of the media as well, were primarily concerned with managing emotions, with hindering panic and creating a feeling of security, even though there were not sufficient numbers of intensive care beds to treat all severe cases.

Around 1990, though, medical science and epidemiology began committing more resources to researching newly emerging infectious diseases, a turn that was initially triggered by the HIV/AIDS epidemic of the 1980s and then bolstered in the 1990s by viroarchaeological studies of the Spanish flu. Virologists' and

---

⁹³ For instance, Marco Evers, Veronika Hackenbroch, Beate Lakotta and Katja Thimm, 'Weltbund der Virenjäger', *Der Spiegel*, 19, 4 May 2003, 194–204.

epidemiologists' concerns that a new, disastrous pandemic could appear at any moment were taken up early on by the WHO. For its part, the WHO had already given up its optimism that infectious diseases could be eliminated around the world. As in virological labs, the WHO gradually began to adopt the conviction that being prepared for an unpreventable global pandemic was the best approach. As a result, new tools of epidemiological surveillance were established around the world and member states developed plans for the anticipated 'public health emergency of international concern'. Even though SARS, avian flu and swine flu did not turn out to be the global pandemics many had feared were on the horizon, this did not extinguish the logic of preparedness. Thus, the measures set in motion in March 2020 had been planned for years but were significantly intensified under public pressure occasioned by knowledge of Covid-19's potential severity.

Nevertheless, the coronavirus pandemic and the public health measures taken to combat it came as a shock to most people. The history of emotions and experiences related to disease sketched in this chapter help explain why. Only few people in Europe and North America had ever had first-hand experience with severe or fatal infectious diseases. The pandemics of the twentieth century did not leave a serious mark on collective memory. The pandemics of the early twenty-first century primarily affected Asia and Africa. Western media used this fact to cast newly emerging infectious diseases as the progeny of insufficient hygiene and an impermissible proximity between the living quarters of humans and animals, while associating both with an element of disgust. Many believed that Western medicine, Western hygienic standards and Western crisis management would protect them from such pandemics. It was not entirely unknown that virologists and WHO public health officials saw things differently and that all European countries had developed pandemic plans and tested them in simulations. However, most people perceived these plans as overly cautious security measures for an exceptionally unlikely event.

Moreover, during the preceding half century, most people in Europe and North America had become accustomed to the notion that chronic illnesses, and not infectious diseases, posed the greatest health risks, and that the chances of being afflicted could best be reduced through 'self-improvement' and 'working' on one's own behaviours. Thus, the coronavirus pandemic caused a situation of great uncertainty and a loss of control in two senses: individual preventive health measures were mostly irrelevant, and Western medicine initially had nothing more to offer than the centuries-old technique of social distancing. Mark Siemons was right to call this a 'blow to Western feelings of cultural superiority', which, it might be added, was compounded by the sense that an unprecedented, difficult-to-define threat was afoot.[94]

The desire to deny the loss of control and reverse the injury to one's sense of security as if everything could go back to how it was may help explain why conspiracy theories have run rampant. Unable to stigmatize 'risk groups' or project the danger onto Asia, some of these conspiracy theories seek different narratives to produce an imaginary sense of agency and invulnerability.[95] Anti-Semitic conspiracy theories from the age of bacteriology have seen a resurgence. Some have latched onto criticisms of the alleged influence of private economic interests on governments' approaches to the 2009 swine flu pandemic.[96] In retrospect, some people did – for reasons unrelated to conspiracy theories – suspect that the WHO's hasty reaction to the 2009 event was spurred by the pharmaceutical industry's sway over the institution, while some states evidently exploited the 'pandemic' to make gains by imposing import restrictions.[97]

The notion that a virus could be produced in a lab and instrumentalized for geopolitical or economic ends has roots in serious concerns that likewise have little to do with conspiracy theorists' exploitation of the concept. Since the early 1990s, security experts have feared that viruses and other biological weapons manufactured in labs in the former Soviet Union could be wielded by terrorists. The 2001 anthrax attacks fed into this worry, which has been played through countless times in films of the popular virus thriller genre.[98] What the different conspiracy theories that abuse these more defined concerns have in common is their desire to uncover an intention behind every danger and demonstrate its 'foreignness'.

This was one reason why wearing masks became a contested symbol in 2020. Certainly, masks had been worn in Europe in the past and invested with patriotic content, such as during the Blitz on London.[99] But in the recent past,

---

[94] Mark Siemons, 'Corona und der Westen: Die zivilisatorische Kränkung', *Frankfurter Allgemeine Zeitung*, 29 March 2020, https://www.faz.net/aktuell/feuilleton/debatten/coronaund-der-westen-die-zivilisatorische-kraenkung-16700907.html.

[95] Carolin Amlinger and Nicola Gess, 'reality check. Wie die Corona Krise kritische und weniger kritische Theorien auf den Prüfstand stellt', *Geschichte der Gegenwart*, 2020, https://geschichtedergegenwart.ch/reality-check-wie-die-corona-krise-kritische-und-weniger-kritische-theorien-auf-den-pruefstand-stellt/.

[96] Philipp Sarasin, 'Fremdkörper/Infektionen: "Anthrax" als Medienvirus', *Virus! Mutationen einer Metapher*, ed. Ruth Mayer and Brigitte Weingart (Bielefeld: transcript, 2004), 139.

[97] Harrison, 'Pandemics', 139.

[98] Ruth Mayer, ' "Bei Berührung Tod". Virenthriller, Bioterrorismus und die Logik des Globalen', in Mayer and Weingart, *Virus!*, 217–19.

[99] On mask-wearing during the Blitz on London see Jesse Olszynko-Gryn and Caitjan Gainty, 'Why Londoners in the Blitz Accepted Face Masks to Prevent Infection – Unlike Today's Objectors', *The Conversation*, 13 July 2020, https://theconversation.com/why-londoners-in-the-blitz-accepted-face-masks-to-prevent-infection-unlike-todays-objectors-142021.

many have sought to turn them into symbols of an alternately threatening and ridiculous other. Thus, hardly a single German newspaper or magazine article on the SARS pandemic in 2002–3 dispensed with a photo of a Southeast Asian-looking person wearing a mask. Even after months of reporting, mask-wearing in Asia still seemed so exotic and in need of explanation that it was constantly thematized.

Many image captions interpreted the mask as a sign of fear. For instance, one caption for a picture of the 'maskless' Chancellor Gerhard Schröder during a state trip to Asia noted that the Chancellor was not afraid of SARS.[100] Every now and again, photos were printed with the aim of illustrating how the 'fear of SARS [in Asia] sometimes has bizarre results', as the caption beneath a photo of a cat wearing a mask commented.[101] The message was clear: wearing a mask is a sign of fear that borders on the ridiculous and is something that people from Asia do. Since SARS, masks have had the added connotation in the West of signifying potential sources of virus from the East. This historical context underscores why mask mandates in 2020 perfectly symbolized an instance of the aforementioned 'blow to Western feelings of cultural superiority'.

---

[100] Matthias Schepp, 'SARS und der Kanzler ohne Maske', *Stern*, 15 May 2003. Image captions that associate masks with fear can be found in articles like: 'Abschwächung von SARS bei jeder Übertragung?', *Stern*, 15 April 2003; 'Hongkong will zu drastischen Maßnahmen greifen', *Stern*, 13 April 2003; 'Wirtschaftswachstum in Asien durch SARS beeinträchtigt', *Stern*, 1 April 2003; 'SARS – weltweit 1610 Erkrankte', *Stern*, 30 March 2003.
[101] 'Vierter Todesfall in Kanada', *Stern*, 31 March 2003.

Datafication and knowledge production

Commentary

A psychiatric clinic in Switzerland in the middle of the twentieth century; a New York technology company at the beginning of the twenty-first century: both institutions focus on affectivity as the cause of mental disorders or diseases, and both refer to scientific knowledge. The following two chapters uncover how this scientific knowledge about affects and emotions is produced. They trace how the complexity of the affective lived experience of human beings is translated into research data. In each case a specific logic is at work, composed of previously valid emotional knowledge and the respective technical or technological settings of knowledge production and therapy: in Kirsten Ostherr's chapter the algorithms behind virtual healthcare interventions; in Marietta Meier's chapter the conventions of psychiatric case histories. In this way, both create their 'data subject', as Kirsten Ostherr calls it, a subject in which certain layers of experience are not taken into account because they do not seem relevant for the emotion model or cannot be translated into this specific kind of data.

What is striking, despite all the differences between the historical cases, is that the construction of both 'data subjects' is predominantly based on the bodily dimension of the emotional. In the Burghölzli in Zurich, affectivity is read from behaviour; today's apps use physiological biomarkers such as heart rate to detect emotions. Increasingly, so-called digital biomarkers are also included, which, as at Burghölzli, evaluate behaviour (in this case smartphone use) to identify traces of emotional disturbances. Both chapters thus refer to a trend in Western medicine: the scientific observation of the emotional on the physiological and moving body, simultaneously with systematic underestimation of introspection, narratives and lived experience.

In both chapters, however, a certain uneasiness about this exclusion is apparent on the part of the parties involved, which the psychiatrist Balthasar Staehelin at Burghölzli counters with an attempt at psychoanalytic therapy for his schizophrenia patients, and the app Happify counters with the promise of including the patient voice through AI-supported conversation and its evaluation by means of text mining.

Kirsten Ostherr shows, however, that even the app user who is made to speak remains a subject constructed from binary data. Happify searches for predefined affective keywords in the 'conversation', to which a positive or negative value is assigned. This results in a kind of 'obstinacy' of the app, as Ostherr illustrates with some app dialogues that seem downright absurd. The app reacts only to these keywords and excludes any more complex user narratives or those that contradict the binary positive-negative code from its calculations. As a behaviour modification app, it is thus not only *based* on the model of a certain emotional 'data subject' but also *models* this on the living consumer, until the user corresponds to this new reduced form of emotional expression.

Unlike Ostherr, Marietta Meier's chapter focuses on the medical expert and their role in the production of knowledge of the affective. Meier draws our attention to how observation and paper technologies interact with emotional styles in the production of knowledge about the affective. Painstakingly, she reconstructs how the character of the affective changes when medical records are transformed into psychiatric case histories. Key here is the preconceived concept of the affective in mental illness that is linked to animal psychology. But at least equally important is how the psychiatrist, the 'reporter' of the case history, writes himself as emotional being in or out of the story. Each paper technology goes with a different emotional style, as Meier convincingly demonstrates. The psychiatric case history requires a third-person perspective: a distant, emotionally non-involved observer. In contrast, the psychoanalytical case history requires constant contemplation of one's own emotional involvement. Drawing on unique source material including both psychiatric and psychoanalytical case studies of the very same patients, Meier unearths the repercussions of these distinct emotional styles on the production of knowledge about the affective.

Both chapters thus expose the mechanics of the emotional that lie behind the polished surface of case history and behaviour modification app. They show how new reduced narratives of the emotional are constructed through the 'knowledge product' in specific ways. Often, context, lived experience and complex narratives are ignored in this construction. Writing histories of affective experiences might be a way to counter these reductionist views and to ask incessantly how to integrate them into our knowledge of dis-ease.

4

The binary logic of emotion in the sensorium of virtual health: The case of Happify

Kirsten Ostherr

The shifting boundaries between human and technological sources of meaning in medicine have raised new questions about how patient experiences are mediated by computational interfaces, both inside and outside of traditional clinical settings. New services that use information and communication technologies to deliver 'virtual health care' present a valuable opportunity to examine the ways that health and illness are being redefined through digital practices. A key feature of virtual care is the emphasis on quantifiable aspects of health and illness, which become more prominent in these systems than those aspects which might resist easy conversion into numerical data. While the trend towards virtual health had been under way for several years, especially in North America, Europe and Asia, the Covid-19 pandemic rapidly accelerated the shift to virtual care worldwide in the effort to prevent exposure to the highly contagious virus.[1] As the pandemic spread, healthcare systems scrambled to 'virtualize', in order to maintain ambulatory and outpatient health services through telephone calls, video visits (using Vidyo, FaceTime, Skype, Zoom and other commercially available platforms), electronic messaging (email), asynchronous communication through patient portals in electronic health record (EHR) systems and SMS text messages (including WhatsApp and WeChat).[2] Healthcare providers sometimes called these services 'telehealth' or 'telemedicine', but the broader concept that these practices represent, which includes the techniques listed above as well as

---

[1] Deloitte, '2019 Global Health Care Outlook' (2019), 41; Devin M. Mann, Ji Chen, Rumi Chunara, Paul A. Testa and Oded Nov, 'COVID-19 Transforms Health Care through Telemedicine: Evidence from the Field', *Journal of the American Medical Informatics Association*, 27 (2020): 1132–5.
[2] James Shaw, LaPrincess C. Brewer and Tiffany Veinot, 'Recommendations for Health Equity and Virtual Care Arising from the COVID-19 Pandemic: Narrative Review', *JMIR Formative Research*, 5 (2021): e23233.

use of wearable devices, virtual reality/augmented reality (VR/AR) headsets, artificial intelligence/machine learning (AI/ML) systems, video games, chatbots, mobile apps and websites, is widely called 'virtual health'.

Through this shift to the virtual, the Covid-19 pandemic has produced a new data archive of healthcare interactions around the world, resulting in widespread adoption of simulated forms of care and increased construction of 'data subjects' as recipients of care.[3] The process of datafication, originally defined as 'the effect of individual actions, sensory data, and other real-world measurements creating a digital image of our reality', has grown in lockstep with the rise of virtual care.[4] As virtual health amplifies quantifiable signals, it excludes more elusive forms of evidence, such as the expression of emotions through complex narratives. In the process, new kinds of patients emerge. This chapter will explore how the exclusion of less quantifiable forms of sensory and affective data transforms our definitions of health and disease, through a case study of a specific virtual health care intervention, the behaviour modification app called 'Happify'. Through close examination of the interfaces and algorithms that structure Happify's approach to emotional improvement, this chapter will explore how virtual care is shaping new and reductive forms of emotional expression. As the case of Happify will demonstrate, virtual healthcare interventions like this app are premised on the idea that the human body – and human emotion – is fully knowable through the digital signals that our bodies emit. Yet, the analysis will show that a binary affective logic results from computational approaches to virtual health. I explain how that logic is constructed through sensors that capture data, transform them into 'digital biomarkers' and convert them into new kinds of data-driven narratives. While these new narratives reduce the range and complexity of acceptable emotional styles, they may also preserve hidden histories of emotion that are rejected by the algorithms of happiness.

Narrating emotion through digital biomarkers

Narratives have come to play important, albeit constrained roles in the construction of data subjects in virtual health ecosystems. While the

---

[3] Paul Webster, 'Virtual Health Care in the Era of COVID-19', *Lancet* 395 (2020): 1180–1; Jacob Metcalf and Kate Crawford, 'Where Are Human Subjects in Big Data Research? The Emerging Ethics Divide', *Big Data & Society*, 3 (2016): 1–14.
[4] Viktor Mayer-Schönberger and Kenneth Cukier, *Big Data: A Revolution That Will Transform How We Live, Work, and Think* (New York: Houghton Mifflin Harcourt, 2013).

unstructured text of patient stories was long neglected as an unwieldy form of evidence, developments in computer science, notably in natural language processing (NLP), have opened the possibility for narratives to be treated as forms of data.[5] This method of text mining has allowed some healthcare and technology companies to claim that they are capturing and restoring the 'patient voice' in medicine but these rhetorical gestures often result in practices designed to reduce the complexity of patients' experiences to the quantitative frameworks of 'biocapitalism'.[6] When patient narratives are elicited and reproduced in digital health apps such as Happify, they are decontextualized from lived experience and their broader significance is typically reduced to a binary logic (positive or negative). The analysis of Happify below will consider the ways that user data, including narratives (unstructured text), demographics and biometric data, are captured, analysed and represented to produce what Dror and colleagues call emotional styles: 'Assuming emotions are intelligible and culturally learned, we extend the notion of emotion to include a nonintentional and noncausal "emotional style", which is inscribed into (and can reciprocally be generated by) technologies, disease entities, laboratory models, and scientific texts.'[7] By arguing that emotional styles 'interrelate with broader emotional cultures and thus can contribute to and/or challenge grand historical narratives', Dror and colleagues present a useful construct for considering the narrative dimensions of virtual health, particularly as those textual forms intersect with data signals from the bodies of their narrators. The analysis of Happify will argue that the emotional style of digital health apps and interfaces produces new narratives of illness that describe and interpret the human body through the digital signals it emits.

The technological construct that enables the digital narration of the body through sensors is called a 'digital biomarker'. Prior to the digital era, a biomarker was defined as 'a substance or process that can be measured in a biological specimen that is reliably correlated to a patient's disease state and/or clinical response'.[8] Examples include blood cholesterol as a biomarker of risk for coronary heart disease, body temperature as a biomarker for fever or prostate-specific antigen as a biomarker for prostate cancer. The term has been extended through

---

[5] Kirsten Ostherr, 'Artificial Intelligence and Medical Humanities', *Journal of Medical Humanities* (2020).
[6] Olivia Banner, *Communicative Biocapitalism: The Voice of the Patient in Digital Health and the Health Humanities* (Ann Arbor: University of Michigan Press, 2017).
[7] Otniel E. Dror, Bettina Hitzer, Anja Laukötter and Pilar León-Sanz, 'An Introduction to History of Science and the Emotions', *Osiris*, 31 (2016): 1–18.
[8] Molly E. McCue and Annette M. McCoy, 'The Scope of Big Data in One Medicine: Unprecedented Opportunities and Challenges', *Frontiers in Veterinary Science*, 4 (2017).

the concept of 'digital biomarkers' to mean 'objective, quantifiable physiological and behavioral data that are collected and measured by means of digital devices such as portables, wearables, implantables or digestibles'.[9] The data collected from digital biomarkers are typically used to predict health-related outcomes, especially those which may validate the efficacy of a digital health intervention. For this reason, the search for digital biomarkers has accelerated in tandem with the rise of digital health technologies, despite a lack of evidentiary standards for ensuring that sensors actually measure what they claim to measure.[10]

The ambiguity of the linkage between digital devices and digital biomarkers is illustrated by an example of a project sponsored by the US Department of Defense, called Warfighter Analytics using Smartphones for Health (WASH). The project's stated aim is to research and develop 'machine/deep learning algorithms that synthesize reliable smartphone biomarkers for the detection of ailments', with a specific focus on traumatic brain injury (TBI) and infectious diseases that may affect soldiers. Smartphone diagnosis of these conditions will be facilitated through 'continuous, real-time assessment … enabled by mining data unobtrusively captured from smartphone sensors'.[11] The researchers state their plan to test and deploy their 'smartphone biomarker detector' on a cohort of millions of smartphone users. The project description demonstrates how a smartphone, worn on the body of a soldier, could detect a TBI fall through the phone's accelerometer and gyroscope to identify the moment of impact. Notably, these indicators would be the same whether the body of the soldier fell to the ground or only the phone fell to the ground. Once a fall is detected, smartphone features could sense subsequent symptoms such as irritability, sleep disturbances, depression and tiredness. For example, the study argues that depression can be validated through indicators of social isolation, as measured by location sensors that compare the maximum radius from home that the soldier travels before and after the accident. A solider with a fulfilling social life that happens to occur in a small radius from their home might be flagged for depression under this protocol. Both depression and sleep disturbance can be tracked through late-night browsing activities, evident in smartphone data on calls (tracking to, from and duration) as well as app usage data. Here, too, a soldier on night watch might be flagged for sleep disturbance due to assigned duties, not inability to sleep.

---

[9] Karger Journal Editorial Board, 'Digital Biomarkers. About the Journal: Aims and Scope', accessed 12 June 2020, https://www.karger.com/Journal/Home/271954.

[10] Katie Palmer, 'A New Research Effort Aims to Vet Digital Health Data from Wearables', *STAT* (blog), 22 June 2021, https://www.statnews.com/2021/06/22/digital-biomarkers-evidence-wearables/.

[11] 'WASH: Warfighter Analytics for Smartphone Healthcare', Worcester Polytechnic Institute, 2018, https://wash.wpi.edu/.

These data proxies, when processed through machine learning classifiers, would lead to a Digital TBI Score and, thus, a potentially erroneous diagnosis of TBI that could have serious consequences for the soldier.

While this example points to some of the ambiguities inherent in the concept of digital biomarkers, in practice, these algorithms are nonetheless being widely deployed in a range of digital health interventions. The concept of digital biomarkers integrates smartphones into the bodily assemblages identified as issuing quantifiable signals that can be deciphered like code and used to identify and predict the development of symptoms of disease. This construct not only formalizes the notion of smartphone as prosthesis for the purposes of scientific research but also pathologizes the smartphones and other wearable sensors as sites of hidden injury and illness, much like the wounded soldiers.

In this way, digital biomarkers can be seen as quantifying and medicalizing sensorial experiences and expressions. Examples of digital biomarkers include precisely the sorts of physiological signals that are associated with emotions, such as sweaty palms as a sign of nervousness or excitement, increased heart rate as a sign of anger or passion or a trembling voice as a sign of fear. In another example of digital biomarker deployment, the start-up company called Pear Therapeutics uses voice biomarkers to identify the early onset of dementia and psychiatric disease. In this case, the voice is a signal of mental health, and the company's AI is trained to detect Alzheimer's, depression, insomnia, schizophrenia, opioid use disorder and substance use disorder. The company is also developing a 'library of voice information on people with depression to develop more effective treatments'.[12] This library of recordings will be transformed through AI/ML analysis into an archive of digital biomarkers; but equally, it will represent a digital repository of emotions and their loss. The app works by having the system listen to users through their smartphone microphones and interpret subtle cues in their speech and tone of voice to identify patterns of changes and lead to earlier intervention. In this case, digital biomarkers represent the medicalization of emotion, raising the possibility of 'reverse engineering' the apps and AI systems that utilize digital biomarkers to reveal and make available to researchers the archives of emotions and senses contained therein.

However, it is important to note that, unlike the Pear Therapeutics library of voice samples taken from real users' utterances 'in the wild', many of the frameworks for identifying and interpreting emotion in AI systems (in the

[12] Casey Ross, 'Pear Therapeutics Licenses Voice Biomarkers for Dementia'. *STAT*, 7 January 2020, https://www.statnews.com/2020/01/07/pear-therapeutics-voice-biomarkers/.

field called Affective Computing) – particularly for machine vision and facial recognition AI systems – are in fact drawn from the calculated performance of emotion rather than any situated, lived expression. Demonstrating this point, Crawford and Paglen have described the 'Japanese Female Facial Expression (JAFFE) Database', developed by Lyons, Kamachi and Gyoba in 1998 and widely used in affective computing research and development.[13] The dataset, modelled after earlier studies on the universality of facial expressions of emotion, contains photographs of ten Japanese female models making seven facial expressions that are meant to correlate with seven basic emotional states (happiness, sadness, surprise, disgust, fear, anger and neutral).[14] Although such datasets have been heavily critiqued for their ethnocentrism and artificial performances, these images form the basis for AI training programs designed to detect and codify emotion in images such as those scraped from social media sites or facial recognition scanners at airports or shopping malls.[15] A similarly reductive logic frames the Happify approach to interpreting emotion, suggesting that these outdated logics may remain hidden in the back end of the digital infrastructures of virtual health.

The case of 'Happify'

In the rest of this chapter, I will consider the emotional style of digital health apps as vehicles for producing new narratives of illness, which claim that the human body is knowable through its digital signals. The discussion will centre on a case study of Happify Health, a popular mobile application that claims to increase the emotional well-being of its users. Returning to Dror et al.'s discussion of emotional style as something that can be 'inscribed into (and can reciprocally be generated by) technologies', this section will present a close reading and analysis of the front-end user interface and the back-end algorithms of Happify Health to examine what kinds of cultural instruction are presented through the emotional style of this widely used app.

Happify is a behaviour modification app designed to help users improve their mental health and well-being. It is available around the world in ten

[13] Kate Crawford and Trevor Paglen, 'Excavating AI: The Politics of Images in Machine Learning Training Sets', *Excavating AI*, 19 September 2019, https://excavating.ai.
[14] Paul Ekman, Wallace V Friesen, Maureen O'Sullivan, Anthony Chan and Irene Diacoyanni-Tarlatzis, 'Universals and Cultural Differences in the Judgments of Facial Expressions of Emotion', *Journal of Personality and Social Psychology*, 53 (1978): 712–17.
[15] Ruth Leys, *The Ascent of Affect: Genealogy and Critique* (Chicago: University of Chicago Press, 2017).

languages and is often provided to users through work-based employee wellness programs. As of February 2021, Happify Health was used by over four million employees, health plan subscribers and pharmaceutical consumers worldwide.[16] In its business-to-business promotional materials, the app is also marketed as a tool that can help companies reduce the preventable costs associated with employee inefficiency and absenteeism due to depression and other mental health issues among workers.[17] The product advertises: 'Overcome stress and negative thoughts. Build resilience. Happify is the single destination for effective, evidence-based solutions for better mental health and wellbeing in the 21st century.' Situated within the nexus of the happiness industry and the politics of happiness, Happify Health presents a compelling example of what Illouz has called 'emotional capitalism', expressed through a range of techniques that Boddice has located within government and corporate mandates.[18]

Emphasizing its science-based approach, the Happify website validates emotion as a component of well-being, asserting, 'How you feel matters! Whether you're feeling sad, anxious, or stressed, Happify brings you effective tools and programs to help you take control of your feelings and thoughts.'[19] By examining the algorithms that provide the digital infrastructure for Happify's approach to emotional improvement, we can begin to disentangle the linkages between emotion and virtual care for chronic health conditions. By analysing the process by which Happify converts the sensorial and emotional experiences of illness into data that are available for intervention and modification, we will uncover the process by which an archive of feelings associated with chronic conditions is erased, but perhaps preserved within the data archive of the app, as those emotions are converted into binary code.

Screenshots of Happify posted in a sponsored research study and on the iTunes App Store display how the app offers 'science-based activities and games to elevate happiness', on five tracks called 'Savor', 'Thank', 'Aspire', 'Give' and 'Empathize'.[20] As described in further research sponsored by the company, these

---

[16] 'Happify Health Expands Global Capabilities with 10 Language Offerings', 9 February 2021, https://www.businesswire.com/news/home/20210209005365/en/Happify-Health-Expands-Global-Capabilities-with-10-Language-Offerings.

[17] Eliane Boucher, Judith T. Moskowitz, Gina M. Kackloudis, Julia L. Stafford, Ian Kwok and Acacia C. Parks, 'Immediate and Long-Term Effects of an 8-Week Digital Mental Health Intervention on Adults with Poorly Managed Type 2 Diabetes: Protocol for a Randomized Controlled Trial', *JMIR Research Protocols*, 9 (2020): e18578.

[18] Eva Illouz, *Cold Intimacies: The Making of Emotional Capitalism* (Cambridge: Polity, 2007); Rob Boddice, *A History of Feelings* (London: Reaktion, 2019).

[19] Happify, 'Happify: Science-Based Activities and Games', *Happify.Com*, accessed 27 April 2021, https://www.happify.com/.

[20] Allison L. Williams, Acacia C. Parks, Grace Cormier, Julia Stafford and Ashley Whillans, 'Improving Resilience among Employees High in Depression, Anxiety, and Workplace Distress' (Cambridge,

five tracks include activities focusing on mindfulness, gratitude, optimism, goal setting, finding meaning and purpose, kindness, forgiveness, prosociality, self-compassion and perspective taking.[21] As a user participates in these games, the significance of the activity becomes redefined through the outcomes-oriented classification of 'Skills' on subsequent screens of the app, where users are asked to 'Choose a personalized happiness track created by experts'. One demonstrated track is called 'Conquer your Negative Thoughts' and features activities titled 'The Power of the Positive' and 'Today's Victories', with the bottom of the screen showing progress bars for the skills developed in the games. The next page of the app offers to 'Reduce stress and anxiety through guided relaxation/meditation' and features video clips of peaceful scenes such as waterfalls and placid lakes surrounded by trees. One of the visual environments that the program uses to help reduce stress and increase well-being is a low-fidelity computer-generated animation called 'Reef', presenting an underwater scene with dolphins, a sunken treasure chest, coral reefs and underwater plants. Below the imagery, a biometric data dashboard displays heart rate, a stress thermometer, a countdown timer and an inhale/exhale cycle tracker. The final screen allows users to 'Gain insights and track your progress over time' on a page called 'My Stats – Happiness Index', which measures progress on three key metrics: overall happiness, life satisfaction and positive emotion. Finally, user testimonials showcase the emotional style set forth by the app, with its aim of increasing pleasurable feelings and eradicating hurt or negative feelings. For example, one user states, 'I adore this app. It has trained me to be more mindful of the good things in life and has allowed me to enjoy happy moments even more than before.'[22] Another user commented, 'I love this app! All that negative energy that contributes to self-doubt and feeling incapable and/or sad – well this app seems to address this and it really helps – really!!'[23] As I will discuss below, however, not all reviews are positive, and the criticisms are instructive.

The imagery and language from the front end of Happify demonstrate the emotional style of the app. For further analysis of how those styles are constructed through user interactions with the computer system, I will examine

---

MA: Harvard Business School, 2018); 'Happify: For Stress & Worry', Apple App Store, accessed 1 April 2021, https://apps.apple.com/us/app/happify-for-stress-worry/id730601963.

[21] Acacia C. Parks, Allison L. Williams, Gina M. Kackloudis, Julia L. Stafford, Eliane M. Boucher and Ryan C. Honomichl, 'The Effects of a Digital Well-Being Intervention on Patients with Chronic Conditions: Observational Study', *Journal of Medical Internet Research*, 22 (2020): e16211.

[22] Melaniekorourke, 'Happify: For Stress & Worry – Ratings and Reviews', Apple App Store, 9 December 2016, https://apps.apple.com/us/app/happify-for-stress-worry/id730601963#see-all/reviews.

[23] G. Batsi, 'Happify: For Stress & Worry – Ratings and Reviews', Apple App Store, 27 August 2017, https://apps.apple.com/us/app/happify-for-stress-worry/id730601963#see-all/reviews.

the back end of the application. The design logic of the Happify app and its 'science-based' techniques for identifying and modifying users' emotions can be seen as an example of the broader health ecosystem in which this technology operates. Intricate details of the scientific framework of Happify's algorithms are available through the company's patent applications, which include textual explanation, citations of relevant research and wireframe models of the intended user experience with the app, all submitted to patent offices in the United States, Canada, the EU and China to ensure protection of the intellectual property and financial interests of the product's creators.[24] The software claims to perform a health intervention by engaging users through data sensors and structured text exchanges, and in this way, the app draws on the logic of digital biomarkers. For this reason, Happify is a provocative site to explore the argument that scientific technologies 'extend the reach of the history of emotions because scientists designed into scientific technologies aspects of the affective logic of their societies'.[25]

In November 2020, Happify Health was issued a US patent encompassing Adherence Fidelity, an algorithm for an AI chatbot (or 'digital assistant') that engages users in structured dialogue designed to produce a predetermined emotional response. The company describes the software as 'a novel algorithm that harnesses the power of AI by using conversational dialog management and natural language processing to detect when a user slips away from the intention of an activity and gently guides them to be more adherent'.[26] The Digital AI assistant named 'Anna' is gendered female and is 'designed to interact with Happify's users in a way that exhibits curiosity and sensitivity, and guides the conversation dynamically to improve health outcomes. This design helps AI to establish deeper relationships with users while maximizing the benefits of our digital interventions'.[27] These behavioural interventions in the form of dialogue with a chatbot show that the app blends the logic of digital biomarkers with that of robot pathographies by utilizing a technique of narrative solicitation and

---

[24] Tomer Ben-Kiki and Ran Zilca, 'Assessing Adherence Fidelity to Behavioral Interventions Using Interactivity and Natural Language Processing', United States Patent and Trademark Office US 10813584 B2, filed 11 July 2018 and issued 27 October 2020, http://patft.uspto.gov/netacgi/nph-Parser?Sect1=PTO2&Sect2=HITOFF&p=1&u=%2Fnetahtml%2FPTO%2Fsearch-bool.html&r=1&f=G&l=50&col=AND&d=PTXT&s1=10,813,584.PN.&OS=PN/10,813,584&RS=PN/10,813,584.

[25] Dror et al., 'An Introduction', 11.

[26] 'Happify Health Granted U.S. Patent for "Adherence Fidelity", a Novel AI Algorithm That Drives Conversational Health Interventions Based on the Detection of Psychological Cues', *BusinessWire*, 19 November 2020. https://www.businesswire.com/news/home/20201119005348/en/Happify-Health-Granted-U.S.-Patent-for-%E2%80%9CAdherence-Fidelity%E2%80%9D-a-Novel-AI-Algorithm-That-Drives-Conversational-Health-Interventions-Based-on-the-Detection-of-Psychological-Cues.

[27] Ben-Kiki and Zilca, 'Assessing'.

revision – that is, the digital assistant aims to persuade users to renarrate their experiences, in conformance with the binary logic of the Adherence Fidelity algorithm. To understand how this algorithm will pursue the stated goal of establishing 'deeper relationships' with users, it will be instructive to examine how the dialogue is constructed.

The patent application explains step by step how an expected interaction between the 'Adherence Fidelity' AI chatbot and a human user would take place. The first step of the invention, as outlined in the patent documents, entails 'interacting with a user in an iterative way (i.e., engaging in a conversation either via text or via voice). For example, an iterative interaction initiated by the computing system may comprise providing a user with a prompt, receiving input data from the user, providing a follow-up prompt to the user, receiving further input data from the user, etc.' The second step of this process is data collection from the user, based on the conversation as well as 'an array of sensors that extract features from the user's responses at key steps of the interaction. For example, the computing system may be in communication (e.g., wired or wireless) with one or more devices configured to collect user information such as a camera, speaker, microphone, heat sensor, motion sensor, fingerprint detector, keyboard, etc.'[28] The data from these sensors are analysed and assigned values corresponding to each activity and are also saved in a continuously expanding repository of personal data unique to the user. Stark has argued, in reference to other mood-tracking apps, that the 'mechanisms of the psycho-computational complex are often proprietary, opaque to users, and increasingly incorporated into comprehensive data profiles'.[29] In addition to the privacy concerns raised by these digital profiling practices, these techniques also enact the logic of digital biomarking, whereby a physiological sensor captures a signal, such as a sweaty palm, and assigns it to an emotional state such as anxiety so that in future interactions with the computing system, any reappearance of that physical signal would be coded as user anxiety.

Based on conversation and sensor data, the Happify algorithm will analyse the current psychological state of the user and subsequently lead them down different branches of the app's logic in response. For example, an activity or a task might be suggested, such as playing a game or engaging in further 'emotional or empathetic' dialogue. The interaction continues in an iterative manner until 'a

---

[28] Ben-Kiki and Zilca, 'Assessing'.
[29] Luke Stark, 'Algorithmic Psychometrics and the Scalable Subject', *Social Studies of Science*, 48 (2018): 204–31.

desired outcome is achieved'. The conversational and sensor data are combined to produce an understanding of the user's emotional state through the technique of sentiment analysis, and all of the data are stored in a repository in the app that constructs, over time, 'a rich description of the user, providing information such as emotional tone, sentiment, semantics, etc.' Sentiment analysis is a subfield of NLP that analyses and classifies text for polarity, from positive to negative.[30] In Happify, sentiment analysis is performed by scanning the body of conversational text for keywords that will be assigned 'positive' or 'negative' values corresponding to positive or negative emotional states. More advanced sentiment analysis would identify more nuanced emotional states, such as 'sad', 'angry' and 'happy', based on the use of specific words that are coded as corresponding to those values. If the Happify conversation occurs through voice instead of written text, the sensors in the smartphone can augment the analysis so that 'the emotional tone of the text can be further identified by recognizing acoustic characteristics associated with different emotions'.[31]

One example of how this dialogue might transpire involves the digital assistant asking the user to 'describe a negative thought that troubles them'. If the user responds with a positive thought, that is, with a body of text that contains words that have 'positive emotion' attribution, instead of 'negative emotion' attribution, as detected by sentiment analysis, then the AI bot will interpret this response as an indication of 'low adherence fidelity' and will prompt the user to try again with a new cue. This approach is notable as it contrasts with the contemporary style of many social technologies that solicit and validate unrestrained expression of feelings.[32] By contrast, Happify only wants users to express the narrow range of emotions that conform to the app's adherence algorithm. An example of a low-adherence conversation from the patent application proceeds as follows:

Computing System: Can you describe a recent romantic dinner you had with your wife?

User: John has been giving me so much work these days that I barely have time to think about anything else.

Computing System: It sounds like you may be talking about your boss at work. Can you try to focus on your romantic life instead?[33]

---

[30] Anastazia Zunic, Padraig Corcoran and Irena Spasic, 'Sentiment Analysis in Health and Well-Being: Systematic Review', *JMIR Medical Informatics*, 8 (2020): e16023.

[31] Ben-Kiki and Zilca, 'Assessing'.

[32] Luke Fernandez and Susan J. Matt, *Bored, Lonely, Angry, Stupid: Changing Feelings about Technology, from the Telegraph to Twitter* (Cambridge, MA: Harvard University Press, 2019).

[33] Ben-Kiki and Zilca, 'Assessing'.

In this example, the digital assistant detects the 'boss' entity based on information previously solicited from the user. The chat bot will iteratively attempt additional conversations focusing on the same emotional state as the previous prompt, and if the user persists in non-adherence, they will receive a low score on that task and will not 'unlock' new activities and games in the app until they receive a high enough score. The logic of applying a penalty to users who disengage from the discussion bot demonstrates a central tenet of the politics of happiness, which 'not only obliges us to be happy, it blames us for not leading more successful and fulfilling lives'.[34] This 'obligation to be happy' is embedded in the rhetoric of 'adherence', a term that was adopted in medicine to move away from the more overtly paternalistic connotations of 'compliance', yet still suggests a value system imposed by external authorities rather than the patients themselves.[35]

Notably, some users find that it is the AI, not the user, that fails to fulfil the desired conversational performance. A user on the Google Play app store commented, 'You know something is wrong when the AI gets off topic and doesn't understand what the patient is saying. Instantly irritating and not worth the effort to continue on when the AI just goes around in circles.'[36] Another user similarly complained, 'The inability of the bot to understand very simple answers outside its expected scenario completely kills the usefulness of this app and makes it work against its purpose. Instead of making me feel better, it makes me feel frustrated. Do not recommend.'[37] A third reviewer commented, 'A stress reducing app should not stress you out. Went through several questions no less than 6 times, get to the same point and the system goes back to the login page.'[38] These complaints highlight a fundamental flaw in the logic of many digital health apps; they presume that automated digital interactions can replace human interactions in health care, when in fact, beyond simple, formulaic

---

[34] Edgar Cabanas and Eva Illouz, *Manufacturing Happy Citizens: How the Science and Industry of Happiness Control Our Lives* (Cambridge: Polity, 2019).
[35] Pablo A. Herrera, Laura Moncada and Denise Defey, 'Understanding Non-Adherence from the Inside: Hypertensive Patients' Motivations for Adhering and Not Adhering', *Qualitative Health Research*, 27 (2017): 1023–34.
[36] Jack Taylor, 'Review of Happify – Apps on Google Play', 6 April 2021, https://play.google.com/store/apps/details?id=com.happify.happifyinc&hl=en_US&gl=US&reviewId=gp%3AAOqpTOEF6GJ5UWYmxEFSoKBLYYVe701S51wJMPxMzys1COI7syrCZ3F2PypV9VZcqhROmpaqdlLUZgSqJFU_xg.
[37] Daniel, 'Review of Happify – Apps on Google Play', 6 February 2021, https://play.google.com/store/apps/details?id=com.happify.happifyinc&hl=en_US&gl=US&reviewId=gp%3AAOqpTOGW0hsRwJYJXbE53VeezE-XDffRn4ic_ONCFYzEn-6-CjbX5cg_VTkr6-a_eLWOilTeJkYJ0uh0eRCKxQ.
[38] N. Heckert, 'Review of Happify – Apps on Google Play', 21 January 2021, https://play.google.com/store/apps/details?id=com.happify.happifyinc&hl=en_US&gl=US&reviewId=gp%3AAOqpTOEtfJW69AzO4fG1G3OZR_cWH203L4Um_obsrIlj1rq-ZVn7ABegSBYXbqKu6lo2RPaQUp1dtiTXTAS34A.

exchanges of information, digital assistants or chatbots are not capable of the sustained, complex, contextually aware conversations that patients require, perhaps most especially in the realm of mental health. The complaints also speak to the implicit privileging of the app's intended audience: corporate decision makers. As noted above, the primary users of the app are 'employees, health plan subscribers, and pharmaceutical consumers'. These end users have access to the paid subscription version through their workplace wellness programmes or health insurance plans, instead of being limited to the free version of the app. Many of the comments in the Google Play store make clear that the users were accessing the free version because they could not afford the subscription version and were not part of any corporate or medical wellness program.

Close examination of the design materials submitted with the Happify 'Adherence Fidelity' patent application reveals the binary affective logic at the core of this emotional health modification technology. Like the binary logic of digital computers, the wireframe model presented to explain the 'Empathy Exercise' component of Happify's Digital AI assistant follows a narrow linear sequence for the opening of the interaction, followed by a binary branching logic that is responsive (in a limited way) to the user's input. The app thus functions according to the logic that Stark has described in reference to the design of mood-tracking apps: 'Particular design decisions enable the transformation of the individual's subjective felt experience into emotion-as-number, making feelings legible to digital systems and those who design and oversee them.'[39] The interaction opens with the computing system's performance of three steps: 'Greeting', 'Ask for name of other person' and 'Ask how life is for other person'. At this point in the exchange, the options branch to four conditions that classify the expected range of responses to the AI assistant's question about how that person's life is: 'Focus on other (rather than self)', 'Description of person's situation', 'Description of traits of person' and 'Description of person's feelings/emotions'.[40] According to a company press release, during this exchange, 'Anna' the digital assistant 'listens to the existence of various psychological cues, and in turn responds by asking questions that guide the user towards maximized health outcomes, while also expressing curiosity and increasing engagement'.[41] If, based on the user's response to Anna's queries, the Digital AI assistant detects that the

---

[39] Luke Stark, 'The Emotive Politics of Digital Mood Tracking', *New Media & Society*, 22 (2020): 2039–57, at 2042.
[40] Ben-Kiki and Zilca, 'Assessing'.
[41] Happify Health, 'Happify Health Granted U.S. Patent for "Adherence Fidelity"', *Happify Health* (blog), 19 November 2020, https://www.happifyhealth.com/news/fidelity.

user has 'slip[ped] away from the intention of an activity', it will ask refocusing questions to guide the user back to the intended activity, such as the 'Empathize' game being played in this example.

A sample 'empathy exercise' dialogue demonstrates a non-adherent response, the chatbot's redirection and a successful resolution to the exchange:

Computing System:	Hi John! Think of a person you know, what is the person's name?
User:	Joe.
Computing System:	Thank you. What can you say about Joe's situation? About how Joe feels, and the way he handles things?
User:	I am a nice person.
Computing System:	Try to focus on things from Joe's perspective. What is Joe's situation, virtues and emotions?
User:	Joe is a resilient individual who is dealing with a heavy workload and feeling sad about it.
Computing System:	Thank you for walking in Joe's shoes![42]

This minimal, one-sentence description of Joe is coded as sufficient input for successful completion of the exercise, allowing the user to progress through the 'Empathize' track. Adherence enables movement through each of the app's five tracks and is associated with successful improvement of the user's emotional state, according to Happify's (sponsored) research. Notably, that research also states clearly the bottom line of these interventions, as seen by the corporate decision makers who invest in employee or patient access to Happify: 'Improving subjective well-being is important for individuals with chronic conditions because it can help improve their physical condition, thereby reducing the associated costs.'[43] This emphasis on reduced costs clarifies the function of the app's attention to the emotional states of its users; their indoctrination into the binary logic of affective computing is meant to make them better employees. Moreover, the concept of non-adherent conversational response demonstrated here ('I am a nice person') shows that the computational framework classifies any departure from its predetermined narrative logic as an illogical non-sequitur. While the AI might code those responses as non-adherent, they are nonetheless preserved in the data repository for that user, suggesting that the data profile stored in the back

---

[42] Ben-Kiki and Zilca, 'Assessing'.
[43] Parks et al., 'Effects of a Digital'.

end of the app might present a rich resource for examining the discarded emotions of virtual health.

The AI assistant's rigid refusal of any nonconformist expressions of negative emotion in the app validates the argument of Cabanas and Illouz, who observe, 'It is noteworthy that the scientific approach to happiness and the happiness industry that emerges and expands around it contribute significantly to legitimizing the assumption that wealth and poverty, success and failure, health and illness are of our own making. This also lends legitimacy to the idea that there are no structural problems, but only psychological shortages.'[44] The logic of Happify clearly conforms to this approach. By only accepting a narrowly prescribed set of emotions expressed by their users, the researchers at Happify exclude the environmental, social and structural dimensions of illness. Although the app has been studied in patients with chronic conditions including arthritis, diabetes, insomnia, multiple sclerosis, chronic pain, psoriasis, eczema and 'psychological problems', the app does not allow for situated expressions of feeling about any of those conditions.[45] The status of an employee's chronic condition, and whether it is well-controlled or an active source of suffering, is presented as less important than whether that employee is expressing negative emotions about that condition. Moreover, the emotional impact of employment circumstances was specifically examined in another Happify-sponsored study seeking to prove that use of the app could reduce feelings of 'workplace distress'.[46] The relative benefit of such a study to employers – as opposed to their employees – further underscores the corporate framing and objectives of this happiness improvement app.

By training users to modify their responses to 'Anna' the conversational AI, Happify reduces and redefines the emotional and sensorial expressions of its users until they reach a state of adherence fidelity. In this way, the app transforms the paternalistic logic of medication adherence into a paternalistic logic of algorithmic adherence and, in doing so, trains users to articulate a narrow, binary range of emotions, with reinforcement of the 'positive' emotions as the only responses coded as acceptable for completion of the digital exchange. The prescription for any 'negative' or non-adherent affect, within this logic, is a return to the screen, to reabsorb oneself into the world of computer-generated dolphins and coral reefs, where users continue generating archives of erroneous

[44] Cabanas and Illouz, *Manufacturing*.
[45] Parks et al., 'Effects of a Digital'.
[46] Williams et al., 'Improving Resilience'.

emotional responses until their personal data profile achieves fidelity to the binary logic of computational emotion.

Conclusion

The emotional style of Happify, like the structure of virtual health more broadly, presents a public-facing interface and a less visible back-end digital architecture. The front-end interface trains users to accept adherence to the 'positive' emotions encoded into the app, and by extension, to embrace the happiness industry of which these users are now a part. The front end narrates the user's success (or failure) at becoming the kind of emotional data subject that Happify Health's corporate clients wish to employ. By contrast, the back end of the app contains a hidden repository of the data collected by the sensors and the textual input of the user, which, if recovered, would present an archive of emotions, coded as adherent or non-adherent by the digital AI assistant. When Happify users register for the app, they must agree to the terms and conditions that provide Happify Health and its third-party partners access to a wide range of data sources about its users: 'Information that we collect about you also may be combined by us with other information available to us through third parties for research and measurement purposes, including measuring the effectiveness of content, advertising, or programs. This information from other sources may include age, gender, demographic, geographic, personal interests, product purchase activity or other information.'[47] This degree of personal health data aggregation and mining raises serious privacy concerns, particularly as regards the broader implications of the 'emotive politics' of these systems.[48] At the same time, this trove of data presents an archive that, if decoupled from the exploitative practices of data mining, might reveal important insights about the emotional styles of users that are discarded by virtual health. The challenge for future researchers will be to devise new methods and new ethical frameworks for preserving and protecting these abandoned emotional histories.

---

[47] Parks et al., 'Effects of a Digital'.
[48] Stark, 'Emotive Politics'.

5

Third person: Narrating dis-ease and knowledge in psychiatric case histories

Marietta Meier

In psychiatry, emotions play a central role.[1] According to the internationally renowned Swiss psychiatrist Eugen Bleuler (1857–1939), who created the clinical picture of 'schizophrenia', affectivity is the 'decisive factor of all mental events'. In the first edition of his widely used textbook from 1916, which was repeatedly revised and published in various languages until the 1980s, he describes affectivity not only as the driving element of human actions but also as the main cause of mental disorders.[2] Bleuler was no exception. 'Affects', as it says in a 1967 article of the handbook *Psychiatry of the Present*, had always been 'highly valued' by 'all psychiatric schools' because, along with drives, they represented 'the strongest motivations of behaviour and psychic life' and the 'cause of neurotic and psychotic disorders'.[3]

The theory that affectivity or affects are the main cause of mental illness implies that psychiatrists, as experts on mental disorders, deal primarily with the feelings of others, not with their own. Science and emotion have often been assumed, by scientists and lay people alike, to represent a pair of opposites, with science based on a purely rational engagement with the world. According to this view, emotions must not crop up in scientific research and practices as they represent disturbing factors that should be avoided.[4]

---

[1] Apart from the term 'emotion', the 'feeling words' in this paper are source terms. Instead of defining them, I am trying to understand what the historical actors understood by these terms and how they evaluated them.
[2] Eugen Bleuler, *Lehrbuch der Psychiatrie* (Berlin: Springer, 1916), 16.
[3] Richard Jung, 'Neurophysiologie und Psychiatrie', *Psychiatrie der Gegenwart: Grundlagenforschung zur Psychiatrie*, Part A, Vol. 1/1, ed. Hans W. Gruhle et al. (Berlin: Springer, 1967), 325–928, at 555.
[4] See, for example, Uffa Jensen and Daniel Morat, eds, *Rationalisierungen des Gefühls: Zum Verhältnis von Wissenschaft und Emotionen 1880–1930* (Paderborn: Fink, 2008).

In contrast to this common opinion, in recent decades various disciplines have come to the conclusion that emotions are not the counterpart of human reason, but that cognitive and emotional processes are interdependent.[5] Thinking about emotions in historical perspective, it therefore makes sense to analyse the reciprocal relationship between emotion and science, in this case psychiatry, which established itself as an academic discipline from the 1860s onwards.[6] What role did emotions play when psychiatrists produced knowledge? How were emotions conceived, perceived, described, interpreted and evaluated in this medical discipline?

These questions will be examined using the example of a psychiatric case study from 1953, enriching its analysis with further research findings on the production of knowledge in clinical psychiatry. In psychiatry, analysis of case histories was the usual form of producing knowledge until the second half of the twentieth century. Cases were used in two ways, which were also combined. They served either as a material basis from which one drew overriding conclusions or as examples to prove or illustrate something. As a rule, a whole series of case histories was presented, so the aim was not – as in psychoanalysis, for example – to describe a case in as much detail as possible.

Scientific contributions to psychiatry are thus based on the observation of cases and an explorative methodology. Case studies were used to collect information about specific patients and their complaints, which were then processed into knowledge about diseases, diagnoses, therapies and ultimately medical knowledge. The assumption was that only the experienced, objective clinical view brought the decisive insights to light.[7] Therefore, case-based knowledge was knowledge that was presented in the third person. It was the knowledge of a doctor about one or more patients and their illness or, more

---

[5] See, for example, Nina Verheyen, 'Geschichte der Gefühle, Version: 1.0', *Docupedia-Zeitgeschichte*, 18 June 2010, http://docupedia.de/zg/verheyen_gefuehle_v1_de_2010, doi: http://dx.doi.org/10.14765/zzf.dok.2.320.v1, 2–3.

[6] Paul White, 'Introduction to Focus Section: The Emotional Economy of Science', *Isis*, 100 (2009): 792–7; Frank Biess and Daniel M. Gross, eds, *Science & Emotions after 1945* (Chicago: University of Chicago Press, 2014). Jensen and Morat (ed.), *Rationalisierungen des Gefühls*; Otniel E. Dror et al., eds, 'History of Science and the Emotions', *Osiris*, 31 (2016).

[7] The case study method plays an important role not only in medicine but also in law, theology and ethics. Much research has been done on thinking in cases and the production of case-based knowledge in the last two decades. On the (history of) case history, especially in medicine, psychiatry and psychology, see among others Carol Berkenkotter, *Patient Tales: Case Histories and the Use of Narrative in Psychiatry* (Columbia: University of South Carolina Press, 2008); Gianna Pomata, 'The Recipe and the Case: Epistemic Genres and the Dynamics of Cognitive Practices', *Connecting Science and Knowledge*, ed. Kaspar von Greyerz, Silvia Flubacher and Philipp Senn (Göttingen: Vanderhoeck & Ruprecht, 2013), 131–54; Susanne Düwell and Nicolas Pethes, eds, *Fall – Fallgeschichte – Fallstudie: Theorie und Geschichte einer Wissensform* (Frankfurt am Main: Campus, 2014); Monika Class, ed., 'Medical Case Histories as Genre', *Literature and Medicine*, 32 (2014): 1–236.

abstractly, knowledge of doctors and finally of medicine about the prevention, recognition and treatment of diseases. The author had no place in such texts. However, knowledge does not arise by itself, it is produced. So, what is the role of the people who wrote specialist articles? To what extent did they write themselves into their texts while simultaneously trying to avoid subjectivity? And how did the way they perceived and talked about patients, their emotions and their illnesses, influence the production of knowledge?

The clinical view: Case-based knowledge production

In 1953, Balthasar Staehelin, an assistant doctor at Burghölzli, the Psychiatric University Hospital in Zurich, wrote an article entitled 'Rules of Community Life of Seriously Mentally Ill Persons', which was published in the most important psychiatric journal in Switzerland. The paper presents in twenty pages the results of a study on severely psychotic patients in the so-called 'unruly' ward. Most of the fifty women had been ill for years, and approximately two-thirds were considered chronically schizophrenic.[8]

Up until the 1970s, hundreds of case studies were published in psychiatry, all of which originated in a similar way. So why focus on this particular contribution from Burghölzli? The example is particularly suitable because further source material exists that allows for the reconstruction of the context in which the case study was produced. First, I had access to the medical records of most of the patients presented in the text.[9] Second, there are sources that contain information about the corresponding department and the clinic staff working there, which were also included in my analysis. Third, Staehelin was, at the same time, conducting psychoanalytic therapy with two severely schizophrenic patients. With this method, there was no objective perspective on mentally ill people; the way a disorder manifested itself depended not least on the doctor. In this way, the therapist's own motives, emotions and behaviour also came into focus. The notes that Staehelin and other doctors made in the context of psychoanalytic therapies are therefore different from the texts written in the usual clinic setting, where the persona of the individual author was negligible. For that reason, they

---

[8] Balthasar Staehelin, 'Gesetzesmässigkeiten im Gemeinschaftsleben schwer Geisteskranker', *Schweizer Archiv für Neurologie und Psychiatrie*, 72 (1953): 277–98.

[9] The medical record is the patient's file. The term 'medical history' refers to that part of the file in which doctors made continuous notes. In Staehelin's study, the cases are marked with initials. In addition, the case histories contain information such as age, year of hospital admission and diagnosis. Six of the eight patients presented could therefore be identified.

can serve as a kind of negative foil for the type of knowledge production that is the focus of this chapter.

Staehelin's study is based on experiences he gained during a year and a half of working in the 'unruly' women's ward. From 1951, the assistant doctor was responsible for that department and was 'in close contact with the ill and the nursing staff on a daily basis'. In 1952, he recorded his observations three times a day for four months. He noted 'individual aggressions and all other antisocial and noticeable behaviour', as well as all the places in the ward and in the yard where the individual patients were spending time.[10]

Staehelin therefore gathered a great deal of material in the course of his study. He did not consider it appropriate to evaluate this information statistically. Rather, he wrote, 'It seemed necessary to describe in detail several conspicuous patients and behaviour patterns in order to illustrate the results of our observations with these examples.'[11] Accordingly, Staehelin condensed his observations into eight case histories, which he analysed, and drew a conclusion on this basis.

The first and longest case history, covering about four pages, dealt with a schizophrenic patient with pronounced catatonic symptoms. She had lived in the ward for ten years and always sat in the same two places: one in the day room and one in the garden. If someone else sat there, she became very aggressive and, according to the doctor, 'conquered back her territory'. She was far more brutal towards weak women who were lower in the social hierarchy than patients who knew how to assert themselves. 'In accordance with animal psychology', Staehelin therefore assigned her a 'so-called alpha position in the social hierarchy' of the community. In order to test how the patient behaved towards someone she 'perceived as a clearly superior rival', he sat in her seat and did not leave it, even when the patient tried various methods to move him away from her seat. She finally fell into a stereotypical behaviour and circled the seat three times. 'Then she stands in front of me again, more relaxed in posture and facial expressions, as if the stereotype had an inherent affective relaxation.'[12]

Staehelin concluded from this attempt that the patient obviously was compelled to act in this way, just as 'the animal has to act in certain situations'. In addition to the spatial fixation, he also noted a temporal fixation. For example, the patient refused to bathe when the schedule was changed and hit the nurses. She even 'broke through her mutism' and said that it was too early to bathe.

---

[10] Staehelin, 'Gesetzesmässigkeiten', 279.
[11] Staehelin, 'Gesetzesmässigkeiten', 281.
[12] Staehelin, 'Gesetzesmässigkeiten', 281–3.

Staehelin concluded that the patient exhibited 'primitive biological phenomena' that 'would hardly ever show themselves with such clarity in a healthy person'.[13] Comparing the record of the aforementioned patient with the case history published in 1953, it is noticeable that Staehelin portrayed her more negatively in the study than in the medical history, where he was responsible for all six entries made in 1952. The case history states that the woman was 'generally feared as sinister and threatening'.[14] In the medical history, however, there are no such references between 1950 and 1953. Instead, it is repeatedly stated that the patient did not answer, did not want to shake hands with the doctor, refused 'any approach' and was 'always dismissive, though not hostile'. Since Staehelin also wrote in one entry that the patient herself was apparently satisfied, the notes in the medical history above all give the impression that the clinic staff struggled with the woman's 'pronounced autism'.[15]

Moreover, the comparison shows that the study mentions only acts of aggression that could be explained by the patient's spatial and temporal fixation; other violent acts were apparently not of interest. Staehelin also brought up only those coercive behaviours that could lead to problems on the ward. For example, the patient obviously wanted to clean the tables after each meal, which the doctor described in the medical record as a 'stereotypical but useful' 'act of will' but does not mention it in the case history.[16]

Finally, it seems remarkable that doctors reported only such compulsions in the medical history from 1949 onwards. At that time, the patient had already been living in the 'unruly' ward for seven years. Her condition had hardly changed since a lobotomy in 1946. Nevertheless, it was presented as clear that it was the disease that had made the patient a 'slave to biological laws'.[17] External factors, such as the long duration of her stay in the clinic, the conditions in the department or the years of intrusive physical treatments, were not at issue.

Case histories are created based on rules and procedures that are bound to disciplinary conventions; the epistemological figures follow certain formal criteria. As the historical analysis of other examples shows, Staehelin's approach corresponds to the way knowledge has long been produced in clinical medicine.[18] For his study, the doctor drew on numerous, heterogeneous pieces

---

[13] Staehelin, 'Gesetzesmässigkeiten', 284–5.
[14] Staehelin, 'Gesetzesmässigkeiten', 282.
[15] State Archives of Zurich, Z 100.36852, 26, 2 January 1952; 27, 3 April and 17 June 1952.
[16] State Archives of Zurich, Z 100.36852, 27, 17 June 1952.
[17] Staehelin, 'Gesetzesmässigkeiten', 297.
[18] Marietta Meier, 'Die Konstruktion von Wissen durch Fallgeschichten: Psychochirurgische Studien in den 1940er und 1950er Jahren', *Wissen. Erzählen: Narrative der Humanwissenschaften*, ed. Arne Höcker, Jeannie Moser and Philippe Weber (Bielefeld: Transcript, 2006), 103–14; Sophie Ledebur,

of information, most of which he had recorded himself. From this, he filtered out certain information with the help of his 'directed perception'.[19] He then put the selected information in a certain order and reformulated it. In this way, he formed short, focused case histories that corresponded to completely different criteria than the medical records and observation protocols on which they were based. With the case history, something new was created; only from summary, simple, coherent and consistent narratives could unambiguous conclusions be drawn; only at this point could practical knowledge be transformed into 'science'. The case history genre thus determined not only the presentation but also the contents of perception and the results of Staehelin's research.

Affects and feelings in psychiatry: An evolutionist concept of emotion

Readers of academic texts assume that author and narrator are identical. In Staehelin's contribution, this unity is reinforced by the author's use of the first-person singular and plural in addition to the third person. The study is written from the eyes of an observer who looks at the ward from the outside and reports on what is happening from a temporal, spatial and emotional distance. The frequent use of the first-person plural, with which the author inscribes himself in the collective of the medical profession, further consolidates the impression of detachment. Phrases like 'our study' are reminiscent of an authorial narrator. Occasionally, the narrative perspective is changed. When the doctor discusses his own procedure, he describes it in the third-person singular, calling himself 'reporter': a turn of phrase that was also used in medical histories when impersonal formulations such as passive constructions could not be used. The narrator only switches to the first-person singular, which is also rarely found in medical histories, in two longer passages. There he describes an experiment he is conducting with a patient. Here he not only observes but also interacts with

---

'Schreiben und Beschreiben: Zur epistemologischen Funktion von psychiatrischen Krankenakten, ihrer Archivierung und deren Übersetzung in Fallgeschichte', *Beiträge zur Wissenschaftsgeschichte*, 34 (2011): 102–24; Marietta Meier, 'Geschichten aus der Klinik: Die Produktion wissenschaftlicher Erkenntnisse in der Psychochirurgie', *Fall – Fallgeschichte – Fallstudie*, ed. Susanne Düwell and Nicolas Pethes, 60–81; Marietta Meier, *Spannungsherde: Psychochirurgie nach dem Zweiten Weltkrieg* (Göttingen: Wallstein, 2015), 238–47.

[19] Fleck understands directed perception as the willingness to perceive phenomena that correspond to the thinking style or to overlook phenomena that contradict the thinking style. Ludwik Fleck, *Erfahrung und Tatsache: Gesammelte Aufsätze, Mit einer Einleitung*, ed. Lothar Schäfer and Thomas Schnelle (Frankfurt am Main: Suhrkamp, 1983), 112.

the patients; when he speaks of himself, however, he only describes what he has done as the experimenter.

While the narrator does not seem to be emotionally involved in the events depicted, a lot of weight is given to the patients' affectivity. However, it is not verbalized feelings that are mentioned but the behaviour of the patients, from which Staehelin deduced their affectivity. Furthermore, he attributed only sensations and affects to the patients he observed, not 'Gefühle' (emotions).[20] He understood affects as physiological, automatic stimulus-reaction patterns to which the patients were, in his opinion, helplessly exposed. This was linked to a mechanistic, hydraulic concept of tension and discharge: the patients had developed compulsive behaviour due to their spatio-temporal fixation, which the doctor attributed to biological laws. If for some reason they could not give in to these compulsions, an 'affect congestion' occurred and finally an 'affect discharge' manifested itself in aggression or stereotypical behaviours.[21]

According to Staehelin, 'mutually exclusive valences' also led to 'affective tension'. In a case history, he describes a patient whose only wish was to go home. The medical record shows that the woman was constantly rushing out through the door.[22] The study does not mention these escape attempts. It says that the woman 'often stood for hours at the door' in the hall and waited 'motionlessly' for her wish to be fulfilled. In the garden, after breakfast, she regularly walked up and down for a quarter to half an hour in front of a large, wide iron door, 'which led in the direction of imagined freedom'. Staehelin claimed that the door symbolized the way to freedom for the woman and therefore had a 'positive affective value' or 'positive valence', as in animal psychology. At the same time, however, the door also had 'negative valence' because it remained closed and prevented the patient from carrying out her thoughts of escape. The 'mutually exclusive valences' led to 'affective tension', whereupon the patient fell into the movement stereotype, through which the 'affective congestion' could be released.[23]

In accordance with the ideal of emotional balance, psychiatry understood emotional life as a constant struggle between drives, affects, feelings and an

---

[20] Staehelin does not use the term 'Gefühl' or 'Emotion' (emotion). He does speak once of a patient who suffers from 'emotional levelling', but here he only uses the adjective with which he wants to characterize the term 'levelling' more closely. Therefore, this exception fits the result that an opposition between affect and emotion is constructed in the text. See Staehelin, 'Gesetzesmässigkeiten', 286.
[21] Staehelin, 'Gesetzesmässigkeiten', 284. See also the description of the first case study on page 106, this volume.
[22] State Archives of Zurich, Z 100.45222, letter from the clinic director to the patient's husband, 8 September 1952.
[23] Staehelin, 'Gesetzesmässigkeiten', 293-4.

inner controlling force. Social-norm violations occurred when this resistance force failed to regulate emotions. A lack of drive and affect control therefore no longer simply led to a disturbance of an ideal equilibrium and to illness as in earlier concepts. In a hydraulic concept of emotion, as advocated by psychiatry from the end of the nineteenth century, the system regulated itself. If something was suppressed in one place, sooner or later it came up again in another place and discharged.[24]

Although mental illnesses could in principle also be associated with a lack of tension, from the turn of the twentieth century tension in psychiatry usually meant an increased tension or too high a tension. Insane people were unable to regulate their affects or else they regulated them too little and therefore they suffered from an extraordinarily high tension that sooner or later exploded. This figure of thought finally condensed into the medical term 'affective tension', which emerged in the 1940s. 'Affective' or 'emotional tension', as it was later also called, was considered a symptom and was always related to a mental disorder.[25]

The predominant emotion Staehelin observed in the patients of the 'unruly' ward was fear, which he calls an 'affect'. He also mentions mistrust and indifference, which were actually only a façade hiding the fear of not being able to assert oneself in the ward. Furthermore, he emphasizes never having observed a 'real' friendly relationship between these women, at most short-term erotic physical approaches.[26] In contrast to the clearly negatively connotated affects that the doctor thought to identify in the seriously ill patients, sane people could feel interpersonal emotions. They would feel respect, compassion and affection, provide help and cultivate friendships. In a community of the healthy, 'the differentiated play of human-ethical relationships' comes into play.[27]

Staehelin thus classified affects on a lower level than feelings. According to him, animals also had affects, but only people on a higher level of development had feelings.[28] Many of the seriously ill women on the 'unruly' ward were, he

---

[24] Marietta Meier, 'Auf der Kippe: Spannungskonzepte an der Wende vom 19. zum 20. Jahrhundert', *Entgrenzungen des Wahnsinns: Psychopathie und Psychopathologie um 1900*, ed. Heinz-Peter Schmiedebach (München: De Gruyter Oldenbourg, 2016), 63–78, at 75.
[25] On the concept of (affective or emotional) tension in psychiatry, see Meier, 'Spannungsherde', 68–74; Meier, 'Auf der Kippe', 63–78.
[26] Staehelin, 'Gesetzesmässigkeiten', 287–9.
[27] Staehelin, 'Gesetzesmässigkeiten', 277, 292.
[28] For the history of ideas about what sensations animals have in comparison to humans, see Rod Preece, *Brute Souls, Happy Beasts, and Evolution: The Historical Status of Animals* (Vancouver: UBC Press, 2005); Pascal Eitler, 'The "Origin" of Emotions: Sensitive Humans, Sensitive Animals', *Emotional Lexicons: Continuity and Change in the Language of Feeling 1700-2000*, ed. Ute Frevert et al. (Oxford: Oxford University Press, 2014), 92–117.

concluded, 'prisoners of primitive biological laws', their behaviour was neither free nor did it depend only on 'individual psychopathological events'.

In Staehelin's eyes, the patients had originally belonged to the 'human society of healthy people' and only became 'slaves to biological compulsions' as a result of the illness. This is evidenced by expressions such as 'enslaved', 'no longer free' or 'falling back', as well as the reference to the 'ruly' ward being 'closer to specifically human behaviour than the more originally biologically oriented unruly ward for the most seriously ill'.[29] In addition, the doctor mentioned that certain patients sometimes had better phases in which they lost their 'obsessive fixation' and then showed neither physical nor verbal aggression related to the social hierarchy but gave 'the impression of a free person moving by her own decision'.[30]

The idea of linking the behaviour of severely psychotic patients with research results from animal psychology probably came to Staehelin when he attended the lectures of two zoologists at Burghölzli. In his text, he not only explicitly refers to papers by these scientists, which were mainly based on studies on zoo and circus animals, but also uses terms from animal psychology, such as territory, social ranking or attack and flight distance, to interpret the behaviour of the patients. However, possible parallels between conditions in the 'unruly' ward and in animal enclosures were not considered. Although Staehelin briefly mentions the cramped situation on the ward, the question of whether the patients' emotional practices as well as the other doings and sayings could also be related to the conditions in the clinic is not addressed.[31]

Staehelin's comparison between the mentally ill and animals is based on the idea that severe mental illness leads to regression. Assuming that mental illness inevitably changed the human personality, psychiatry in the nineteenth century suggested that mental disorders could impair this development, leading to regression and, in the worst case, to a 'defect state': the final state of a person without personality. In other words, because of mental illness, the development

---

[29] Staehelin, 'Gesetzesmässigkeiten', 277, 290, 292, 295–6.
[30] Staehelin, 'Gesetzesmässigkeiten', 291–2.
[31] Staehelin, 'Gesetzesmässigkeiten', 278; according to Monique Scheer, emotional practices are 'manipulations of body and mind to evoke feelings where there are none, to focus diffuse arousals and give them an intelligible shape, or to change or remove emotions already there'. Monique Scheer, 'Are Emotions a Kind of Practice (and Is That What Make Them Have a History)? A Bourdieuian Approach to Understanding Emotion', *History and Theory*, 51 (2012): 193–230, at 209; Benno Gammerl has pointed out that spaces and emotional styles are interrelated. For example, emotions are shaped by the type of space in which they are performed. Benno Gammerl, 'Emotional Styles: Concepts and Challenges', *Rethinking History*, 16 (2012): 161–75, at 164–6.

process went backwards instead of forwards.[32] According to Staehelin, this had the consequence that pathological behaviour could no longer be explained individually but only by 'primitive biological laws'.[33]

The concept of a disease-induced reversal of evolution became widely accepted in psychiatry at the beginning of the twentieth century. Mental health was equated with the progression of higher functions, which were located at the top of an evolutionary pyramid, while illness was seen as the collapse of such higher functions. Chronically mentally ill people, especially schizophrenics, were, therefore, thought to be at a lower stage of development than other adults in the same cultural group. Although they were not discursively excluded from the human community, they were often described as people who had lost their humanity.[34] After the Second World War, this was especially true for schizophrenic patients. Four decades after the introduction of the schizophrenia concept in psychiatry, the view dominated that schizophrenia was a biologically determined, inexorably progressing disease process and that no conclusions about the disease could be drawn from the life history of the patients.[35]

The practical conclusions Staehelin drew from his results were in line with the idea of a disease-related reverse process of development. According to the doctor, violence, stereotypes and other undesirable ways of behaving could often be avoided if one considered that these were rooted in 'elementary social instincts'. In the case of certain aggressive patients, for example, it was sufficient to respect their territorial claims in order to avoid aggression. The 'main therapeutic demand', however, was to 'contain the effectiveness of the lower … drives over and over again by bringing into play all possibilities of more differentiated and human reactions'.[36] The aim, therefore, was to promote the emotions and behaviours of patients who were assigned to a higher level of development.

---

[32] Andreas Heinz, *Anthropologische und evolutionäre Modelle in der Schizophrenieforschung* (Berlin: Verlag für Wissenschaft und Bildung, 2002); Andreas Heinz and Fatima Napo, 'Fallstricke evolutionärer (Selbst-)Bewusstseinsmodelle', *Funktionen des Bewusstseins*, ed. Detlev Ganten, Volker Gerhardt and Julian Nida-Rümelin (Berlin: De Gruyter, 2008), 245–65; Andreas Heinz and Ulrike Kluge, 'Anthropological and Evolutionary Concepts of Mental Disorders', *Journal of Speculative Philosophy*, 24 (2010): 292–307; Marietta Meier, 'Stufen des Selbst: Persönlichkeitskonzepte in der Psychiatrie des 20. Jahrhunderts', *Historische Anthropologie*, 19 (2011): 391–410.

[33] Staehelin, 'Gesetzesmässigkeiten', 278.

[34] Staehelin, 'Gesetzesmässigkeiten', 278.

[35] For an overview of the changes in the concept of schizophrenia 1945–80, see Sandra Schmitt, *Das Ringen um das Selbst: Schizophrenie in Wissenschaft, Gesellschaft und Kultur nach 1945* (München: De Gruyter Oldenbourg, 2018).

[36] Staehelin, 'Gesetzesmässigkeiten', 297.

To achieve this goal, work therapy and 'psychotherapeutic guidance' were used, which was understood to mean educational efforts. Sometimes attempts were made to transfer a patient to a 'better' ward in the hope that she would adapt to the level there.[37] Basically, however, severely psychotic patients, as Staehelin describes them in his article, were no longer given any opportunities for development. If the available therapies had no effect or only a short-term effect, patients were considered 'incurable'. The hierarchical concept of emotion as well as the ideas of affect regulation and a disease-related regression thus had serious consequences for psychiatric diagnostics, prognostics and therapeutics.[38]

'Emotional Devotion': The psychoanalytic therapy of psychoses

Staehelin's contribution repeatedly emphasizes that the behaviour of the patients could not be explained only by the 'individual disease process'.[39] The psychoanalytic therapy of psychoses took a completely different approach. In contrast to Europe, where analysts concentrated on the therapy of neuroses, after the end of the Second World War some psychiatrists in the United States began to treat schizophrenic patients psychotherapeutically as well.[40] Various methods were used. However, all approaches were based on the assumption that schizophrenics had been exposed to severe trauma in their early childhood. The therapy was intended to give the patients some of the love and care that their parents had denied them and, thus, heal them.[41]

Manfred Bleuler, the son of Eugen Bleuler, who had taken over the directorship of Burghölzli in 1942, was probably the first European psychiatrist after the Second World War to try psychoanalytic therapy of psychoses in a state hospital. In 1951, he published a widely acclaimed, comprehensive overview of schizophrenia research in the 1940s, which strongly influenced the

---

[37] Staehelin, 'Gesetzesmässigkeiten', 278, 285, 292–3.
[38] See Meier, *Spannungsherde*.
[39] See, for example, Staehelin, 'Gesetzesmässigkeiten', 288, 292, 295–6.
[40] Although analytical psychotherapy for psychoses experienced a peak after the Second World War, the first attempts had already been made at the beginning of the twentieth century. Towards the end of the 1920s, several doctors began working with hospitalized schizophrenic patients, but not in state institutions. Michael Stone, 'The History of the Psychoanalytic Treatment of Schizophrenia', *Journal of the American Academy of Psychoanalysis*, 27 (1999): 583–601, at 585.
[41] On the history of psychoanalytic therapy of psychoses see Nathan G. Hale Jr, *The Rise and Crisis of Psychoanalysis in the United States: Freud and the Americans 1917-1985* (New York: Oxford University Press, 1995), 245–56; Yrjö O. Alanen et al., eds, *Psychotherapeutic Approaches to Schizophrenic Psychoses: Past, Present and Future* (London: Routledge, 2009).

development of German-language psychiatry.[42] The article concluded that the many contributions on physical treatment methods could not hide the fact 'that hopes ... had shifted from physical treatment to psychotherapy'. For a long time, it was thought that schizophrenics could not be influenced in this way, but now the approach was also being used to treat psychoses. Therapists concentrated on a few patients and dedicated a lot of time to them. The 'emotional devotion' of the doctor was an important, perhaps even 'the most essential part of the whole therapy'.[43]

In 1951, individual, analytically orientated psychotherapy for schizophrenics began to be pursued at Burghölzli and the first therapies were taken. Under the guidance of Marguerite Sechehaye, an internationally known, freely practising psychologist and psychoanalyst from Geneva,[44] Staehelin and some other assistant doctors tried psychotherapeutically to influence selected severe schizophrenic patients. In addition, Bleuler was also in contact with American therapists. All the clinic's residents were introduced to psychotherapy. Finally, at the end of 1952, a doctor was employed who treated several schizophrenics psychotherapeutically every day and supervised the therapies carried out by other staff members. A woman and a male nurse supported the psychotherapeutic efforts.[45]

Since the psychoanalytic therapy of psychoses assumed that the social factors of a disease process were revealed in the relationship between doctor and patient, the personality of the therapist came into focus. According to this approach, the way in which a disorder manifested itself depended in no small part on the doctor. Therefore, the vision of an objective perspective on mentally ill people disappeared. The intensive work with individual patients and the attempt to understand their illness on the basis of their individual life stories also enabled the therapist to establish a relationship, develop compassion and perceive the patient as a personality. Instead of emphasizing the differences between schizophrenics and healthy people, as was previously the case, commonalities were discovered.[46]

---

[42] Kurt Schneider, 'Zur Frage der Psychotherapie endogener Psychosen', *Deutsche Medizinische Wochenschrift*, 79 (1954): 873–5, at 873.
[43] Manfred Bleuler, 'Forschungen und Begriffswandlungen in der Schizophrenielehre 1941–1950', *Fortschritte der Neurologie und Psychiatrie*, 19 (1951): 385–452, at 427–9.
[44] Sechehaye had developed the 'Réalisation symbolique', a method based on the symbolic satisfaction of basic needs. She had treated a young, severely schizophrenic girl with this method for ten years and had cured her. See Meier, *Spannungsherde*, 264.
[45] The attempts at the Psychiatric University Hospital Zurich were presented in publications and lectures that met with great international interest. See Meier, *Spannungsherde*, 265–6.
[46] See Meier, *Spannungsherde*, 267–70.

What was fascinating about the psychoanalytically oriented therapy of schizophrenics, as Bleuler put it in 1957, was that one often found access to patients about 'whom it was previously assumed that they were no longer human beings, indeed of whom Forel still emphasised that they had become mere vegetative beings, like plants':

> Such 'vegetative beings' become people ..., whom one thinks to understand as well as healthy friends, indeed to recognise oneself. The insurmountable wall that seemed to be erected between the healthy and the demented schizophrenics can dramatically crumble in this psychotherapy and – at least temporarily – instead of a person consumed by a pathological process, we are faced with a fellow human being who is like ourselves.[47]

Therefore, one opponent of the approach criticised the method for disregarding the common dividing line between doctor and patient and warned of 'very embarrassing and very real conflicts [as well as] human chaos'.[48]

Psychiatrists who were engaged in analytical psychotherapy of psychoses thus developed a different understanding towards the mentally ill. Madness was no longer just something strange or different. For this reason, a doctor could no longer distance himself, or treat and describe patients in the same way as before. This is evident in the case histories as well as in the medical histories of schizophrenic patients who were treated with the method.

In contrast to other medical records, Staehelin often wrote in the first person when making notes in the medical histories of the two schizophrenic patients whom he treated psychotherapeutically. Presumably at the request of Sechehaye, who accompanied the therapies, he also recorded his own emotions. For example, when one patient was 'scared to death' by another patient and clung to the doctor, screaming, but shortly afterwards 'fell back into her hebephrenic-catatonic protective mechanism' and became sexually suggestive towards him, he wrote: 'My own reaction: deepest human resonance, dismay to experience such things. Afterwards, only pity again for this strange, dispatched world.' 'Important', it says on a handwritten note by Staehelin next to an arrow pointing to 'My own reaction'.[49]

The fact that the doctors at Burghölzli who carried out analytically orientated psychotherapies critically reflected on their behaviour, built up a closer

---

[47] State Health Services of Zurich, 12.06.2, Burghölzli, Activity reports by director and administrator, Lecture by Manfred Bleuler to the Society of Physicians in Zurich, 24 January 1957, 14.
[48] Schneider, 'Zur Frage', 875.
[49] State Archives of Zurich, Z 100.45455, n.p., 18 February 1952.

relationship with the respective patients and learned to mention such aspects in the medical history is shown by notes such as, 'I want to give him the impression that I can wait patiently until he says more of his own accord' or 'I was afraid at the time that he might relapse [into the old state]'.[50] When the condition of a patient improved in the course of the therapy, which lasted a total of about 300 hours, he could be discharged. In his last entry in the medical history, the doctor who had treated him asked to be contacted if the patient was to return to the clinic, even if he no longer worked there.[51]

The case histories of psychotherapies for schizophrenic patients are also very different from other case studies in clinical psychiatry. As in psychoanalysis, usually only one case was presented, but in great detail. The authors spoke of themselves only in the first-person singular or plural, addressed the feelings that the patient being treated triggered in them, explained the patient's illness and symptoms from the individual life story and consequently also produced different knowledge.[52]

For example, a twenty-page article on the psychotherapy of a schizophrenic patient, published by Balthasar Staehelin in 1955, goes into detail about the woman's biography, problems and therapy and also brings up the relationship between therapist and patient. According to the author, the case history not only provides 'important insights into the peculiarities and necessities' of such therapy but also significant findings about schizophrenic phenomena. In the conclusion, it is said that the family, education and milieu did not allow the woman to 'unfold' according to her 'actual destiny'. The illness was therefore 'a last possibility of existence'.[53]

It would be problematic to build up a dichotomy between the texts that were commonly written in clinical psychiatry before the 1970s and those that were written in the context of psychoanalytic therapy for psychoses. In notes and publications written in the context of intensive psychotherapies, there were also expressions such as 'In the ward he [the patient] complies well'.[54] Here too there

---

[50] State Archives of Zurich, Z 100.441821, part 2, special report, 22, 9 March 1952.
[51] State Archives of Zurich, Z 100.46222, 19, 31 December 1952.
[52] See, for example, Robert P. Knight, 'Psychotherapy of an Adolescent Catatonic Schizophrenia with Mutism: A Study in Empathy and Establishing Contact', *Psychiatry*, 9 (1946): 323–39; M. Schweich, 'La psychothérapie des schizophrènes: A propos d'un cas clinique aperçu général du problème', *L'Encéphale*, 42 (1953): 63–87; Gaetano Benedetti and Christian Müller, eds, *Internationales Symposium über die Psychotherapie der Schizophrenie, Lausanne, Oktober 1956/Symposium international sur la psychothérapie de la schizophrénie, Lausanne, Octobre 1956* (Basel: Karger, 1957).
[53] Balthasar Staehelin, 'Aus der Psychotherapie einer Schizophrenie', *Acta Psychotherapeutica, Psychosomatica et Orthopadeagogica*, 3 (1955): 341–60, at 341–2, 357–9.
[54] State Archives of Zurich, Z 100.441821, part 2, special report, 16, 22 February 1952.

were limits: patients who were felt not to be amenable to psychotherapy, where therapy was not worth starting or continuing.⁵⁵ Moreover, the approach was also characterized by a clear power asymmetry: doctors explained the patients' illness and symptoms and knew what was good for them. Finally, the texts of Staehelin and other employees of Burghölzli prove that one and the same doctor could observe, describe, evaluate and interpret patients' affects and behaviour differently. Depending on whether one took the role of departmental doctor or that of psychotherapist, different expectations had to be fulfilled and different knowledge produced. Thus, in a scientific discipline, different, sometimes even contradictory, emotional concepts and styles could coexist at the same time.⁵⁶

However, the sources on psychoanalytic therapy for psychoses also show that a new language was created and learned within the framework of this approach, even in state psychiatric clinics. Or, as a representative of psychoanalytic therapy for psychoses put it in 1958: 'Whereas in the past it was a matter of course to cultivate the driest objectivity and to frown upon the personal touch in case reporting ... today we are more careless and freer in this respect.'⁵⁷ Different emotional styles thus not only result in different emotional practices, languages and narratives but also affect the knowledge produced, which in turn influences the former.

Conclusion: Othering and surplus meaning

The 'Rules of Community Life of Seriously Mentally Ill Persons' was based on dichotomies: healthy–sick, human–animal, culture–nature, freedom–compulsion, individuality–collective, civilization–primitivity. The pole with

---

⁵⁵ See, for example, State Archives of Zurich, Z 100.43763, 20, 14 November 1951; Z 100.44885, 17–18, 30 September, 14 October and 4 December 1950; Z 100.45506, 36, 4 and 26 November 1953.

⁵⁶ The concept of emotional style that the editors of 'History of Science and the Emotions' propagate

  aims at a specific emotional *haltung* – an ethos, mindset, and attitude – that the researcher of a certain group, discipline, or science in general had internalized and is reenacting every time he or she is doing research. The emotional style ... can determine how the researcher deals with emotions in general or with specific ones, how he or she acts and interacts, and what techniques or instruments he or she uses. It is tied to and trained through practices and techniques that are part of his or her field. ... The emotional style, moreover, ... is not necessarily emphatically emotional nor does it necessarily emphasize certain expressive emotions or emotionality as such.

  Otniel E. Dror et al., 'An Introduction to History of Science and the Emotions', *Osiris*, 31 (2016): 1–18, at 14.

⁵⁷ Christian Müller, 'Die Pioniere der psychoanalytischen Behandlung Schizophrener', *Der Nervenarzt*, 29 (1958): 456–62, at 461.

the negative connotation was mentioned far more often than the pole with the positive connotation. In addition, several poles with the same connotation were connected with each other. According to the author, the female patients, for example, showed 'slave-like and automaton-like' behaviour because they were seriously ill. They were 'addicted' to compulsions that reflected 'the most primitive biological phenomena' and resembled animals for that reason.

One of the dichotomies Staehelin uses is the dichotomy of doctor–patient.[58] Since the doctor appears in the text only as a distanced observer, this dichotomy remains more or less hidden. Nevertheless, the roles are clearly assigned, and a role reversal seems unthinkable. There are, on the one side, the patients of the 'unruly' ward, the examinees. According to the author, in contrast to healthy people, these seriously ill women showed no feelings of pity, appreciation or affection for each other. Instead, he perceived fear and mistrust, emotional charge and discharge and antisocial, conspicuous behaviour, which he attributed to biological-affective laws.

On the other side was the doctor. He observed the patients in a case study and drew general conclusions from it, which were to gain scientific status. The publication seems even more distanced than the entries in the medical histories of the patients presented, where Staehelin, for example, once spoke of a 'tragic defective state'.[59] Since the doctor was responsible for the ward, he knew the patients and was very involved with their care. Nevertheless, the text gave the impression that it could also have been written by someone who followed the everyday life of the department from the outside. The author himself hardly appeared in the text but functioned, so to speak, as a medium through which the most objective knowledge possible was generated. In one experiment, he even maintained his observer position when he violated the 'territory' of a patient. Although the woman held a high social position in the ward, she felt he was clearly superior to her. She did tell him to leave the seat but did not use force against him.

In the second experiment, it became obvious that the doctor was not simply an observer, either in the daily routine of the clinic or in research, but intervened in the field of his observations, thereby shaping it. Here it came to physical aggression: Staehelin approached a patient with a lower position in the social

---

[58] Another important dichotomy that cannot be pursued here is that between men and women. On the gender-specific perception, treatment and representation of female patients in psychiatric clinics, see Meier, *Spannungsherde*, chapter 7. On the importance of gender norms in medical case histories, see Regina Schulte and Xenia von Tippelskirch, eds, 'Fall – Porträt – Diagnose', *L'Homme: European Review for Feminist History*, 30 (2019).

[59] State Archives of Zurich, Z 100.16072, part 2, 42, 3 April 1952.

hierarchy who was visibly afraid of him but could not escape: 'On crossing the distance of 30 cm, as I offer her my hand, the behaviour of the sick woman, pent up with fear, changes, she lunges at me with the most aggressive intent.'[60] The woman thus literally came close to the doctor. It is obvious that at this moment he had to give up his role as observer and fight back, perhaps feeling fear, anger or shame. In the text itself, however, there is a break: the event is not retold. Instead, after the semi-colon, the level is changed and the patient's behaviour is interpreted as a 'critical reaction' in accordance with animal psychology.[61]

Such passages indicate that in addition to the many dichotomies with which the article worked, there was the element of distinction. This third party did not hold a position of its own, but it related both sides of the distinction by simultaneously connecting and separating them. In Staehelin's contribution, the 'primitive biological laws' were the third: they connected the healthy with the sick because they applied to all people, but they also separated the two groups. Severely psychotic people were 'addicted' to these laws, whereas healthy people were autonomous.

This is most evident in the final passage, where the terms individual, collective, slave and freedom were used for both humans and animals. There, it said:

> The animal knows no freedom; it is a slave to biological laws. Its individual behaviour is largely a manifestation of this biological bondage. These same constraints to which the animal world is subject are also latent in man as a collective compulsive willingness. A psychosis or a psychotic defect state involves the danger of becoming a slave of these latent, primitive biological laws again.[62]

In the mid-1950s, as an assistant doctor, Staehelin managed to incorporate two different scientific selves with different takes on his own emotions and subjective experience.[63] In the context of the psychoanalytical therapies he conducted with schizophrenic patients, he tried consciously to perceive and name the feelings that the patients and their behaviour triggered in him. He also reflected on the

---

[60] Staehelin, 'Gesetzesmässigkeiten', 295.
[61] Staehelin, 'Gesetzesmässigkeiten', 294–5.
[62] Staehelin, 'Gesetzesmässigkeiten', 297–8.
[63] Whether and how the experience of psychoanalytic therapy for psychoses changed Staehelin's psychiatric self in the longer term is difficult to judge. However, psychotherapy played an important role in his further career. In 1955, Staehelin completed the specialist training in psychiatry and opened his own practice in Zurich. In 1957, he became a consultant for the psychosomatic department of the Zurich Medical Polyclinic. In 1963 he founded the Swiss Society for Psychosomatic Medicine with a colleague. Later he developed Basic Psychosomatic Therapy, which countered psychosomatic disorders by building trust in God. Angela Graf-Nold, 'Staehelin, Balthasar', *Historisches Lexikon der Schweiz (HLS)*, version of 30 November 2011, https://hls-dhs-dss.ch/de/articles/046171/2011-11-30/ (2 May 2021).

possible impact of his emotions on his relationship with the patient and the therapy. Furthermore, he probably dealt in depth with his own feelings during the training analysis he began in 1952.[64]

In contrast, when working on the ward and performing his study of the patients' behaviour there, regulating emotional practices dominated. This meant maintaining distance and writing in the third person, from a 'rational' or 'objective' perspective. But this third person not only separated the observing first from the observed second person; it also connected the two with each other. Staehelin's contribution can therefore be understood as a product of certain emotional practices that had epistemic effects. The way in which emotions are conceived and thematicized or faded out affects the material conditions, the narrative forms and the content of the knowledge produced.

Unlike texts on psychoanalytically oriented therapies, 'Rules of Community Life of Severely Mentally Ill Persons' was almost exclusively about the patients. Implicitly, however, here again Staehelin wrote of the fragility of the self, of himself, of the feelings the patients triggered in him and probably also of the fear of being helplessly at the mercy of his emotions, of losing his personality and of no longer being perceived as an individual. Thus, talking about severely psychotic patients, their disease and behaviour also meant talking about his own 'dis-ease'.

---

[64] State Archives of Zurich, Z 99.261, Marguerite Sechehaye to Manfred Bleuler, 10 December 1952.

Dis-ease narratives: Making and listening

Commentary

This section picks up where the previous one left off. It suggests ways in which the complexity of affective experience can inform our historical and medical knowledge of dis-ease. Narration and narratives play a central role here. Yet neither chapter presents a simple answer, but they rather raise a new set of questions to be addressed and decided.

Both chapters focus on chronic or long-term conditions. Franziska Gygax's chapter is about cancer; Heidi Morrison's text is about childhood trauma. This is no coincidence. Chronic conditions such as cancer or trauma divide the world of those affected into a before and after, profoundly changing what was previously accustomed as life. This makes them affective challenges of a special kind. As a long-term or lifelong presence in the life of the sufferer, they often represent a story of their own, with highs and lows. A quasi-narrative structure is therefore already inscribed in them. So are narratives only suitable for this section of 'feeling dis-ease'? Undoubtedly, such narratives of chronic or life-threatening illness exist in far greater numbers and are clearly more present in medicine and the medical humanities. However, the opening chapter of this book, Emmanuel King Urey Yarkpawolo's Ebola story, points out that narratives can also tap into otherwise overlooked dimensions of 'feeling dis-ease' when considering diseases of other kinds, such as epidemics.

Narratives in both chapters are the result of the attempt to find an expression for what has wounded and still wounds the body. They revolve around the relationship between (disintegrating or dismembered) body, illness and expression. This is more visible in Franziska Gygax's chapter. She devotes herself to literary texts that were created during the cancer illness of their authors. These texts navigate between the bodily sensations and the emotion words chosen or avoided in the determination to transform them into art; the narrative strategies that in their brokenness and non-linearity seek to express this experience outside the frame of reference of what was previously experienced. The struggle to express what seems to elude pre-existing language is not only evident but is often also the very subject of these texts. Writing here can be both emotional expression and emotional refuge from the body's feelings.

Heidi Morrison's chapter is about the trauma inflicted on West Bank Palestinian children growing up during the second intifada between 2000 and 2006. So even though psychological trauma is the 'disease' here, the body occupies a central position. The story of Mustafa portrayed by Morrison shows that trauma is inscribed in the body and gradually dismembers it. Impressively, Morrison makes clear that the emotional experiences of these traumatized children threaten to escape expression in several ways. Above all, the symptom-oriented language of psychiatry, as offered by the American-dominated DSM or the Trauma History Questionnaire (THQ), proves inadequate. Unlike Gygax's chapter, however, here it is not the traumatized children themselves, now grown up, who struggle on their own impulse to find an adequate expression of their trauma experience. Instead, Morrison engages them as an historian employing the method of 'portraiture', developed by Sarah Lawrence-Lightfoot, in order to tell and understand their story.

The use of this method points to the relationship between art, medicine and history that Franziska Gygax's chapter also raises. In 'portraiture', the depth and complexity of human experience is captured by paying special attention to aesthetic and sensory expressions. In 'life writing', as Gygax addresses it, it is literary writers who transform their experiences into art because everyday language cannot capture them. Both forms of narrativity involve listening from the outset. Many of the authors cited by Gygax reflect on their intended audience in their writing. The 'portraiture' used by Morrison is intended to give voice to the experiences of the traumatized. It thus contains – like life-writing – a moment of agency in a situation of exposure or powerlessness. What methodological conclusions should historians draw from this? Does this entail a readjustment of their position?

Gygax and Morrison give art and aesthetics a firm place in their literary and historiographical examination of 'feeling dis-ease', albeit in different ways. Both are concerned with the sources on which they draw, how these sources are generated and how they are read in a methodologically reflective way. Heidi Morrison goes beyond this: 'portraiture' also transforms writing about the history of 'feeling dis-ease'. Perhaps, then, it is time to contemplate new forms of historiographical writing about the history of affective experience. This also means thinking about the position of history and determining how and in what ways the narratives of a history of emotions and experiences related to 'feeling dis-ease' differ from the narratives of patients, victims and survivors, which they nonetheless include as sources. This seems all the more important as history has recently become increasingly central to processes of coming to terms with traumatic experiences.

6

Feeling (and falling) ill: Finding a language of illness

Franziska Gygax

Introduction

The future flashed before my eyes in all its preordained banality. Embarrassment, at first, to the exclusion of all other *feelings*. But embarrassment curled at the edges with a weariness, the sort that comes over you when you are set on a track by something outside your control, and which, although it is not your experience, is so known in all its cultural forms that you could unscrew the cap of the pen in your hand and jot down in the notebook on your lap every single thing that will happen and *everything that will be felt* for the foreseeable future. Including the surprises.[1]

Confronted with the diagnosis of cancer Jenny Diski describes four crucial aspects of her feelings: first, the emotional response of feeling embarrassed (of having become a cancer patient); second, the instant realization of the cultural knowledge of cancer that triggers future feelings; third, feelings in reaction to unknown things ('surprises'); and fourth, she mentions engaging with these feelings through writing. In this short paragraph, set at the beginning of her illness narrative, Diski highlights emotions,[2] as illness is intertwined with its

---

[1] Jenny Diski, *In Gratitude* (London: Bloomsbury, 2016), 2 (my emphasis). All subsequent page references refer to this edition and are given in the text.

[2] I neglect the still controversial differentiation between emotions, feelings and affects. I am using both the terms 'emotion' and 'feeling'. For a discussion of differences and explanations of the different terms, see for example the introduction to *Emotion, Affect, Sentiment: The Language and Aesthetics of Feeling*, ed. Andreas Langlotz and Agnieszka Soltysik Monnet (Tübingen: Narr Verlag, 2014), 11–16. See also Rob Boddice, 'The History of Emotions: Past, Present, Future', *Revista de Estudios Sociales*, 62 (October 2017): 12; Bettina Hitzer, *Krebs fühlen: Eine Emotionsgeschichte des 20. Jahrhunderts* (Stuttgart: Klett-Cotta, 2020). Hitzer explores the historical dimensions and changes regarding emotions related to the experience of cancer.

associated emotions. Narrating the suffering of a disease, especially a serious one, goes hand in hand with writing about ensuing anxieties, hopes, desperation and pain. Moreover, being ill not only evokes specific feelings of fear and hope simultaneously, it also generates an emotional upheaval for the seriously sick writer, which is often explored through narrative.

My discussion focuses on contemporary texts. My examples, written by well-known writers, are representative of what in life-writing studies are classified as literary texts that challenge fundamental notions of experience, existence, knowledge and ethics. They often do so in demanding imaginary and aesthetic ways. I mainly selected these illness narratives because their authors all thematize their search for and their struggle with a language to express their feelings as sick writers. The two women and the two men come from different cultural and national backgrounds. Illness narratives, especially autobiographical ones, have gained attention in the past twenty years, not only in the field of literature but also on the book market and, above all, in the fairly new academic fields of the medical humanities and health humanities (including various subdisciplines like disability studies, narrative medicine and literature and medicine).[3] It is self-evident that not all scholars from these fields share the same theoretical background, yet most of them underline the connection between illness and narrative, between suffering and narrative. There are vast differences in such narratives depending on the cultural, social and medical context, but each individual illness experience incorporates an emotional response.[4]

When suffering writers record their anxieties and pain, they draw upon norms and ideas in order to reach their readers, who equally rely on such norms to be able to interpret the narrative.[5] Thus, it is vital to remember

---

[3] More recently, there is also the field of the critical medical humanities which is concerned with

> (i) a widening of the sites and scales of 'the medical' beyond the primal scene of the clinical encounter; (ii) greater attention not simply to the context and experience of health and illness, but to their constitution at multiple levels; (iii) closer engagement with critical theory, queer and disability studies, activist politics and other allied fields; (iv) recognition that the arts, humanities and social sciences are best viewed not as in service or in opposition to the clinical and life sciences, but as productively entangled with a 'biomedical culture'; and, following on from this, (v) robust commitment to new forms of interdisciplinary and cross-sector collaboration.

William Viney, Felicity Callard and Angela Woods, 'Critical Medical Humanities: Embracing Entanglement, Taking Risks', *Medical Humanities*, 41 (2015): 2–7, at 2.

[4] As it is impossible to provide a clear and generally accepted definition of narrative, I will refrain from such a task. Different academic disciplines conceptualize narrative within their own traditions, and different questions are asked, as Paul John Eakin demonstrates: 'What is narrative? A literary form? A social and cultural practice? A mode of cognition? An expression of our most basic physiology?', 'Travelling with Narrative: From Text to Body', *The Travelling Concepts of Narrative*, ed. Matti Hyvärinen, Mari Hatavara and Lars-Christer Hydén (Amsterdam: John Benjamins, 2013), 83.

[5] Cf. Judith Butler, 'Giving an Account of Oneself', *Diacritics*, 31, no. 4 (Winter 2001): 22.

that such a narrative neither transports nor triggers unique or essentialist feelings, although a certain illness and accompanying pain and anxiety may be experienced in similar ways. My focus is on the specific ways in which these emotions are represented in the narrative, and, furthermore, if and how the sick autobiographer theorizes his or her search for language to express these emotions. It is conspicuous that many of these writers not only express their need and even urge to write but also explore the narrative act and their search for language more closely as they are often confronted with the traumatic experience of learning of their serious illness.[6] As Shlomith Rimmon Kenan also maintains, 'a disintegrating body may threaten the very possibility of narration. ... Texts that struggle with its disturbance invite both a challenge and an expansion of the category of "narration".[7]

Narrating suffering: Feeling and writing, reading and feeling

Literary autobiographical texts express emotions of all kinds. Anxiety, hope, pain, shame and so on dominate in autobiographical narratives about experiences of different illnesses. It is necessary to explore the specific narrative discourse in which they are embedded. Both critical emotion research and the critical medical humanities emphasize that emotions are not just marked by physical and mental experiences, but they are also ideologically and socially marked. Sara Ahmed speaks of emotions as cultural practices because emotions 'do' something: They relate to our bodies, to objects and to spaces, and being relational they are not restricted to the individual or the social but produce 'the very surfaces and boundaries that allow the individual and the social to be delineated as if they are objects'.[8] The performative implication of this description illustrates how emotions can create proximity and distance between people and (sick) bodies, a dynamics that is crucial in a sick person's relationships.

---

[6] For a detailed exploration of the relation between trauma and autobiography see Leigh Gilmore's study *The Limits of Autobiography: Trauma and Testimony* (Ithaca, NY: Cornell University Press, 2001).

[7] Shlomith Rimmon-Kenan, 'What Can Narrative Theory Learn from Illness Narrative?', *Literature and Medicine*, 25 (2006): 241–54, at 245.

[8] Sara Ahmed, *The Cultural Politics of Emotion* (Edinburgh: Edinburgh University Press, 2004), particularly 1–19, quote at 10. All page references in the text refer to this edition. See also Monique Scheer, 'Are Emotions a Kind of Practice (and Is That What Makes Them Have a History? A Bourdieuian Approach to Understanding Emotion', *History and Theory*, 51 (2012): 193–220. Scheer speaks of 'emotional practices' (194), emphasizing that 'practice is action' (200).

With these theoretical observations in mind, it is still necessary to decide how to describe and analyse emotional responses to illness in autopathographies when their writers struggle with different illnesses and write in an individualistic style, with different backgrounds and aesthetic agendas. Are there similar processes of subjectivity when sick autobiographers learn of their diagnosis or when they are confronted with intensive technological treatments?[9] And does such a focus reveal an emotional response? How can we ascribe an emotional expression to a writer's use of a highly sophisticated metaphor? Why should a prosaic, rather dry description of an everyday routine activity by a sick autobiographer *not* express any emotion of a writer's health condition? Ahmed aptly states that 'words that name a specific emotion do not have to be used for texts to be readable in terms of that emotion'.[10] Furthermore, emotion words can create different effects depending on their relation to other words, to past experiences, past histories, in short, to all kinds of contexts. Ahmed speaks of a 'circulation of words for emotion' indicating that these words are not stable and can acquire different meanings.[11]

Linguistic research with its reliance on a word corpus can provide evidence for a speaker's/narrator's use of emotional words such as feel, upset, worry, anger and so on., and conclusions can be drawn from the quantity and frequency of such words.[12] Recently, combined efforts of linguists and neuroscientists have yielded results in emotion semantics.[13] But literary texts employ a complex and constructed language and narrative. Such quantitative approaches do not (yet) give us great insight into the composition of a writer's creative text, and they neglect cultural and historical contexts. Therefore, I direct my attention to the narrative strategies that express, allude to or only hint at emotional responses, and to the relation between the personal, the social and the cultural. Focusing on emotions in a selection of autopathographies I pay attention to explicit uses of words and phrases connoting emotions, but specific cultural and social representations of illness regarding emotional responses are much more revealing. I take into account how an autopathographer's narrative strategy may downplay a certain experience and ironize it. Evading the topic of illness

---

[9] See Renata Kokanović and Jacinthe Flore, 'Subjectivity and Illness Narratives', *Subjectivity*, 10 (2017): 332.
[10] Ahmed, *Cultural Politics*, 19.
[11] Ahmed, *Cultural Politics*, 13.
[12] See, for example, Miriam Locher, 'How Medical Students Handle Emotions', *Emotion, Affect, Sentiment*, 215–36.
[13] Joshua Conrad Jackson et al., 'Emotion Semantics Show Both Cultural Variation and Universal Structure', *Science*, 366 (20 December 2019): 1517–22.

and creating distance to it may well point to an extreme experience of anxiety and worry. Such a reading can be based on additional discursive practices that demonstrate emotional responses. Structural characteristics equally need to be considered: non-linearity, for example, and even incomplete paragraphs, may hint at a potential loss of orientation or an utter despair, and these narrative strategies emphasize the impossibility of coherence, whether in life or in writing.

Another characteristic that features prominently is the theorizing of illness in autobiographical writing. Many autobiographers express their urgent need to write about their emotional and intellectual response to this sudden change of their lives, since writing, for them, is the only possible antidote against the illness and they want to document and comprehend its different physical, mental and emotional states. In this case, positioning themselves as patient, writer and theorist, the formation of the subject becomes a complex process. How does illness transform the writing subject and create new, unusual forms of writing? What about coherence/disruption and chronology/non-linearity? Studies on illness narratives call them 'broken narratives' because traditional discursive practices often cannot express the traumatic experience of a serious illness and the self appears shattered and disoriented in time and space, which, in turn, influences the narrative form.[14] Other scholars speak of 'narrating the unnarratable': the disturbing experiences with which any such writer is confronted.[15]

Suffering, creativity, and aesthetics

Christoph Schlingensief, a German artist, author and theatre director, who died of lung cancer in 2010, explicitly thematizes his need to express emotions by proclaiming his emotional turmoil directly. In his cancer diary *So schön wie hier kanns im Himmel gar nicht sein! Tagebuch einer Krebserkrankung* (It can't possibly be as beautiful in heaven as it is here! A diary of cancer), he explains that his speech act represents the necessity of not wanting to silence his extreme fear of illness, dying and death:

> They [people] should let out their emotions! I don't give a shit about this roleplay of security, hiding from other people. I don't give a damn about these metre-long

---

[14] See, for example, *Health, Illness and Culture: Broken Narratives*, ed. Lars-Christer Hydén and Jens Brockmeier (New York: Routledge, 2008), 10.
[15] Rimmon-Kenan, 'What Can Narrative Theory Learn from Illness Narratives?', 249.

bandages people wrap around their wounds. I want to encounter another human being in the very state I am now ...[16]

This passage illustrates how the autobiographer's emotional upheaval is transformed into a provocatively prescriptive agenda to deal with suffering and anxieties (his own and in general), and at the same time, the mere fact of being so direct and honest creates a pleading narrative, even though his language cannot be called poetic or literary. The fact that his published narrative is based on daily recording his thoughts into a Dictaphone may explain this seemingly unpolished form of language. In her recent book on writing illness, Nina Schmidt emphasizes that this explicit act of going public dissolves the boundaries between high and low culture and ultimately between life and art.[17] By addressing readers/audiences and encouraging them to give vent to their own experiences in such a manner, Schlingensief establishes a link between his own suffering and that of his fellow human beings. On the one hand, his imploring sentences underline his emotional and physical pain; on the other hand, they evoke in readers a reconsideration of their own emotions regarding suffering. Schlingensief, a provocative activist in the theatrical and operatic worlds, who in this narrative is primarily a patient dying of incurable lung cancer, still writes as someone who is deeply embedded in the context of his professional life. His sense of self as an artist, therefore, is torn between his plans and aspirations to stage a big opera, and the realization of his more or less imminent death. This triggers bouts of anger, which empower him to move on and to keep writing and hoping. Anger, as Ahmed theorizes in her reading of feminist authors, can be creative and 'hence moves us by moving us outwards'.[18] Although Ahmed's argument is embedded in feminist theory and politics, I argue that Schlingensief's anger similarly expresses a critique of normative attitudes towards and behaviour in relation to illness. It opens up new possibilities, in this case for the patient *and* the artist Schlingensief, even if it is for a short time only. Other autopathographers also express their anger towards their suffering, but Schlingensief's direct, unfiltered way of recording his thoughts and emotions into a Dictaphone endows his emotional outbursts with even more power.[19] As with a feminist position that

---

[16] Christoph Schlingensief, *So schön wie hier kanns im Himmel gar nicht sein! Tagebuch einer Krebserkrankung* (Köln: Kiepenhauer & Witsch, 2009), 243. All page references refer to this edition. All translations from German into English are mine.
[17] Nina Schmidt, *The Wounded Self: Writing Illness in Twenty-First-Century German Literature* (Rochester, NY: Camden House, 2018), 130.
[18] Ahmed, *Cultural Politics*, 176.
[19] A well-known autopathography expressing a lot of anger is Fritz Zorn's *Mars* from 1977. Bettina Hitzer expands on Zorn's anger in more detail in her *Krebs fühlen: Eine Emotionsgeschichte des 20. Jahrhunderts*, 89–90.

demands public activism and must be 'loud' in order to be heard, he goes public with his anger and is not afraid of criticizing those who do not want to show their wounds: 'Those people all have their incisions, wounds. Why don't we show them to each other?'[20]

Schlingensief's text is a direct and at times aggressive reply to his accusing question, although other passages reveal a suffering, desperate and disillusioned diarist/writer when, after a chemotherapy session, he feels utterly lost and sees no hope for the future. It is intriguing that in one such passage, recorded a few days after a devastating experience of hopelessness, he suggests the necessary but fruitful interaction between art and medicine – one of the main postulates of medical humanities – because it is the only way of comprehending a human being holistically: 'And I really believe that we should start thinking about the ways in which art and medicine are connected.'[21] As he puts it, his soul is intricately related to his artistic creativity, and this existential communication has almost been cut during this phase of utter despair. His statement illustrates the emotionally destructive force that the horrors of the chemotherapy session triggered, and yet, having overcome this state, a new insight evolved helping him to move on to the next session. Whereas the present tense dominates in most other sections, the passage describing Schlingensief's anguish and wretchedness appears in the past tense: a distancing strategy chosen to deal with the extremeness of the situation.

Christopher Hitchens, writer and journalist who died of oesophageal cancer in 2011, also used the present tense more often than the past tense, yet he employed different narrative strategies to express his emotional responses in his *Mortality* (2012).[22] Although his narrative is infused with ironic comments that tend to create distance and detachment much more often than Schlingensief's, Hitchens's emotions are frequently expressed in more bodily ways. Descriptions of his body's reactions to his illness and treatments construct a self that becomes a writing body or, literally, an embodied self: 'I don't *have* a body, I *am* a body.'[23] It is 'like a return to the body', as Ahmed explains.[24] In particular, sensations of pain and the experience of a serious illness in general intensify embodied existence, while in ordinary times the body tends to be 'absent' because of its entanglements with so many other people and objects. Yet pain is not a private

---

[20] Schlingensief, *So schön*, 197.
[21] Schlingensief, *So schön*, 227.
[22] Christopher Hitchens, *Mortality* (London: Atlantic Books, 2012). All page references refer to this edition.
[23] Hitchens, *Mortality*, 41.
[24] Ahmed, *Cultural Politics*, 26.

experience. On the contrary, one's pain is always also connected to others in a relational way. Others witness our pain and, providing they have the cultural tools to access it, can 'authenticate its existence'.[25] By sharing his pain explicitly, readers witness Hitchens's pain, and it becomes acknowledged, although it may be impossible for us to ever feel it exactly in the same way as he does. The daily focus on the body as 'being a foe' that makes him feel weak and resigned further triggers emotions of despair and disillusionment, which are described in an elaborate and ironic manner:

> On a much too regular basis, the disease serves me up with a teasing special of the day, or a flavor of the month. It might be random sores and ulcers, on the tongue or in the mouth. Or why not a touch of peripheral neuropathy, involving numb and chilly feet? Daily existence becomes a babyish thing, measured out not in Prufrock's coffee spoons but in tiny doses of nourishment, accompanied by heartening noises from onlookers, or solemn discussions of the operations of the digestive system, conducted with motherly strangers. On the less good days, I feel like that wooden-legged piglet belonging to a sadistically sentimental family that could bear to eat him only a chunk at a time. Except that cancer isn't so ... considerate.[26]

This passage describes a daily experience of terminal cancer with a whole number of side effects often not taken into account by medical care, which nevertheless create immense emotional distress for patients. The emotional reaction to these daily challenges is expressed with verbal irony, intensified by the precise account of seemingly unimportant yet disturbing bodily discomfort ('numb and chilly feet') and of insensitive conversations with medical-care professionals about his digestion.

Hitchens's narrative style becomes more elliptical and fragmentary the more his physical state deteriorates. The last chapter consists of short paragraphs and elliptical sentences: 'Banality of cancer. Entire pest-house of side-effects. Special of the day' or 'See Szymborska's poem on torture and the body as a reservoir of pain'.[27] They do not establish narrative coherence. We are reading short observations as if jotted down in a journal often without the autobiographical 'I'. Considering the entire narrative context of the sick autobiographer these fragmentary sections intensify the severity of the writer's fragile health state and

---

[25] Ahmed, *Cultural Politics*, 31. See also Rob Boddice, *Pain: A Very Short Introduction* (Oxford: Oxford University Press, 2017), 59–60.
[26] Hitchens, *Mortality*, 40, 46.
[27] Hitchens, *Mortality*, 92.

emanate a sense of urgency that carries great emotional weight and contributes to our understanding of the individual suffering from life-threatening cancer.

Hitchens's emotional response to his terminal illness is mirrored in another unusual manner. He thematizes the readerly response to autothanatographies and refers to a potential voyeuristic implication.[28] He comments on John Diamond, the journalist, who had a weekly column on his experience of throat cancer:

> Like many other readers, I used to quietly urge him on from week to week. But after a year and more ... well, a certain narrative expectation inevitably built up. Hey, miracle cure! Hey, I was just having you on! No, neither of those could work as endings. Diamond had to die; and he duly, correctly (in narrative terms) did. Though – how can I put this? – a stern literary critic might complain that his story lacked compactness toward the end ...[29]

Hitchens ironically reflects on his own, past reaction while making his reader emotionally uncomfortable when reading about his own dying. His own 'narrative expectation' regarding Diamond's text was not fulfilled because he was waiting for Diamond's end, which did not occur as expected. Are we also waiting for the writer's end? This intriguing meta-text is inserted between those short passages, which accelerate the reading on the one hand while, on the other hand, the reading process is interrupted to make us reflect on the time that may be left to Hitchens. Besides having this emotional impact on the reader (reading about dying), for Hitchens the passage serves as a means of critically reflecting on his own writing while at the same time creating some comic relief for himself from suffering – and for the reader perhaps as well. This narrative strategy contributes to a critical stance towards the complex concept of authenticity and its relation to the reader's empathy. By outing himself as one who has eagerly waited for the weekly account on dying by a fellow writer, and by virtually performing the same writerly act, Hitchens simultaneously critiques such intense and immediate autobiographical writing and legitimizes its urgency and necessity, but without diminishing its emotional impact. Retrospectively analysing his own critical reading of an autopathography while being terminally sick Hitchens draws his

---

[28] The term 'autothanatography' has been used in life writing studies in the past years for autobiographical accounts of the experience of a terminal illness, although an autothanatography as such 'reports an experience that can be rendered possible only through an unthinkable *sur-vivre*', as Ivan Callus points out in his discussion of such texts. See his '(Auto)thanatography or (auto)thanatology? Mark C. Taylor, Simon Critchley and the Writing of the Dead', *Forum of Modern Language Studies*, 41 (2005): 427–39 at 427.

[29] Hitchens, *Mortality*, 89.

readers' attention even more closely to his writing and suffering. Jenny Diski in her illness narrative also thematizes the public's potential voyeuristic attitude towards cancer memoirs suggesting that readers expect the sick writer to die: 'It's a delicate balance, this publicising of one's cancer. The public's interest is fixated on when each of them will die. For some reason cancer is the disease of choice for public tongue-wagging.'[30] Like Hitchens, she refers to a writer (Clive James) who, thanks to a new medication, did not die according to his own forecasts or his readers' expectations. Despite this critical awareness, she decided to write on, and '[n]o cure is expected, just a slowing down of the deadly events going on inside me.'[31]

British writer Diski, who died from lung cancer in 2016, wrote a monthly column for the *London Review of Books* and candidly reported on the stages of her illness and pain. Besides sharing her anxieties and painful memories of her troubled childhood and teenage years, there are also cheerful accounts of happy times. These collected columns were published under the title *In Gratitude* (2016). Her narrative is a striking example of an illness experience that triggers an exploration of a painful phase or event that, it seems, was not possible before. After the short section entitled 'Diagnosis' the entire first chapter of about a hundred pages is dedicated to her disturbing relationship with Doris Lessing, the famous British-Zimbabwean writer, who took her in when Diski was a teenager. Diski's engagement with the painful issues of this relationship is a strategy to deal with the dreadful diagnosis. Concentrating on a crucial phase of her past enables her to deal with the disruptive experience of illness and vice versa. Both experiences are emotionally charged.

In a later section concerned with Diski's life-threatening illness, she describes feeling dumbstruck at the idea of ceasing to be: 'The prospect of extinction comes at last with an admission of the horror of being unable to imagine or be part of it, because it is beyond the you that has the capacity to think about it. I learned the meaning of being lost for words; I came up against the horizon of language.'[32] And yet, even in spite of the recognition and insight that being dead cannot be approached through language – or put differently, language does not provide the means to describe being dead – Diski keeps on writing in the process of dying; the sheer act of writing is a means of coping with her deep distress, and her narrative not only proves to be culturally and socially but also aesthetically

---

[30] Diski, *In Gratitude*, 157.
[31] Diski, *In Gratitude*, 159.
[32] Diski, *In Gratitude*, 141.

productive because she explores her role as a creative writer in the last chapter. Continuing her search for a way to express her anxiety in language, Diski experiences an even stronger emotional upheaval; it concerns her husband and not herself: 'When the Poet [her husband] expresses his sadness and forthcoming grief, it hits me as if I were him and suffering his loss of me … The pain and sadness that engulfs me at his distress is projection, a mirroring of another soul.'[33] The description of this emotional bonding reveals what not only Ahmed theorizes with regard to pain (see above) but also what in life writing studies is called the 'relational self'. Paul John Eakin, in his groundbreaking study *How Our Lives Become Stories: Making Selves*, elucidates how in autobiographies the autobiographical self and identity are always relational. Our lives and identities are intricately entangled with others, and notions of an autonomous or singular self are a myth.[34] Attempting to describe her anguish about her terminal illness and her imminent death, Diski includes her partner's suffering and even makes his ordeal her own. The limitation of language to the living made her turn to an other self in her exploration of her own, as if she were already dead.

Diski's memoir ends with a cryptic passage consisting of seemingly unrelated painful memories of her mother's harsh reaction to her first menstruation and of a reference to a scene with the caring mother figure from Louisa May Alcott's *Little Women*. This caring mother figure from a fictional work stands in stark contrast to her own mother's cold reaction to her daughter's pain, and the memories of this traumatic experience seem to be triggered by her traumatic experience of dying. Diski's use of the phrase '[u]nwell, after all, is not ill' – 'unwell' is the euphemism used by her mother for menstruation – to describe the hurtful experience of her menstruation must be read in relation to her terminal illness and to its severe pain.[35] Knowing that she is going to die of her illness and at the same time remembering her traumatic experience of her first menstruation, with its accompanying stomach pains, confers a dramatic effect on this enigmatic narrative combination. It not only affects the reader, but it also implicitly describes Diski's suffering from her past life as a teenager in a fractured family. This passage again reminds us of the strong cultural and social context in which pain is embedded, and, additionally, of the gender-related impact of childhood experiences. Furthermore, this difficult passage reflects the relationality of pain, the ways in which it 'shapes the relationships we have

---

[33] Diski, *In Gratitude*, 142.
[34] Paul John Eakin, *How Our Lives Become Stories: Making Selves* (Ithaca, NY: Cornell University Press, 1999), particularly chapter two, 43–98.
[35] Diski, *In Gratitude*, 250.

to our bodies and with others'.³⁶ This final passage in Diski's narrative shares a further, crucial characteristic of creative autobiography. It emits an aesthetic and imaginary power because of its unusual narrative strands expressed in poetic language, triggering contextual and intertextual associations.

Swiss writer Ruth Schweikert, who has been diagnosed with an aggressive kind of breast cancer, calls her illness narrative *Tage wie Hunde*³⁷ ('Days like Dogs') 'an investigation into specific motifs; fragments and experiences, which I want to recollect with the help of an abstract diary'.³⁸ Like Diski and Hitchens, she does not want to write another heroic warrior story like 'an "I have conquered my breast cancer" triumphal march'.³⁹ The disconcerting sentence, written after her operation and treatments, explaining that she sometimes 'really misses THE CANCER as an inner vis-à-vis' illustrates how the cancer experience made certain forms of her written explorations possible, in particular concerning emotions unknown to her before.⁴⁰ Diverse narrative strands from very different phases of her life are woven into her account of her illness, in-between email messages or quotes from other people's statements. The multivocality of her text mirrors the writing self's search for form and answers to her numerous questions, or, more precisely, figures the relationship between questions and knowing, which she can explore only through writing: 'The longer I am writing this text, the more precisely I remember; the more precisely I remember, the more questions come up, which I explore writing: writing, narrating as a recherche *vers l'inconnu*, as an expedition to the *terrae incognitae*, no longer only to one's own memory.'⁴¹ Being confronted with a serious illness, Schweikert's exploration of the unknown realm may refer to death, 'the index of all alterity' that cannot be expressed in speech, as the philosopher Michel de Certeau puts it.⁴² On this expedition to what ultimately cannot be known she not only encounters new questions but also faces all sorts of memories, and she describes the complex interrelationships between an autobiographer's personal experience – here serious cancer – and the writer's remembering and those evolving questions that constantly need to be approached anew. Schweikert's explanations underline the intricate connection

---

³⁶ Leigh Gilmore, 'Agency Without Mastery: Chronic Pain and Posthuman Life Writing', *Biography*, 35, no. 1 (Winter 2012): 84.
³⁷ Ruth Schweikert, *Tage wie Hunde* (Frankfurt am Main: S. Fischer, 2019). All references in the text refer to this edition, and all translations into English are mine.
³⁸ Schweikert, *Tage*, 73.
³⁹ Schweikert, *Tage*, 73.
⁴⁰ Schweikert, *Tage*, 161, emphasis in original.
⁴¹ Schweikert, *Tage*, 174.
⁴² Michel de Certeau, *The Practice of Everyday Life*, trans. Steven Rendall (Berkeley: University of California Press, 1984), 193–4.

between her cancer illness, her emotional responses and the ensuing 'research' she undertakes in her autobiographical text.⁴³

The personal diary gives us insight into a number of emotional responses to Schweikert's diagnosis, one of which is shame. The explicit use of the word appears several times and is always connected to cancer, a social and cultural stigma still hovering over her; Schweikert's description painfully and also quite radically expresses her feelings of shame:

> Dogs can smell it; the shame and rot, the tumor, the growth that has formed in me, that I have formed in my left breast; dogs might smell it because of my breath I exhale; as soon as I open my mouth it takes their breath away.⁴⁴

In many instances, shame is related to cancer, the so-called 'C word'. When suffering from teratoma, Jackey Stacey wrote, 'Whatever you say, don't say "cancer". The unspoken word, written on everyone's lips, must not be voiced.'⁴⁵ Although twenty-four years have passed since Stacey made this statement in her illness narrative, which is both an autobiography and a cultural study of cancer, social and cultural taboos around cancer are still dominant. Hitchens, too, comments on 'the big C', referring to its stigma.⁴⁶ One of Stacey's explanations for the associated horrors that cancer evokes concerns its frequent invisibility: 'It silently makes itself at home and waits.'⁴⁷ Describing her shame Schweikert also mentions this feeling of not having noticed what happened inside her body: 'As soon as I open my mouth shame confronts me ... it is as if something had made itself visible, a secret that finally shows itself.'⁴⁸ This 'blindness' towards the distinction between inside and outside is theorized by Stacey. The inability to recognize boundaries between inside/outside, subject/object, normal/abnormal, healthy and well (often before cancer is diagnosed) causes anxieties and even horror.⁴⁹ The inability to recognize clearly definable boundaries is often linked to 'the abject', Julia Kristeva's term, which describes a reaction triggered by the

---

⁴³ In philosophy, psychology, history, trauma studies and more recently in the neurosciences, numerous studies have explored the interface of memory and emotions. In life writing studies, many of which focus on accounts of traumatic experiences, memory is often linked to the body (e.g. in sexual abuse testimonies); affect theorist Patricia Clough suggests, '[t]rauma is the engulfment of the ego in memory. But memory might be better understood not as unconscious memory so much as memory without consciousness and therefore, incorporated, body memory, or cellular memory', in *The Affective Turn: Theorizing the Social*, ed. Patricia Ticineto Clough and Jean Halley (Durham, NC: Duke University Press, 2007), 6–7.
⁴⁴ Schweikert, *Tage*, 41.
⁴⁵ Jackie Stacey, *Teratologies: A Cultural Study of Cancer* (London: Routledge, 1997), 65.
⁴⁶ Hitchens, *Mortality*, 28.
⁴⁷ Stacey, *Teratologies*, 73.
⁴⁸ Schweikert, *Tage*, 41.
⁴⁹ Stacey, *Teratologies*, 77.

threat of not distinguishing between subject and object, self and other and, in this case, between the healthy and the sick body.[50] The fact that Schweikert all of a sudden is confronted with a tumour inside of her that she has not seen or realized intensifies her feelings of horror and shame. The reference to dogs, with their ability to sense cancer, need not necessarily evoke shame (they actually are said to be able to detect some cancerous tumours), but Schweikert's description of her own breath 'poisoning' the dogs' breath ('it takes their breath away') enhances the association of disgust with odour.[51]

By writing so bluntly and openly about her emotional state as a cancer patient, Schweikert challenges stigmatizing notions and, in the course of her narrative (and also because of her continuous investigation into her emotional state), the feeling of shame becomes less powerful and overwhelming. Similarly to Schlingensief's insistence on sharing one's emotional response to one's illness, Schweikert minutely analyses her diverse emotional reactions when learning of her diagnosis and creates a complex narrative structure mirroring the turmoil even syntactically. Some of her paragraphs, for example, do not end with a complete sentence and do not have a full stop. Even grammatical normativity is challenged. Furthermore, the visual form of the page expresses the multiple strands of thought and memory that dominate Schweikert's mind. A different font is used for letters and email messages; recollections of direct speech by other people and texts the autobiographer reads or remembers are intentionally put in italics by the author. In some of her email messages we find typos indicating her anguished state when wanting to learn the result of the biopsy as soon as possible. The noun *Befund* (medical findings) is once written with a correct capital letter, another time with a small letter, thus highlighting not only the urgency of the result for the writer but also the horrific confusion such a result can cause for the patient/writer. Leaving such typos in the published book form enhances the writer's emotional state and sharpens the reader's attention to potential explanations for the writer's challenge of normative rules. Furthermore, the author's choice to keep such inconsistencies and to mark different text genres underlines her continuous exploration of the unknown realm mentioned above and create an effect of incompleteness.

---

[50] Julia Kristeva, *Powers of Horror: An Essay on Abjection*, trans. Leon S. Roudiez (New York: Columbia University Press, 1982).

[51] See also Bettina Hitzer, 'The Odor of Disgust: Contemplating the Dark Side of 20th-Century Cancer History', *Emotion Review*, 12, no. 3 (July 2020): 164, and her reference to Ángela Guirao Montes et al., 'Lung Cancer Diagnosis by Trained Dogs', *European Journal of Cardio-Thoracic Surgery*, 52 (2017): 1206–10.

Conclusion

The experience of illness illustrates the immense difficulties the autobiographer/patient is faced with in their search for a language of illness; it is also this painful experience that triggers unusual, disruptive and creative narrative strategies. In all of the four texts I have discussed, different narrative strategies are employed to describe the lived experience of illness, but they all relate to emotional responses by their autobiographers. Representations of a relational self in pain, anguish and hope are present in all these illness narratives. Schlingensief's anger and pain are expressed in a direct address to the reader in an activist manner; Hitchens's writing bears testimony to the tragic and painful relationship between the terminally sick body and the writing self, and yet, it acquires a poetic quality, even in its elliptic and fragmentary style towards the end of his writing (life). Diski's imminent death evokes anxieties and an urge to delve into these. Thus, even philosophical short treatises evolve. But at the same time, she can finally face the painful phase in her life with Doris Lessing, exemplifying the emotional influence of illness on the memory of earlier traumatic experiences. Through her search for form and language, Schweikert creates a formally challenging text that resonates with her emotional response to her illness experience, integrating disconcerting feelings of shame and disgust.

In her canonical essay 'On Being Ill', Virginia Woolf emphatically insists on the relation between a new language of illness and the emotions:

> He [the sufferer] is forced to coin words himself, and, taking his pain in one hand, and a lump of pure sound in the other … so to crush them together that a brand new word in the end drops out … Yet it is not only a new language that we need, more primitive, more sensual, more obscene, but a new hierarchy of the passions; love must be deposed in favor of a temperature of 104; jealousy give place to the pangs of sciatica …[52]

Woolf prophetically claims that emotions not only shape the language of illness but that emotional responses to illness are as worthy of being written about as is the topic of love. More than ninety years later, autopathographers still boldly share their emotions in new languages. Exploring their experiences of illness in and through creative writing is bound to engender new forms.

---

[52] Virginia Woolf, *On Being Ill* (Ashfield, MA: Paris Press, [1930] 2002), 7.

7

Beyond symptomology: Listening to how Palestinians conceive of their own suffering and well-being

Heidi Morrison

The prominent Palestinian activist Hana Ashrawi begins the poem 'From the Diary of an Almost-Four-Year-Old' with the heartbreaking words of a little Palestinian girl imagining what the world will look like now that she has lost an eye from an Israeli soldier's bullet. 'I wonder will I see half an orange, half an apple, half my mother's face with my one remaining eye?'[1] The poem concludes with this same little girl worrying about a nine-month old who she recently learns has also lost an eye from an Israeli bullet. The little girl pities the helpless baby and says: 'I'm old enough, almost four, I've seen enough of life, but she's just a baby, who didn't know any better.'

This poem holds significance for many reasons, one of which is the spotlight it places on contextualizing childhood trauma. The four-year-old no longer sees herself as a child due to her life experience, which outmeasures her age. Palestinians commonly claim that Israeli violence robs them of a childhood.[2] Palestinian blogger Yasmeen El Khoudary writes that some Palestinian children

---

I would like to thank the National Endowment of the Humanities (NEH), the Palestinian American Research Center (PARC), the Fulbright Scholar Program, the University of Wisconsin, La Crosse, UCLA's Center for Near Eastern Studies, Tampere University's Center of Excellence in the History of Experiences and Birzeit University's Ibrahim Abu-Lughod Institute of International Studies. For critical feedback, thanks to the Middle East Studies Association meeting (2019), the Social Psychology Days conference at the University of Helsinki (2021) and to Penny Mitchell, Rita Giacman, Nadera Shalhoub-Kevorkian, Rob Boddice and Bettina Hitzer.

[1] From Salma Khadra Jayyusi, ed. *Anthology of Modern Palestinian Literature* (New York: Columbia University Press, 1994), 340.

[2] Heidi Morrison, 'Unchilding by Domicidal Assault: Experiences of Childhood and Home during the Second Intifada', *Jerusalem Quarterly*, 84 (2020): 70.

do not define their age by years but by the number of wars they have lived through.³ Poet Mourid Barghouti describes how

> the Occupation has created generations without a place whose colors, smells, and sounds they can remember; a first place that belongs to them, that they can return to in their memories in their cobbled-together exiles. There is no childhood bed for them to remember, a bed on which they forgot a soft cloth doll, or whose white pillows – once the adults had gone out of an evening – were their weapons in a battle that had them shrieking with delight.⁴

Palestinian academic Nadera Shalhoub-Kevorkian coined the term 'unchilding' to refer to Zionists' deliberate and wholesale stripping of Palestinian children of their childhood as an essential pillar to building, maintaining and growing the state of Israel.⁵

In a situation where violence systematically prevents children, generation after generation, from having a proper 'childhood' (as enshrined in the near universally ratified Convention of the Rights of the Child, adopted by the United Nations in 1989), how do we understand and measure childhood trauma? This chapter argues that conventional psychological and psychiatric behavioural and medical experiments and assessments do not suffice for understanding Palestinian childhood trauma. The widely used Trauma History Questionnaire (THQ), for example, uses a simple yes/no checklist to assess the types of trauma a person has been exposed to, as well as the severity. Charts of mental health symptoms based on the Diagnostic and Statistical Manual (DSM) refer to individual patients, not general populations, let alone populations enduring multigenerational trauma. Further, the DSM is shaped by American culture, but symptoms are couched in context and may vary from one time and place to another. Also, feelings derived from exposure to trauma change over time, particularly for children. Trauma 'symptoms' may not appear until decades later, or may worsen or get better with time. Symptoms are a snapshot of time- and place-bound realities. Scholars are increasingly turning to the humanities (historical, artistic and literary analysis) to expand trauma research.⁶ This is part

---

³ Yasmeen El Khoudary, 'Gaza Child: Three Wars Old', *Aljazeera*, 16 July 2014, retrieved from http://www.aljazeera.com/indepth/opinion/2014/07/gaza-child-three-wars-old-2014716505446437.html.
⁴ Mourid Barghouti, *I Saw Ramallah*, trans. Ahdaf Soueif (New York: Anchor Books, 2003), 62.
⁵ Nadera Shalhoub-Kevorkian, *Incarcerated Childhood and the Politics of Unchilding* (Cambridge: Cambridge University Press, 2019).
⁶ Nigel Hunt, *Memory, War, and Trauma* (Cambridge: Cambridge University Press, 2010); Nigel Hunt, *Landscapes of Trauma: Psychology of the Battlefield* (London: Routledge, 2019); Ville Kivimäki and Peter Leese, eds, *Trauma, Experience and Narrative in Europe during and after World War II* (London: Palgrave Macmillan, 2022).

of a larger trend towards interdisciplinarity in the field of medicine (medical humanities and narrative medicine).

This chapter uses 'portraiture' to capture the experience of Palestinian childhood war trauma in the recent past.[7] It looks specifically at the experience of Palestinian children who grew up during the second intifada, 2000–6, providing a sample portrait (abbreviated from its original version) as well as an analysis of that portrait.[8] My portraits are based on oral histories, and to a lesser extent on photos, journals, Facebook posts and observations I have collected in Palestine for the last decade while following the lives of ten young adult Palestinians. In my research, I have sought to understand the impact of violence, and memories of it, on Palestinians' well-being. More generally, I have asked what their life stories tell us about mental health in Palestine and how academics, particularly those of us in the humanities, can advance trauma studies. The chapter pushes the bounds of conventional psychological studies as well as conventional war history in its use of portraiture. In terms of the former, my research questions symptomology in understanding trauma, and instead accounts for context. In terms of the latter, my research moves away from battlefields and armies and into the intimate spaces of war.

Note on methodology

To broaden our understanding of children's experiences with violence, past and present, we need to ask questions about the human condition, illness and suffering and perceptions of oneself. Sarah Lawrence-Lightfoot's method of 'portraiture' can be one effective tool for achieving this. The goal of portraiture is to blend artistic expression with systematic empirical research to capture the complex and subtle dynamics of human experience.[9] The portraitist paints with words a person's life story. Portraiture is a method employed by anthropologists

---

[7] Sarah Lawrence-Lightfoot and Jessica Hoffmann Davis, *The Art and Science of Portraiture* (San Francisco, CA: John Wiley, 1997). Historical study of the very recent past is a vital project. As Renee Romano argues, 'It is the past that people draw on for analogies, and it is this past that proves a "fertile breeding ground for crude myths", which can gain power only when scholarly work doesn't exist to test their credibility.' For a historiographical analysis of writing the very recent past, see Renee Romano, 'Not Dead Yet: My Identity Crisis as a Historian of the Recent Past', *Doing Recent History*, ed. Claire Bond Potter and Renee Christine Romano (Athens: University of Georgia Press, 2012), 23–44.
[8] In my larger work I rely on multiple portraits to tell the story with which this chapter engages through only one.
[9] Lawrence-Lightfoot and Davis, *Art and Science of Portraiture*.

and sociologists who reject the constraints of ethnography and biography to capture contemporary human experience. Historians, like myself, are well suited to apply portraiture to their work on the past. Portraiture requires the historical method, namely systematic and empirical description based on primary sources and contextualization. To a certain extent, portraiture is similar to microhistory, in that they both ask larger questions in small places. History emerges from the intimate spaces in which humans function. However, the distinguishing feature of portraiture is its use of aesthetics (metaphors, rhythms, tone, etc.) to capture what it means to be human, as well as its attention to sensory experiences (of the subject *and artist*). These distinguishing features do not belie the historian's craft. The historian who seeks to capture the way people felt in the past can benefit from imbuing their and their subjects' feelings in the method of writing itself.

The historian is not neutral but instead always has a stake in the production of knowledge. There is no such thing as an unmediated reality.[10] Lawrence-Lightfoot and Davis explain how portraiture makes room for subjectivity in academic writing:

> The portraitist's voice, then, is everywhere – overarching and undergirding the text, framing the piece, naming the metaphors, and echoing through the central themes. But her voice is always a premediated one, restrained, disciplined, and carefully controlled. Her voice never overshadows the actors' voices (though it sometimes is heard in duet, in harmony and counterpoint.) The actors sing the solo lines, the portraitist supporting their efforts at articulation, insight, and expressiveness.[11]

Although some historians define their discipline in opposition to literature and art, there is a long legacy of academics and artists crossing boundaries to try to present a more complete reality. Feeling motivates reason more than opposes it.[12] Joan Scott advocates for historians to engage in more 'literary' readings of the past, to not confine oneself to single meanings of words and ideas.[13] This is a way to free the historical actor from ossified, one-dimensional categories of existence. Historians' use of portraiture is a way to engage in more 'literary'

---

[10] H. Porter Abbott, *The Cambridge Introduction to Narrative* (Cambridge: Cambridge University Press, 2014).
[11] Lawrence-Lightfoot Davis, *Art and Science of Portraiture*, 85.
[12] Piroska Nagy and Damien Bouquet, 'Historical Emotions, Historians' Emotions', *Emma*, 5 March 2011, https://emma.hypotheses.org/1213.
[13] Joan W. Scott, 'The Evidence of Experience', *Critical Inquiry*, 17 (1991): 796.

writings about the past, to go beyond singular modes of historical representation, which in turn can expand our understanding of historical trauma.

Note on context

According to UNICEF's Chief of Child Protection, nearly one billion children today live in countries and territories affected by war and conflict.[14] This harsh reality is not necessarily a result of children carrying AK47s – as the iconic child soldier image might lead us to believe – but instead a result of bedrooms, schools and playgrounds becoming targets in warfare.[15] The twentieth- and twenty-first-century historical phenomenon of adults conducting wars against children constitutes the larger backdrop to this chapter.[16] I tell this story through the case study of West Bank Palestinian children's experiences in the second intifada. Scholars such as Rashid Khalidi, Sara Roy and Ramzy Baroud have written about the larger political and economic landscape that initiated the second intifada, yet no scholar has sought to seriously understand what children experienced in their daily lives and how that experience lives in their memory today.[17] The few academic studies that exist on Palestinian children in the second intifada are quantitative in nature.[18] Focusing on numbers and statistics, they measure instances of bedwetting and nightmares and make generalized statements about symptoms of post-traumatic stress syndrome.[19]

[14] As quoted in Robin Wright's 'The New Way of War: Killing the Kids', *New Yorker*, 3 July 2014.
[15] Attacking children in war is not an entirely new invention of the modern era, but what is new is the significant growth in the frequency and intensity over the last one hundred years. Other differences are the existence of global standards of war and also the imbalanced geographical distribution of the victims (mostly residing in the non-West).
[16] James Marten, ed., *Children and War: A Historical Anthology* (New York: NYU Press, 2002); Kim Huynh et al., *Children and Global Conflict* (Cambridge: Cambridge University Press, 2015).
[17] Rashid Khalidi, *The Iron Cage: The Story of the Palestinian Struggle for Statehood* (Boston, MA: Beacon Press, 2007); Ramzy Baroud, Kathleen Christison, Bill Christison and Jennifer Loewenstein, *The Second Palestinian Intifada: A Chronicle of a People's Struggle* (New York: Pluto Press, 2006); Sara Roy, *Failing Peace: Gaza and the Palestinian-Israeli Conflict* (New York: Pluto Press, 2007).
[18] My article 'Unchilding by Domicial Assault' provides an exception, looking at the ways in which Israeli violence during the second intifada permeated the beds, rooftops and kitchens of Palestinian children.
[19] See the work of Ziad Abdeen, Rawdan Qasrawi, Shibli Nabil and Muhammad Shaheen 'Psychological Reactions to Israeli Occupation: Findings from the National Study of School-Based Screening in Palestine', *International Journal of Behavioral Development*, 32 (2008): 290–7; A. Sagi-Schwartz, 'The Well-Being of Children Living in Chronic War Zones: The Palestinian-Israeli Case', *International Journal of Behavioral Development*, 32 (2008): 322–56; Muhammad M. Haj-Yahia, 'Political Violence in Retrospect: Its Effect on the Mental Health of Palestinian Adolescents', *International Journal of Behavioral Development*, 32 (2008): 283–9; Brian Barber, 'Political Violence, Social Integration, and Youth Functioning: Palestinian Youth from the Intifada', *Journal of Community Psychology*, 29 (2001): 259–80.

The second intifada, coming in the wake of the first intifada and subsequent decade-long failed Oslo Peace Talks, resulted in yet another generation of Palestinian children hit by violence in their daily lived space.[20] Palestinian family homes were the object of Israeli-led demolitions, occupations, lockdowns and raids. Many children lost their lives on their journey to or from school or while tending farmland.[21] In 2002, the second year of the second intifada, one-third of documented Palestinian children's deaths took place in or around the home.[22] At the height of the intifada, Israel turned some Palestinian schools into interrogation and detention centres to hold detainees, including children.[23] Due to such factors as the shelling of populated areas, most children died in daily-life activities and not in violent confrontations.[24] The West Bank city of Jenin, which is the site of the events discussed in this chapter, was one of the hardest hit areas of the second intifada. During the notorious ten-day 2002 Battle of Jenin, Israeli forces levelled hundreds of buildings, leaving one quarter of the population homeless.[25] Until today, Jenin remains under a brutal Israeli military occupation.

My research cohort of ten Palestinians represents a cross-section of the West Bank. I began talking to these Palestinians in 2010 when they were in their late teens and early twenties, and they are now in their mid to late twenties and early thirties. The quantity of my cohort is intentionally small so that I could do in-depth life histories, which required multipart interviews with my subjects and also shorter interviews with their families, friends and associates.[26] Numerous in-country visits allowed me to develop a working alliance with my interlocutors. Rich communication takes time to emerge. That my research does

---

[20] For a survey of the near century of violence Palestinian children have experienced at the hands of Zionists see Nadera Shalhoub-Kevorkian, *Incarcerated Childhood*.

[21] Catherine Hunter, Annelien Groten and Ayed Abu-Qtaish, *Children of the Second Intifada: An Analysis of Human Rights Violations against Palestinian Children* (Palestine: Defence for Children International, 2003), 46.

[22] Hunter et al., 'Children of the Second Intifada', 19.

[23] Hunter et al., 'Children of the Second Intifada', 46.

[24] Defence for Children International/Palestine Section, 'Surviving the Present, Facing the Future: An Analysis of Human Rights Violations against Palestinian Children in 2004', April 2005, 14.

[25] https://www.unrwa.org/where-we-work/west-bank/jenin-camp.

[26] I am inspired in my research by the works of scholars like Edmund Burke III, Dina Matar, Laetitia Bucaille and Leyla Neyzi, who similarly seek to understand Middle Eastern history and society through a biographical and life story approach. For good examples of oral history projects that include interviews with the larger network of the subject, see Kathryn Nasstrom, *Everybody's Grandmother and Nobody's Fool: Frances Freeborn Pauley and the Struggle for Social Justice* (Ithaca, NY: Cornell University Press, 2000); Valerie Yow, *Bernice Kelly Harris: A Good Life Was Writing* (Baton Rouge: Louisiana State University Press, 1999); Valerie Yow, *Recording Oral History: A Guide for the Humanities and Social Sciences* (3rd edition, Lanham, MD: Rowman & Littlefield, 2014); Irum Shiekh, *Detained without Cause: Muslims' Stories of Detention and Deportation in America after 9/11* (Houndmills: Palgrave Macmillan, 2011).

not focus on Israelis and Palestinians of all ages does not in any way imply that suffering was not widespread.[27]

Portrait of Mustafa

When I arrived in Jenin in March 2014, I could not find Mustafa in his normal hangout location; nor could I reach him on his cell phone. Mustafa's absence was concerning, especially in light of his words to me two years prior: 'If there were some medicine in this world that made a human lose his memory and be a new human being, I am ready to try it.' Where was Mustafa? Had Mustafa locked himself again in his room in a sedated stupor? Had Israel reimprisoned him? Did he finally get a visa to Norway? Was Mustafa dead?

Mustafa once shared with me a childhood memory which embodies the story of his life. 'When I was a child, we used to try to catch birds in the mountains. I spent two years trying, before I finally caught one. Then, it died.' In many respects, Mustafa's life mirrors that of the bird. As a child, Mustafa visited and explored freely in the villages around Jenin, until suddenly a fatal force caught him in its grip. That force was the Battle of Jenin, a brutal, ten-day Israeli assault on the Jenin refugee camp and surrounding areas which included documented Israeli war crimes that left one quarter of the camp homeless, fifty-four Palestinians dead (half of which were thought to be civilians), hundreds wounded, and about two hundred captured. Mustafa suffered bullet injuries to the knee and eye that left long-term nerve damage. Mustafa lost his best friend in the invasion, as well. Jenin fell back under Israeli occupation, which Mustafa had seen subside during the Oslo years. (He was nine years old when the Israeli government turned Jenin over to the Palestinian Authority (PA).)

After the invasion, Mustafa felt that the world had 'flipped upside down'. Mustafa stopped being a happy, obedient child who loved school, swimming, playing soccer and running in the mountains. Instead, he became an armed militant. In his words: 'We started carrying weapons, simple ones in front of the

---

[27] In paying special attention to children, this in no way is meant to imply that killing and destruction of other age groups of Palestinians is not equally horrific. As Maya Makdashi warns, massifying the plight of Palestinian children (and women) runs the risk of leaving out Palestinian men from public mourning, and hence deeming the men dangerous (Maya Makdashi, 'Can Palestinian Men Be Victims? Gendering Israel's War on Gaza', *Jadaliyya*, 23 July 2014). Generally speaking, it could be argued that studying issues related to violence in the Middle East risks fuelling the flame of cliché about the region. Laleh Khalili makes clear that scholarly conversations about violence and the Middle East should move 'beyond the terrain of prejudice and paranoia'. Laleh Khalili, 'Thinking about Violence', *International Journal of Middle East Studies*, 45 (2013): 791–4.

tank and the airplanes, not because we wanted to carry weapons. But without weapons you will die ... We did not have any choice. We could not immigrate to Norway and America, no one helped us.' Mustafa said global events at the time intensified his desire to pick up arms. He related his Palestinian experience to the plight of the innocent civilians suffering in the war in Afghanistan. Further, US propaganda about spreading democracy in Iraq angered Mustafa.

Mustafa spent five years in Israeli prison, beginning at seventeen years of age (in 2003). In prison, Mustafa was diagnosed with migraines, anxiety and depression. He became dependent on sedatives and painkillers prescribed by Israeli prison doctors. When he came out of prison, he felt once again that the world had turned upside down on him. He was twenty-two years old and without a high school diploma (Tawjihi). He came to learn about friends and family who had been injured, killed or arrested while he was in prison. Also, the PA's leadership, which he so admired in the Oslo years, diminished even more. All these changes, compounded by the memories of the invasion and prison, weighed heavily on Mustafa. He did not leave the house or see anybody. Mustafa wanted to erase his past. 'I don't see any benefit in remembering death', he says.

Unfortunately, for as much as Mustafa wanted to forget the past, he could not. The nightmares he had in prison returned. Mustafa describes them: 'I dream that I am falling in a place that is very dark. I am between the sky and the earth. I feel that I am suffocating. I see strange creatures. I dream that the sea is swallowing up Jenin. The people are drowning in the sea and I am with them.' During the day, Mustafa suffered from bursts of rage. He would break glasses in the kitchen or flip tables upside down. Mustafa felt isolated in his turmoil. He explains, 'There is nobody to listen because everybody has their own worries and problems.' Mustafa resumed taking the pills he had relied on in prison. He slept for twelve hours straight during the night and felt numb during the day.

In his darkest days, Mustafa's mother was his only source of hope (his 'refuge'), but he did not want to trouble her with his problems. Mustafa began regular therapy sessions at the Treatment and Rehabilitation Center for Victims of Torture in Jenin. A Palestinian therapist suggested that Mustafa think about something positive, such as the beach, before going to sleep at night.[28] Mustafa said he found this useless. He felt that seeking therapy was making family and friends also perceive him as 'crazy'. He stopped going.

---

[28] At the Middle East Studies Association (MESA) annual conference in 2019, Dr Said Shehadeh argued in his paper presentation that the work of Palestinian mental healthcare workers complements Zionist settler colonialism. He is seeking to decolonize Palestinian mental health and chart an indigenous framework for repair.

In 2013, at twenty-seven years of age, Mustafa set out to begin a new life in Europe. He used his savings, which normally would have been used at this age for marriage, buying a house and establishing a life. Mustafa got as far as Turkey but missed his connecting flight to Russia when airport police accused him of having a forged passport. Mustafa came back to Jenin on edge, angry and with depleted resources. His brother called him a donkey, shaming him for what happened.

A few months later, in January 2014, the Israeli military came to Mustafa's home in Jenin in the middle of the night. They blindfolded and arrested him. For this reason, I could not find Mustafa in March 2014. Mustafa was released from prison after fifteen months, at twenty-nine years of age. When I went to Jenin to visit Mustafa in 2019, he failed to show up at our arranged appointment. Mustafa's friends told me this was typical behaviour for him. On the rare occasions when Mustafa met with friends, he often left suddenly and without explanation. Mustafa only left the house to work the night shift as a garbage collector for the municipality.

Time seems to be gradually erasing Mustafa's existence, just as his nightmares forebode. As a child, war injuries took away feeling in parts of his body. Violence killed friends and loved ones. Mustafa emerged from prison as a ghost only to be submerged again. He hides now in his room. From many perspectives, Israel has treated Mustafa as the discarded trash he so dutifully picks up each night.

Portrait analysis

What does portraiture reveal about childhood trauma in Palestine? My goal in using portraiture is not to create a new diagnostic tool (another 'how damaged are you on a scale of 1–10' tool). The objective is not to prove that Palestinians are traumatized. My goal is also not to create yet another method of analysis that reduces trauma to one dimension (another 'what did Israel do to you?' tool.) It is a given that the Israeli occupation is primarily at fault in creating endless cases of childhood trauma. The distinguishing feature of portraiture is its use of aesthetic and sensory expression (metaphors, rhythms, tone, etc.) to capture what it means to be human. Thus, portraiture captures the experience of trauma, which takes the focus away from symptoms, diagnosis and singular causations of illness. Portraiture puts the focus instead on context. Portraiture presents a three-dimensional view of trauma. In the case of Mustafa, portraiture elucidates that (1) trauma is embedded in intimate spaces that can escape medical classification; (2) there are local and global structures in addition to the occupation that are causing and perpetuating trauma; and (3) children who experience trauma can grow up to have agency (of multiple forms, including through narration).

First, listening to the experience of Mustafa tells us that trauma is embedded in his life and memory. Trauma is not something that is short-lived and temporary, like a gunshot or a high-pitched scream. It is something that lives in the intimate spaces and objects of daily life. It is in the scars on Mustafa's body as well as in his soccer ball, his bedroom, his table, his friendships. The portrait shows this by paying attention to the subject's situated affective and embodied experience, including his actions, the tone and intensity of his moods and emotions and his social interactions, all of which often escape medical classification or terminology. The portrait captures situated experience through descriptive gestures, poetic narratives and allegories about the subject. The bird that Mustafa tries to catch in the hills is one such example. The bird is a metaphor of Mustafa's own search for freedom and for life other than that which is available. The references to the sea are about Mustafa's search for a new horizon to emerge. Often people, particularly children, do not consciously process stimuli and instead react in seemingly unrelated ways. Children may be haunted by traumatic experiences that escape linguistic designation and get unclearly bound up over time in other aspects of life.

Second, the portraitist takes a life story approach, letting the event under question fall where it may.[29] The desire is to move the zone of attention away from the epicentre of the subject's trauma to a whole set of issues around the edges. This portrait shows that Mustafa is a multidimensional being. Mustafa's trauma is interlocked with more than the second intifada. It is a function of cultural, economic, political, local, national, global and temporal phenomena, as well as memory and physical and mental development over time. Trauma is never just about one event, such as personal suffering, social unrest or rupture.[30] Trauma is cumulative and can be felt over the life course, depending on intensity, chronicity and so on. Portraits are palimpsests, or points where otherwise unrelated phenomena interweave.[31] The portrait allows us to look at the entire context of a person's experience with trauma, and not just the symptoms. Mustafa's trauma

---

[29] Mary Marshall-Clark, 'Herodotus Reconsidered: An Oral History of September 11, 2001, in New York City', *Radical History Review*, 111 (2011): 79–89.
[30] Christina Zarowsky, 'Writing Trauma: Emotion, Ethnography, and the Politics of Suffering among Somali Returnees in Ethiopia', *Culture, Medicine, and Psychiatry*, 28 (2004): 189–209.
[31] Sarah Dillon, *The Palimpsest: Literature, Criticism, and Theory* (London: Bloomsbury, 2013).

is part of the matrix of war, multigenerational loss (the Nakba), the fledgling authority of the PA in the post-Oslo years, prison torture, family poverty, injustice in Afghanistan and Iraq and Israeli state-led surveillance, racism and settler colonialism. Political rights and freedoms are the key domains of good functioning for Palestinians.[32] Additionally, the difficulty of local, daily living conditions can even at times trump larger abstract concepts such as collective national identity.[33] Mustafa's trauma emerges from and through a context. The trauma is not a pathology to be treated with sedatives, like the Israeli doctors did in prison. Sedatives numb feelings for a while, which then re-emerge, sometimes larger than before if the trauma is unresolved.

Mustafa's portrait shows the gradual dismemberment of a human being. We see Jaspir Puar's concept of the right to maim being carried out.[34] Physical and mental pain and injury make Mustafa debilitated and unable to function. He tells me that he is not living, and that ten years from now he will still just be 'sitting, drinking coffee, waiting to die' in Jenin. We see Sherene Razack's concept of disposability, or Mustafa as undeserving of full personhood and dignity.[35] Doctors prescribe Mustafa addictive drugs under the guise of healthcare. The therapist tells Mustafa to imagine scenes of the ocean to relax, even though he cannot even get a permit to visit the ocean in real life. We see Nadera Shalhoub-Kevorkian's 'unchilding', or 'a violent racial regime of control that actively maintains the machinery of dismemberment, always and everywhere'.[36] During Mustafa's initial imprisonment at seventeen years of age, he was held for sixty days in a room without light or family contact. As an adult, Mustafa rarely leaves the bedroom in his house. The regime of control sucked his body in and spat it out in pieces. Thus, Mustafa's childhood trauma cannot be reduced to bedwetting and crying. His trauma was born in a place and time that regarded his body as waste. What Mustafa says he wants is justice and recognition.

Third, for all his trauma, Mustafa is more than a victim. The portrait seeks to unflatten the voice of a child under occupation. Narration itself is a form

---

[32] Brian Barber et al., 'Politics Drives Human Functioning, Dignity, and Quality of Life', *Social Science of Medicine*, 122 (2014): 90–102.
[33] Diana Allan, *Refugees of the Revolution: Experiences of Palestinian Exile* (Palo Alto, CA: Stanford University Press, 2014).
[34] Jasbir K. Puar, *The Right to Maim: Debility, Capacity, and Disability* (Durham, NC: Duke University Press, 2017).
[35] Sherene H. Razack, *Dying from Improvement: Inquests and Inquires into Indigenous Deaths in Custody* (Toronto: University of Toronto Press, 2015); Sherene H. Razack, 'Stealing the Pain of Others: Reflections on Canadian Humanitarian Practices', *Review of Education, Pedagogy and Cultural Studies*, 29 (2007): 375–94.
[36] Nadera Shalhoub-Kevorkian, *Incarcerated Childhood and the Politics of Unchilding* (Cambridge: Cambridge University Press, 2019).

of power for Mustafa. Vernacularizing, or Mustafa's choice to use words and concepts such as the sea, horizon, bird, allows him to tell his story 'his way'. Further, Mustafa resists in daily life 'his way'. He picks up weapons to reassemble his home, homeland and self. He finds refuge in his mother's love. Mustafa hides in his room, existing in the only way he knows possible to survive the pain. Mustafa tells me there is no such thing as love and that most religious people are hypocrites. He is critical of cultural customs, rejecting the sacred which has left him behind. At one point, Mustafa told me my research would not amount to anything important for the Palestinian people or him. He shuns me as another invader in his life, keeping himself protected. Mustafa finds dignity in the trash he picks up. His salary helps his parents, who are both ill. Mustafa's agency cannot be reduced to a binary framework of powerful/powerless. He is both dismembered and refuses dismemberment at the same time.

Conclusion

In Palestine, there is not a system of sustainable public mental health services.[37] Many scholars have pointed out the deficiencies of individualized, Western, medicalized understandings of trauma that extract Palestinians from their context.[38] Mustafa's portrait, along with the others in my collection, brings up broad strokes for enriching conventional approaches to mental health in Palestine. My role as an oral historian has been to make space for Palestinians to tell their stories. Instead of chopping up the interviews into quotes to share with a broader audience, I have chosen to use portraiture as my medium of communication. In my writing and analysis, I have relied heavily on the historical method of contextualization, seeking to understand what my interlocuters say in relation to what other scholars have written on similar topics as well as contemporaneous

---

[37] Rita Giacaman et al., 'Mental Health, Social Distress, and Political Oppression: The Case of the Occupied Palestinian Territory', *Global Political Health*, 6 (2011): 547–59.

[38] Rita Giacaman, 'Reframing Public Health in War Time: From the Biomedical Model to the "Wounds Inside"', *Journal of Palestinian Studies*, 47 (2018): 9–27; Stephen Sheehi, 'The Transnational Palestinian Self: Toward Decolonizing Psychoanalytic Thought', *Psychoanalytic Perspectives*, 15 (2018): 307–22; Brinton M. Lykes and Marcie Mersky, 'Reparations and Mental Health: Psychosocial Interventions towards Healing, Individual Agency and Rethreading Social Realities', *The Handbook of Reparations*, ed. Pablo de Grieff (Oxford: Oxford University Press, 2006); R. W. Srour and A. Srour, 'Communal and Familial War-Related Stress Factors: The Case of the Palestinian Child', *Journal of Loss and Trauma*, 11 (2006): 289–309; David J. Marshal, 'Save (Us from) the Children: Trauma, Palestinian Childhood, and the Production of Governable Subjects', *Children's Geographies*, 12 (2014): 281–96.

events. I approach trauma neither as a traumatologist nor medical specialist of any kind.

Oral historians and portraitists can make contributions to medicine, particularly because of their threefold ability to systematically document (1) the multileveled causes of trauma; (2) trauma's diverse meanings in time and place; and (3) agency (in all its forms). When we listen to Palestinians, we learn that trauma is embedded in their history, memory and daily lives. Childhood trauma functions at a deeply intimate level, and it cannot always be captured by conventional medical terminology and classification. The trauma is multipronged, stemming from local and global structures of violence that seek to unchild, maim and debilitate. Lack of good functioning is not the fault of the individual but is the result of exposure to perpetual danger over long periods of time. Palestinian children's frailties cannot be treated or cured so long as they remain to be seen out of their larger political context.

Just as the four-year-old girl's words remind us to understand her lived experience, and not just slap a label on her based on chronological age, we see through Mustafa's portrait that a biomedicalized approach to trauma creates only half the picture. The four-year-old girl remarks that even with her eyes closed, she can still see clearly the soldier who shot her in her head. She says, 'It could be that inside our heads we each have one spare set of eyes to make up for the ones we lose.' The portrait of Mustafa begs us to see trauma differently. The full view of the apple incidentally (and at times) requires shutting one's eyes to convention.

Expertise, authority, emotion

Commentary

The feelings of the medical encounter are, in these two chapters, acutely unstable. They make for uneasy reading at times, but what emerges is the ambiguity of medico-cultural scripts for how to feel. They are often only partly formed, leading to both conceptual and experiential uncertainty on the part of medical authorities and on the part of the people who find themselves before them. Here, considering the victim-survivors of sexual violence on the one hand, and imprisoned male psychopaths on the other, we are dealing with people who found themselves dramatically out of place, for vastly different reasons, and facing medical authority and the medical gaze to negotiate their suffering. We see the doubts on the part of those medical authorities about how to look at, how to examine, and how to treat the embodiment of dis-ease before them, as well as their own emotional reactions to specific types of suffering and the possibility of its mediation.

Both chapters deal with the subject, broadly, of pain. But they show just how open the category 'pain' needs to be if we are to reach a thorough historical understanding of past (and present) suffering. First and foremost, the subject matter here deals with emotion, the capacity to feel, and feelings out of place. Joanna Bourke's chapter conjures with shame and shaming to examine why those who experience sexual violence feel shame in the encounter with forensic medicine, when there is no ostensible reason to be ashamed. She asks explicitly where this shame comes from and how it emerges through the encounter. Implicated here is the medical gaze itself, which does the shaming work. By extending the rape ordeal to the medical examination that follows, Bourke implicates the power embodied by medical personnel in doubling down on the emotional suffering caused by sexual violence. This is vital research in its specific target, but it also serves as a reminder that it is not enough to talk about bioculturally situated and constructed emotional experiences like shame without careful contextual consideration of what it means and how it comes to be.

Marcel Streng's account of the changing fortunes of 'Leidensdruck', both on the part of psychotherapists and their potential patients, is a further reminder of the highly situated status of suffering. Not only is the concept difficult to translate, Streng's account shows the course of a short-lived concept undergoing change, of the ways in which medical scripts find their way to patient-perpetrators and are re-voiced back to medical authorities. The power dynamic is essential, since this particular capacity to suffer, according to the assessment of medical authorities, was the primary pathway to treatment and recovery for male prisoners deemed psychopathic. To become well first required the would-be patient to know or be able to show that he felt his dis-ease in the correct way. 'Leidensdruck' could only be validated by the expert, which demonstrates an acute example of the politics of pain and the possibility of both psychological and social redemption.

Though the chapters do not braid in their subject matter, they clearly speak to one another. They unmask the relationship between the broad cultural repertoire of attitudes and understandings of criminal violence, and of the ways in which the harm it causes is mediated by the medical refinement of that broad cultural repertoire. The cases are highly specific, highly dynamic, and yet depend upon a general understanding of the social and cultural contexts in which they take place.

8

Forensic sense: Sexual violence, medical professionals and the senses

Joanna Bourke

On 12 June 1993, the editors of the *British Medical Journal* (*BMJ*) published a personal account by a male doctor of being sexually assaulted by a colleague. In light of the sensitive nature of the account, the editors took the unusual decision of allowing the victim to remain anonymous. The doctor described how a male medical friend had sexually abused him when they were sharing a hotel room during a medical conference. Although the doctor was angry, he was also ashamed. He fretted about whether he was partly culpable for what had been done to him. After all, he admitted, he had been drinking alcohol and, during the attack, had frozen instead of fighting his abuser. He noted that the attack had left no physical scars; psychologically, though, he was still in turmoil.[1]

A month later, the *BMJ* published a response from psychiatrist Donald John Brooksbank, a senior medical officer in the Department of Health. He advised the upset doctor to contact the voluntary organization Survivors, which had been founded in 1986 to support male victims of sexual assault.[2] SurvivorsUK (as it came to be called) had been established to deal with the fact that male rape was imbued with tremendous shame and stigma but was being ignored by most of the specialist assault services (particularly feminist ones) that had been set up to support female victims.[3]

However, not all medical professionals who read the anonymous doctor's harrowing account were sympathetic. The editors of the *BMJ* found themselves having to defend their decision to protect the victim's anonymity, informing

---

[1] Anonymous, 'Male Rape', *British Medical Journal*, 306, no. 6892 (12 June 1993): 1620–1.
[2] Donald John Brooksbank, 'Male Rape', *British Medical Journal*, 307, no. 6899 (31 July 1993): 323.
[3] Michael King, 'Male Rape. Victims Need Sensitive Management', *British Medical Journal*, 301, no. 6765 (15 December 1990): 1345.

readers that 'we accepted that the author might suffer unnecessarily if the article was signed'.[4] But a particularly vicious response came from Stephen Due of the Medical Library at Geelong Hospital in Victoria (Australia). Due began by sneering that the unnamed author 'apparently believes that his self revelations will benefit readers', before suggesting that the doctor's wish to remain anonymous was really because he was ashamed. Due maintained that the doctor's shame was an appropriate response since the letter was a 'sorry tale of childish behavior which reflects no credit on him, for he claims to have been indecently assaulted while in a drunken stupor at an international conference'. The *BMJ* was beginning to read 'like a lonely hearts club', Due complained, adding that 'sordid personal confessions add nothing to our understanding of a subject, but they do demean a scholarly, professional journal'.[5]

These 1993 exchanges between an anonymous doctor, a kindly psychiatrist, the editors of the journal published by the prestigious British Medical Association and an unforgiving medical librarian address some of the themes of this chapter. These include the role of medical professionals in debates about sexual violence, contested understandings about the emotional aftereffects of sexual abuse, anxieties about the gendered nature of assault (particularly when it involved male victims), victim culpability and the powerful impact of shame on victims. Such issues would resonate with millions of people worldwide. The statistics are startling. In times of societal conflict, sexual violence against women, girls, men and boys routinely reaches extreme levels.[6] But even in those societies that only rarely experience war on 'home soil' (and these are the societies I will be focusing on in this chapter), levels of sexual abuse are high. For example, according to Rape Crisis, in England and Wales today, eleven people are raped every hour, affecting approximately 85,000 women and 12,000 men; another half a million adults are sexually assaulted.[7] In the United States, thirty-three residents over the age of twelve are raped and sexually assaulted every hour. That makes 288,820 legally acknowledged victims annually.[8] These figures do not include the millions of victim-survivors who never report their assault.

---

[4] The Editors, 'Anonymity in the BMJ', *British Medical Journal*, 307, no. 6899 (31 July 1993): 323.
[5] Stephen Due, 'Anonymity in the BMJ', *British Medical Journal*, 307, no. 6899 (31 July 1993): 323.
[6] See discussions in Raphaelle Branche and Fabrice Virgili, eds, *Rape in Wartime* (Houndmills: Palgrave Macmillan, 2012); Elizabeth D. Heineman, ed., *Sexual Violence in Conflict Zones: From the Ancient World to the Era of Human Rights* (Philadelphia: University of Pennsylvania Press, 2011); Gaby Zipfel, Regina Mühlhäuser and Kirsten Campbell, eds, *In Plain Sight: Sexual Violence in Armed Conflict* (New Delhi: Zubaan, 2019).
[7] Rape Crisis England and Wales, at https://rapecrisis.org.uk/get-informed/about-sexual-violence/statistics-sexual-violence/, viewed 10 December 2019.
[8] US Department of Justice, Office of Justice Programs, Bureau of Justice Statistics, *National Crime Victimization Survey, 2010–2014* (Washington, DC, 2015).

Understanding reactions to sexual abuse requires a critical historicization of medical responses to sexual abuse and the historization of the emotions. I will do this in the context of British and American discourses from the late nineteenth century to the 1980s. Historical framings of sexual violence have tended to focus on important questions of law enforcement, legal outcomes and public responses. The public health dimensions have been neglected, which is significant given that only a small proportion of abuses then (as well as now) are ever reported to the police, let alone reach the courts. As a result, the negative health outcomes for victim-survivors who remain silent about their experiences of violation are an important topic of enquiry. This chapter will argue that an analysis drawing on the history of the emotions can illuminate some of the harms of sexual violence. In particular, I will focus on the complex emotion of shame and cognate feelings and experiences, exploring its situated constructions and meanings in relation to a neglected field of power: that is, the pivotal role played by medical discourses in the production of victim-shame. Although many of these arguments are relevant to the experience and treatment of rape victims today, this chapter focuses on the late nineteenth century to the 1980s, the period before the dramatic (although, in retrospect, ineffectual) revisions of legal procedure and introduction of feminist-led crisis interventions. The first section begins by examining ways that physicians have contributed to the shaming of victims. Medical and forensic textbooks used by police surgeons, hospital physicians and other medical examiners are saturated with shaming tropes. I ask why even medical professionals who are sincerely dedicated to caring for ailing and distressed people, and who are also accustomed to visceral sights that untrained observers usually find upsetting, might respond negatively to victims of sexual abuse. In caring for victim-survivors of sexual abuse, why have medical professionals been complicit in shaming practices?

The second section directly addresses the experience of shame for victim-survivors themselves. Given that they are not responsible for the abuse perpetrated against them, why do so many victim-survivors report feeling high levels of shame? How can we understand the embodiment of victim-shame?

Language needs to be addressed first, however. The words used to write about sexual harms are complicated. In this chapter, I use concepts like rape, sexual violence, sexual assault and sexual abuse interchangeably. This is only a shorthand way of referring to a range of harms. It is not intended to imply that these acts are identical – nor that there is a continuum in seriousness, starting with emotional hurt and ending with sadistic violence. I am not concerned with the hierarchies of harms that pervade legal texts and public discussions (e.g.

notions that physical harms are 'worse' than psychological ones or that women can be 'raped' while men are 'assaulted'). Rather, I seek to draw attention to the unique context and quality of suffering for each victim-survivor for whom the physical and psychological are emmeshed. I also use concepts like 'victim' and 'survivor' cautiously. The term 'survivor' is anachronistic for much of the period I am writing about but, in general, the term 'victim-survivor' is helpful.

Shaming

There is a sophisticated literature on why victim-survivors of rape are reluctant to report their abuse to the authorities and, when they *do* go public, on their discriminatory treatment by law enforcement agents (who routinely 'no-crime' or 'unfound' complaints) and court systems (where jurors and judges fail to convict all but a tiny proportion of offenders).[9] Given these failures, exploring the significant health outcomes for the vast majority of victim-survivors whose accounts of abuse remain unheard is imperative.

It is well known that the harms caused by sexual abuse are legion. They include physical injuries, sexually transmitted infections, unwanted pregnancies and psychiatric illnesses. Even those victim-survivors who do not suffer such harms routinely report experiencing debilitating and painful emotions. The most shattering to their self-esteem is shame, which is complex, multiformed and contextually contingent. It is thus an often elusive emotion. Clinical observations and empirical evidence, together with first-person accounts of extreme forms of abuse (such as sexual assault or torture), testify to high levels of personal and social shame.[10] Victim-survivors often refer to feeling culpable and dishonoured.

[9] This is a huge literature. In the British context, see Liz Kelly, Jo Lovett and Linda Regan, *A Gap or a Chasm?: Attrition in Reported Rape Cases: A Home Office Research Study* (London: Home Office Research, Development and Statistics Directorate, 2005); Jennifer Temkin and Barbara Krahé, *Sexual Assault and the Justice Gap: A Question of Attitude* (Oxford: Hart, 2008); Jennifer Temkin, *Rape and the Legal Process* (Oxford: Oxford University Press, 2002).

[10] This is evident in first-person rape accounts. For medical literature about sexual abuse and shame, see Bernice Andrews, Chris R. Brewin, Suzanna Rose and Marilyn Kirk, 'Predicted PTSD Symptoms in Victims of Violent Crime: The Role of Shame, Anger, and Childhood Abuse', *Journal of Abnormal Psychology*, 109 (2000): 69–73; Bolanle Akinson and R. Nicholas Pugh, 'Patients' Perspective Is Also Important', *British Medical Journal*, 324, no. 7350 (8 June 2002): 1397–8; Jonathan I. Bisson, Sarah Cosgrave, Catrin Lewis and Neil P. Robert, 'Post Traumatic Stress Disorder', *British Medical Journal*, 351 (14 April 2007): 789–93; T. J. Gerrald and J. D. Riddell, 'Difficult Patients: Black Holes and Secrets', *British Medical Journal*, 297, no. 6647 (August 1988): 530–2; Paul Gilbert and Beatrice Andrews, eds, *Shame: Interpersonal Behavior, Psychopathology, and Culture* (New York: Oxford University Press, 1998); Sir Basil Henriques, 'A Magistrate's View', *British Medical Journal*, 2, no. 5267 (16 December 1961): 1629–30; Tessa Richards, 'Medicine and the Media', *British Medical Journal*, 289, no. 6458 (8 December 1984): 1658 ; Jan Welch and Fiona Mason, 'Rape and Sexual Assault', *British Medical Journal*, 334, no. 604 (2 June 2007): 1157. For other empirical studies, see Emily

Indeed, feelings of shame are central to many of the *other* harms inflicted by sexual violence. Shame is entangled with powerful feelings, such as sadness, anxiety or self-hatred. It contributes to destructive behaviours, including sexual and social dysfunction, drug and alcohol abuse and self-harm. The emotional distress of the anonymous doctor with whom I started this chapter was typical. He was troubled by an overwhelming sense of shame for what happened to him. Despite being intellectually aware that any feelings of shame rested solely with his attacker, he nevertheless felt culpable. After subtly questioning whether the assault had even taken place ('he *claims* to have been indecently assaulted'), the judgmental interlocuter explicitly contended that the anonymous doctor *should* be ashamed, not only for drinking alcohol and failing to fight off his abuser but also for daring to publicize his 'sordid' tale. The anonymous doctor summoned up emotional and professional resources to make his abuse known to others but, for most victim-survivors, shame was the main reason they were reluctant to report their experiences.

There is a huge corpus of research documenting the numerous ways that victim-survivors of sexual harms are led to feel ashamed. In *Rape: A History from the 1860s to the Present*, I argue that today, as in the past, everyday knowledges, including institutional ideologies and practices within law enforcement, judicial systems and the mass media, attack the self-esteem of victims. Powerful 'rape myths' (including 'no means yes', 'it is impossible to rape a resisting woman', 'women make false accusations', 'no wound, no rape', and 'many kinds of forced sex are not really rape') ensure that victims of sexual violence struggle to make their voices heard, let alone be believed.[11] Sexually abused boys and men face further hurdles. Shouldn't they have been capable of fighting off any attacker? Are they consciously or unconsciously gay? Are they 'real' men anyway?

I will not repeat these issues. Instead, I turn to the contributions made by medical discourses to the shaming of victim-survivors. Textbooks in medical jurisprudence are influential in propagating 'rape myths' that attack the esteem of complainants. These texts became increasingly important from the end of the eighteenth century, starting a process that resulted in the declining role of midwives and local women in medically helping girls and women who had been sexually molested. Male physicians rapidly became the 'experts' responsible for

---

J. Ozer, Suzanne R. Best, Tami L. Lipsey and Daniel S. Weiss, 'Predictors of Posttraumatic Stress Disorder and Symptoms in Adults: A Meta-Analysis', *Psychological Bulletin*, 129 (2003): 52–73; Angela Ebert and Murray J. Dyck, 'The Experience of Mental Death: The Core Features of Complex Posttraumatic Stress Disorder', *Clinical Psychology Review*, 24 (2004): 617–35.

[11] See my *Rape: A History from the 1860s to the Present* (London: Little, Brown, 2007). Also see my *Disgrace: Global Reflections on Sexual Violence* (London: Reaktion Books, 2022).

examining the bodies of victims, assessing their states of mind and adjudicating on their claims. As part of this process, the professional field of medical jurisprudence was introduced and grew in status. By the mid-nineteenth century, all countries in Western Europe and all states in the United States had introduced medical jurisprudence courses in universities. Elsewhere, I have discussed the ways textbooks on medical jurisprudence routinely disparaged women's complaints of sexual assault.[12]

Less frequently analysed is the role of everyday medical practitioners – especially police surgeons and forensic medical examiners – in promoting practices that shamed people who reported having been abused. These medical professionals shared knowledges concerning how to judge 'true' violation. Because they were seen by the police, courts, the media and indeed complainants themselves as providing 'objective' knowledges based on a comprehensive, reproducible analysis of the body, their judgements of victim-survivors of sexual abuse were prescriptive, not merely descriptive. In other words, for a woman's complaint to be taken seriously, victim-survivors were required to comport themselves according to a script that was composed and policed by physicians and other medical professionals.

Medical examiners were taught to cast a formal, forensic eye on complainants' body language. Were they acting like 'innocent' victims of sexual assault, or might they have 'precipitated' their own assault? Did complainants look strong or physically fit? Were there signs that they vigorously resisted? Surely 'true' victims would have visible lesions and bruising to corroborate their accounts? As one commentator quipped in 1967, 'A woman can run faster with her skirt up than a man can with his pants down.'[13] Previous sexual experience was also used to shame victim-survivors: 'It's not been the first time, has it?' asked one medical examiner.[14] Wearing sexy clothes or hitchhiking was condemned as risky behaviour that made victim-survivors at least partly culpable. Might they be unconsciously inviting abuse? This was the view of forensic expert Charles G. Wilber. Writing in 1974, he criticized the 'patterns of behavior, deportment, and dress' of the 'healthy, adult, sexually mature girl … in our modern society'. Such young women 'consciously or subconsciously stimulate a rape response in the susceptible male'. Of course, he hurriedly added, he did not want to 'justify the serious invasion of the personal integrity of one person by another through

---

[12] See my *Rape*.
[13] R. McCaldon, 'Rape', *Canadian Journal of Corrections*, 9 (1967): 39.
[14] Barbara Toner, *The Facts of Rape* (1977; revised edition, London: Arrow, 1982), 176.

the crime of rape'. Nevertheless, he contended, 'it is a fact that many kinds of modern female dress do, in fact, present an image which can trigger the rape response in the susceptible type of male'.[15]

These are not isolated examples. Medical professionals were *taught* to draw inferences about the veracity of assault from the comportment of complainants. The 1978 Royal Commission on Criminal Procedure, for example, instructed physicians to note 'the method of undressing' of the victim. They were advised to observe the 'general appearance and demeanour of the victim', including any 'eccentricity of dress and use of cosmetics'. They should ask themselves, 'Is the woman a shy retiring child, or is she a professional stripper?'[16] In 1974, Irving Root, Wendell Ogden and Wayne Scott issued similar instructions in their article entitled 'The Medical Investigation of Alleged Rape'. Police surgeons should question whether 'the emotional attitude or affect of the patient' was 'appropriate or inappropriate to the history and physical findings?' They maintained that the complainant's comportment was important for police surgeons since victims would have already undergone 'extensive, pointed, and often embarrassing questioning before and after the medical examination'. This would have been a 'very traumatic and emotional ordeal' for any 'innocent' complainant. Therefore, 'if the woman appears to be distraught, emotionally upset or frightened', this increased the likelihood that the rape actually happened. 'Conversely', they continued, 'a casual or almost nonchalant attitude after an alleged vicious and forcible attack might cause some doubt about the truth of the history'.[17]

It might be argued that such suspicions about the post-rape behaviour of victim-survivors would have declined with the increasing acceptance of rape trauma syndrome (RTS) and post-traumatic stress disorder (PTSD) from the 1970s onwards. After all, nurse Ann Wolbert Burgess and sociologist Lynda Lytle Holmstrom had invented RTS in 1974 precisely to teach medical professionals that victims responded in a huge variety of ways to rape. Some were 'hysterical' and teary while others maintained an emotionally blank calm, at least outwardly. It was not uncommon to hear victims nervously laughing. Many delayed reporting having been assaulted for days, weeks, even years. Crucially, Burgess and Holmstrom noted, all these responses were 'normal'.[18] By the 1980s, the

---

[15] Charles G. Wilber, *Forensic Biology for the Law Enforcement Officer* (Springfield, IL: Charles C. Thomas, 1974), 209.
[16] RCCP, *Rape: Police, and Forensic Practice* (London: Royal Commission on Criminal Procedure, 1978).
[17] Irving Root, Wendell Ogden and Wayne Scott, 'The Medical Investigation of Alleged Rape', *Western Journal of Medicine*, 120 (April 1974): 331.
[18] Ann Wolbert Burgess and Lynda Lytle Holmstrom, 'Rape Trauma Syndrome', *American Journal of Psychiatry*, 131 (1974): 981–6, at 981. For a detailed analysis, see my 'Sexual Violence, Bodily Pain, and Trauma: A History', *Theory, Culture and Society*, 29 (2012): 25–51.

varied ways that victim-survivors behaved after rape were widely acknowledged. However, the replacement of a 'trauma script' for the previous 'distress script' brought its own forms of shame. Diagnoses of RTS or PTSD did help victim-survivors understand why they reacted in contrary ways to their abuse, but it retained the focus on the behaviours of victims while also characterizing them as suffering from a mental illness. As educationalists Corrine C. Bertram and M. Sue Crowley explain, 'Labelling is not a socially neutral process.' Victim-survivors of sexual abuse

> may prefer to avoid health-care and counselling services after experiencing sexual violence, since survivors may perceive these institutions not as sources of help or advocacy, but as locations of blame and additional trauma.[19]

The ways in which medical services might be experienced as part of the 'bad event' itself – rousing self-blame, for example – will be explored shortly.

These professional procedures and practices meant that victim-survivors routinely reported feeling shame, anger and distress. In 1983, for example, Gerry Chambers and Ann Millar conducted a survey of rape complainants. They found that 42 per cent made negative comments about their treatment by police surgeons and an additional 18 per cent gave mixed positive and negative views.[20] Typical complaints included the painful nature of the examination, the amount of time they had to wait prior to the examination, inadequacies with the room, the unavailability of a female doctor and the lack of privacy. Some even objected to the fact that male police officers were allowed to sit behind a screen in the medical room during their examination. Women described how their clothes had been taken away, but they were not given alternative garments. Police surgeons were described as 'insensitive', 'unsympathetic' and 'abrupt'. Victims were upset that the collection of samples and the tests took precedence over the treatment of their injuries. They resented being questioned about whether they had resisted sufficiently. One complainant was even asked if she enjoyed it. 'It was as if I was on the slab in the morgue', said another.[21] In other words, the forensic

---

[19] Corrine C. Bertram and M. Sue Crowley, 'Teaching about Sexual Violence in Higher Education: Moving from Concern to Conscious Resistance', *Frontiers: A Journal of Women's Studies*, 33 (2012): 67.
[20] Gerry Chambers and Ann Millar, *Investigating Sexual Assault: A Scottish Office Social Research Study* (Edinburgh: Her Majesty's Stationary Office, 1983), 99.
[21] Gerry Chambers and Ann Millar, *Investigating Sexual Assault: A Scottish Office Social Research Study* (Edinburgh: Scottish Office, Central Research Unit, 1983), 100–1. This was also the conclusion drawn by Robley Geis, Richard Wright and Gilbert Geis, 'Police Surgeons and Rape: A Questionnaire Survey', *The Police Surgeon: Journal of the Association of Police Surgeons of Great Britain*, 14 (1978): 7–14, and reprinted in the journal (October 1984): 56–66.

examination was experienced as part of the rape 'event' itself. In *The Story of Pain* (2014), I argue that it is useful to distinguish between *what* is experienced and the *way* people experience something. Distress is a manner of feeling or a way of perceiving an experience. It is practiced within relational, environmental contexts. For victim-survivors, the forensic examination is evaluated in the context of the rape itself: it becomes part of the pain they experienced.[22]

This point was acknowledged by the London Metropolitan Police. In 1991, they carried out their own survey. Although one-third of all reported rapes in England and Wales took place in the Metropolitan Police district and the Metropolitan police offered training in the medical examination of rape victims, nevertheless, the survey concluded that 'many of the police surgeons who examine rape victims, though professionally competent, are unsympathetic.'[23] Forty per cent of women surveyed who had reported their rape to the police complained that the doctors who examined them had acted in ways that lacked sympathy.[24]

How can we explain the propensity of physicians and other medical professionals to engage in practices that shamed victim-survivors? Obviously, their training in medical jurisprudence, with its pervasive hostility to and mistrust of female complainants, was one reason. But there were others. First, police surgeons were uniquely sensitive to being falsely accused of sexually abusive actions. Unlike other professionals, medical personnel are regularly required to have intimate contact with the sexual organs of strangers. From their first year in medical school, they had been schooled in the risk of false accusations of sexual assault and they were advised to always have a chaperone present when conducting intimate examinations. All would have been aware of cases where fellow practitioners had been (falsely or not) accused of sexually abusing their patients. They were particularly susceptible, therefore, to believing the most powerful of all the rape myths: 'women lie'.[25]

Second, police surgeons were immersed in police culture. This includes a generalized suspicion towards people seeking their services, an awareness of the need to seek collaboration for any witness testimony and a greater familiarity with aggression than most people, especially girls and women, which make

---

[22] Joanna Bourke, *The Story of Pain: From Prayer to Painkillers* (Oxford: Oxford University Press, 2014), introduction.
[23] Caroline White, 'Police Surgeons Are "Unsympathetic" to Rape Victims', *British Medical Journal*, 303 (20 July 1991): 149.
[24] White, 'Police Surgeons Are 'Unsympathetic' to Rape Victims', 149.
[25] For an extended discussion, see my 'Police Surgeons and Victims of Rape: Cultures of Harm and Care', *Social History of Medicine*, 31 (2018): 679–87, at http://doi.org/10.1093/shm/hky016.

them less sensitive to how others might respond to displays of belligerence. In this period, the job of police surgeon was a highly masculine one. As late as 1985, the Medical Women's Federation found that the ratio of female to male police surgeon was a dismal 1 to 7.5.[26] They were also more distanced than most physicians from the usual patient–doctor dynamics. After conducting the medical examination, police surgeons rarely saw the victims again. Victim-survivors almost never became part of their regular medical practice, which meant that physicians were ignorant about their families and communities as well as not being required to forge long-standing duties of care towards them. Victim-survivors were not really conceived of as 'patients'.[27]

These explanations for the failure of medical professionals to exercise more than an abstract, professional variety of sympathy towards the victims they examined contributed to the shaming of rape complainants. But they are insufficient. In order to understand why medical professionals who were sincerely dedicated to caring for ailing and distressed people might respond negatively to victims of sexual abuse, we need to turn to the history of the emotions. In the historiography on sexual violence, the emotional lives of medical professionals have been ignored. There is abundant evidence that many medical professionals disliked examining rape victims. As Wilber frankly admitted in 1974, physicians were 'openly hostile to the idea of becoming involved in a rape case' and their hostility 'extends to their resistance to examining a rape victim'.[28] In the early 1980s, one survey found that physicians and hospital workers believed that working with rape victims was 'dirty' and 'beneath dignity'.[29] Interviews with over 200 professionals who dealt with victim-survivors in 130 organizations in Florida between 1983 and 2004 also showed that there was considerable distaste for the work.[30] In other words, despite the fact that intimate examinations of vaginas and anuses are common practice in medical contexts, the rape exam was regarded as something different. In the words of one male Chief Resident of a hospital obstetrics/gynaecology ward, rape cases

---

[26] Anon., 'Are Doctors Trained to Deal with Rape?', *British Medical Journal*, 291 (7 December 1985): 1655.
[27] Patricia Yancey Martin, Douglas Schrock, Margaret Leaf and Carmen Van Rohr, 'Crisis Work. Rape Work: Emotional Dilemmas in Work with Victims', *The Emotional Organization: Passions and Power*, ed. Stephan Fineman (Oxford: Blackwell, 2008), 54.
[28] Wilber, *Forensic Biology*, 203.
[29] Lynda Lytle Holmstrom and Ann Wolbert Burgess, *The Victim of Rape: Institutional Reactions* (1978; revised edition, New Brunswick: Transaction, 1983), 64.
[30] Patricia Yancey Martin, Douglas Schrock, Margaret Leaf and Carmen Van Rohr, 'Crisis Work. Rape Work: Emotional Dilemmas in Work with Victims', in Fineman, ed., *Emotional Organization*, 53–4. Also see P. Y. Martin and D. DiNitto, 'The Rape Exam', *Women and Health*, 12 (1987): 5–28.

make us all uncomfortable. ... I always had a feeling when I walked into the victim's room that I was not wanted, needed maybe ... but not wanted. I felt like I was an intrusion at a very sensitive time. We all dislike the rape exam; it's a distasteful time.[31]

It was a telling statement, registering both an acknowledgement that he was dealing with a distressed person who might resent and fear his 'intrusion', as well as his own feelings of helplessness in overcoming his own emotions and those of his patients. Rape victim-survivors could not help but register the reluctance of medical professionals to 'deal with' them.

One way to approach this question is to note that the medical professional not only *has* a body, she or he *is* one, to paraphrase Merleau Ponty.[32] As with shame (which I will be turning to soon), disgust is a social emotion. It is a culturally constituted and socially inscribed reaction to the perception of contamination. The doctor's disgust was powerful because the rape victim was perceived as a threat or pollutant. Rape complainants often arrived in a disarranged state. They were typically distraught, stained with blood and semen and barely able to make consistent statements. Many were considered to be the 'dregs of society': drunks, prostitutes and other 'unsavoury' characters. The abused child was too knowledgeable about sex; the raped girl, a seductress; the sexually assaulted older woman, a fantasist who was going through the 'climacteric'. In all cases, cultural anxieties about the boundaries between good/bad, men/women and self/other needed to be policed. It was no coincidence that one of the few other instances where medical professionals openly expressed disgust was in response to intersex children, that is, another category of patient who blurred boundaries.[33]

Of course, it is important to note that disgust was not an attribute of the victim-survivor but was a response or projection of *another* person. In addition, medical professionals might cognitively know that their disgust response was inappropriate and unfair to victim-survivors. But despite being aware that they should feel no more disgust with the victim than they would for any suffering person, they still felt it. As we will see in the next section, this disengagement

---

[31] Cited in Patricia Yancey Martin, Douglas Schrock, Margaret Leaf and Carmen Van Rohr, 'Crisis Work. Rape Work: Emotional Dilemmas in Work with Victims', in Fineman, ed., *The Emotional Organization*, 54.
[32] Maurice Merleau-Ponty, *Phenomenology of Perception* (London: Routledge, 2002), n.p. (Part 1).
[33] Ellen K. Feder, 'Tilting the Ethical Lens: Shame, Disgust, and the Body in Question', *Hypatia*, 26 (2011): 633–50.

between cognition and feelings was mirrored in the emotional lives of victim-survivors and their shame.

Embodying shame

This final section turns to the various ways that victims embodied shame. In the last section, I explored certain medical norms, values and practices that might have *incited* shame in victim-survivors. Although they may have noticed that medical examiners recoiled from their bodies, it is still not at all clear why victim-survivors might have felt *shame* (as opposed to embarrassment or anger, for instance)? What explains the paradox that victim-survivors might *intellectually* have known that responsibility lay solely with the agent of harm and they might have consciously resisted the shaming eye of medical examiners – but were nevertheless ashamed? What does the politics of shame contribute to the harms of sexual abuse?

The gendered element of the recent history of shame makes it of particular interest to scholars exploring the emotional lives of victim-survivors of sexual abuse. When looked at through the lens of sexual violence, many philosophical explanations for shame are highly problematic. Arguments that shame is about policing propriety or that it is an 'enforcer of proper behavior'[34] are unconvincing: after all, given the widespread condemnation of sexually violent men, why do victim-survivors report feeling ashamed immeasurably more frequently than those who offended against them? Evolutionary approaches also stumble when attention is turned to the shame of victim-survivors. For example, humanities scholar Jörg Wettlaufer contends that shame is a 'universal, pan-human emotion' that 'has been selected as part of evolution and thus is a functional adaptation'. He claims that shame 'is elicited by behaviour that is deemed inappropriate in terms of in-group norms'. It 'only works', he insists, 'if everyone agrees on the norms and if the culprit [sic] identifies themselves with the norms of the group'.[35] Of course, Wettlaufer did not have rape victims in mind when he wrote these words nor was he concerned with other communities who report systemic feelings of shame, such as survivors of the holocaust or other atrocities. However, such an explanation cannot address the lived experience of victim-survivors of rape, unless one adopts the view of some evolutionary

---

[34] Eve Kosofsky Sedgwick, 'Queer Performativity: Henry James's *The Art of the Novel*', *GLQ*, 1 (1993): 6.
[35] Jörg Wettlaufer, 'The Shame Game', *RSA Journal*, 161, no. 5564 (2015): 36, 39.

psychologists that rape is an evolutionary adaptation and the rape victims really *are* partially culpable.[36]

Feminist approaches provide more productive tools to think about shame and why victim-survivors might feel it. Many feminist philosophers point to the fact that people are constituted through interactions with other people, objects and institutions. Rather than being a personal or private emotion, shame is fundamentally a *social* response to being-in-the-world: it is an interrelational response to societal values and practices. It is not about what a person has done (which, as Helen Block Lewis argues, is more like guilt)[37] but about how victim-survivors believe *other* people think about them. This way of thinking about shame offers a powerful critique of the liberal view of shame as an *individual* response to having not lived up to ideals that the shamed person agrees with. As ethicist Elisa A. Hurley explains:

> When who we are is partly determined by others' treatment of us and, more specifically, by the evaluations and interpretations of us implicit in their treatment, then the contingency in the relationship between shaming treatment of us and our shame, presupposed by the liberal view, dissolves.[38]

In other words, a relational approach draws attention to the link between 'shaming treatment' and an individual's feeling of being shamed. It insists on the importance of the social contexts in which shaming ideologies and practices take place, or what philosopher Sandra Bartky calls the 'condition of dishonor' that 'is woman's lot in a sexist society'.[39] Accordingly, shame is not a personal attribute but a social emotion that is deeply rooted in historical time, geographical place and a myriad of institutional regimes of power.

Although this approach takes as its focus the diminished lives of women within patriarchal societies, it remains important to acknowledge the vulnerabilities of all bodies. This was one reason why I started this chapter by exploring the experiences of a white, middle-class man. Shame is refracted through people's multiple, intersectional selves, which include a wide range of genders, races, ethnicities, religions, sexual orientations, ages, generations and so on. It is inequitable in its distribution, since it is inculcated through relations

---

[36] Randy Thornhill and Craig T. Palmer, *A Natural History of Rape: Biological Bases of Sexual Coercion* (Cambridge, MA: MIT Press, 2000).
[37] Helen Block Lewis, *Shame and Guilt in Neurosis* (New York: International Universities Press, 1971), 30.
[38] Elisa A. Hurley, 'Pharmacotherapy to Blunt Memories of Sexual Violence: What's a Feminist to Think?', *Hypatia*, 25 (2010): 536.
[39] Sandra Bartky, 'Shame and Gender', in her *Femininity and Domination: Studies in the Phenomenology of Oppression* (New York: Routledge, 1990), 85.

of domination, including sexism, racism, colonialism and economic inequalities. As Ann Cvetkovich explains in *An Archive of Feelings* (2004), 'sexual trauma seeps into other categories' of oppression.[40] Although common, shame is a particularly strong emotion amongst socially subordinate groups.[41]

A person's intersectional identities are also influential in framing *responses* to shaming ideologies and practices. Theorists like Jennifer C. Manion believe shame can be a positive emotion, encouraging reflection in the shamed person and thus enabling her to re-evaluate her life and principles.[42] However, most subordinated peoples do not have access to the personal, emotional and financial resources that would enable such transformations.[43] They are less able to reject external evaluations of their worth, especially when those assessments take the form of systemic degradation. In the words of Ullaliina Lehtinen in her article 'How Does One Know What Shame Is?', too much of the literature assumes 'the moral agent is autonomously free' and is fortunate enough to either 'internalize or to defy the episodic dis-esteem and de-valuation'.[44] Privileged persons might be able to reflect on their shame, transforming it into a moral tale; for the underprivileged, it is either a confirmation of their lowly status or a pervasive, corroding affect. This is not to imply that shaming behaviours cannot inflict serious harm on white, young, elite, Western men, such as the anonymous doctor with whom I started this chapter. But it is to draw attention to a range of different responses to shame. After all, this deeply shamed doctor was able to persuade the editors of the prestigious *British Medical Journal* to publicize his experiences and ensure that his identity remained secret. This did not prevent those same editors from also publishing Stephen Due's shame-endorsing letter in a later edition.

This approach to shame helps explain the common paradox that a person might *feel* shame yet intellectually know that she or he has done nothing to warrant *being* ashamed. There is a term for the kind of shame that a person *feels* despite his or her beliefs conflicting with those feelings: it is called 'recalcitrant shame'.[45] Again, this was the experience of the anonymous doctor

---

[40] Ann Cvetkovich, *An Archive of Feelings: Trauma, Sexuality, and Lesbian Public Cultures* (Durham, NC: Duke University Press, 2004), 36.
[41] Lewis, *Shame and Guilt*; Frantz Fanon, *Black Skin, White Masks* (New York: Grove, 1967).
[42] Jennifer C. Manion, 'Girls Blush, Sometimes: Gender, Moral Agency, and the Problem of Shame', *Hypatia*, 18 (2003): 21–41.
[43] See Kathleen Woodward, 'Traumatic Shame: Toni Morrison, Televisual Culture, and the Cultural Politics of the Emotions', *Cultural Critique*, 46 (2000): 210–40.
[44] Ullaliina Lehtinen, 'How Does One Know What Shame Is?', *Hypatia*, 13 (1998): 62.
[45] For discussions, see Justin D'Arms and Daniel Jacobson, 'The Significance of Recalcitrant Emotion', *Royal Institute of Philosophy Supplement*, 52 (2003): 127–45; Heidi L. Maibom, 'The Descent of Shame', *Philosophy and Phenomenological Research*, 80 (2010): 566–94.

who maintained that he was not responsible for his own abuse but nevertheless felt ashamed for having been victimized. There are several ways to explain this paradox, including claims that victim-survivors of sexual abuse had internalized a self-hating message (and were suffering from false consciousness), were being irrational (and therefore need to realign their cognitive understandings with their emotional responses) or were neurotic (and required treatment). An understanding of shame as interrelational – a social practice – leads to a rejection of such victim-blaming explanations. Crucially, a relational approach does not assume that a person must *share* the values of the Other in order to feel ashamed. Victim-survivors don't have a free hand in choosing the witnesses who can make them feel ashamed, notes philosopher Cheshire Calhoun. All that is needed is that they feel that other people, with whom they share social spaces and moral practices, are disparaging them.[46] Gender scholar Liz Constable concurs, adding that shame is not something 'inner' or intra-psychic since to feel shamed 'is *already* to have encountered others' values and principles, and to have sensed the force and forms of their affective articulation'.[47] Shame is constituted within historical times, geographical places and the full range of communities in which the shamed person cannot help but be emmeshed.

The emphasis on shame as a social emotion allows for the separation of the feeling of shame from the endorsement of harmful belief systems based on prejudices such as misogyny, racism and homophobia (to name just three). This is why ideologies and practices that devalue victims can have devastating consequences even when a person might intellectually reject their fundamental premises. Shame *reveals* a person's felt experience in a world not of her own making.

There is another way to express this: shame is part and parcel of the process of constituting women and other denigrated people *as* subordinate and disrespected. Philosopher Robin S. Dillon explores the 'multiple-layered' frameworks that women employ in their attempts to make sense of the world. These frames 'shape conscious experience and can conflict with avowed beliefs and judgments without themselves being explicitly represented in or even representable to the individual'. To the extent to which these structures of meaning are invisible, a person's 'understanding is resistant to modification through reflection, criticism, or reconceptualization'.[48] Some of these commonplace, free-floating

---

[46] Cheshire Calhoun, 'An Apology for Moral Shame', *Journal of Political Philosophy*, 12 (2004): 127–46.
[47] Liz Constable, 'Introduction – States of Shame', *L'Esprit Créateur*, 39 (1999): 6.
[48] Robin S. Dillon, 'Self-Respect: Moral, Emotional, Political', *Ethics*, 107 (1997): 240. I have silently corrected the typo 'multiply' to 'multiple'.

and sometimes invisible discourses and practices include those 'rape myths' mentioned earlier, especially ones that contend that rape survivors precipitated their own abuse or were 'asking for it'.

Rather than individualizing shame, acknowledging the often obscure yet harmful frameworks of meaning offered to groups within societal contexts draws attention to the historical and institutional structures that create shame. This strengthens critiques of the liberal, individualizing notions of shame that remain welded to ideas of pathology, dissonance (such as between a victim-survivor's cognition and emotions) and irrationality. As Elisa A. Hurley explains:

> When rape is an integral part of a system of oppressive social practices that uphold the subordination of women to men, then, in that society, a woman's experience of shame in response to being raped starts to look not only psychologically understandable and unsurprising, but reasonable and, indeed, appropriate.[49]

Dillon takes this argument further, contending that the 'divergence of emotions and beliefs' is simply a mirror image of the 'ambiguities in the sociopolitical valuings of women', including the 'contradictions between the official story of equality and the devaluation actually instantiated in the myriad circumstances of women's lives'. She devastatingly concludes that women 'believe that they are supposed to believe about themselves, but they also feel what they are supposed to feel'.[50] The victim-survivor of rape dwells in social worlds that convey the message that she is esteemed while making her feel the opposite.

Conclusion

The shame-making world is not inevitable. It can be changed, in part because victim-survivors are not wholly constituted by violence. Shame bears witness to injustice and, like anger and contempt, can be employed in political ways. Shame is a particularly powerful emotion because it is constructed in societal contexts that deny the pervasiveness of sexual harms. In other words, victim-survivors feel ashamed because the silence around victimization conveys the message that they are not like other, more 'normal' people. This feeling of invisibility makes them reluctant to speak about their experiences and more likely to assume that

---

[49] Elisa A. Hurley, 'Pharmacotherapy to Blunt Memories of Sexual Violence: What's a Feminist to Think?', *Hypatia*, 25 (2010): 537.
[50] Robin S. Dillon, 'Self-Respect: Moral, Emotional, Political', *Ethics*, 107 (1997): 247.

others hold them in lower regard because of their abuse. In Sedgwick's words, shame is a feeling 'whose very suffusiveness seems to delineate my precise, individual outlines in the most isolating way possible'.[51] In contrast, publicizing the extent of sexual abuse in our societies conveys the message that victim-survivors are everywhere. It creates a visibility that makes the internalization of the values of harm-supporters less likely. As Amanda Holmes argues in an article entitled 'That Which Cannot Be Shared: On the Politics of Shame' (2015), shame

> seems to dissipate when it is made public or when it is shared. That is, the negative and isolating qualities that are constitutive of the affect of shame are negated when it is confessed. To confess one's shame is to destroy it.[52]

Indeed, the 'public reclamation of shame' turns it into the opposite. After all, shame varies according to its audience. A victim-survivor may feel ashamed to speak in a room full of harm-ignoring, violence-minimizing or rape-excusing people – but not ashamed in a room full of feminist, activists and angry survivors. For male victim-survivors as well as gender-nonconforming ones, this has created additional concerns given the reluctance of many women's consciousness-raising groups and feminist organizations (including most rape crisis centres prior to the 1980s) to admit male victims. Their shame and distress was effectively sidelined by anti-rape, feminist activisms until the 1990s.

I have attempted to set out some of the issues relating to sexual violence. I argue that understanding the mechanisms of shame can help reverse its pernicious effects for both victim-survivors and those who harm. Shame is dependent upon witnesses who 'do' the shaming; but those witnesses equally have the power to *deny* shame. Jettisoning the power/sex dichotomy and paying more attention to intersectionalities can deepen and productively complicate our understanding of sexual violence. The chapter calls for closer attention to be paid to the bodies and emotions of victim-survivors as well as to those who have the task of caring for them. Understanding of the mechanisms of disgust and shame can help reverse their pernicious effects for both victim-survivors and those who (often unintentionally) harm. An emphasis on the emotions does not simply reveal underlying human experiences: it suggests political responses to the harms of sexual abuse.

---

[51] Eve Kosofsky Sedgwick, 'Queer Performativity: Henry James's *The Art of the Novel*', GLQ, 1 (1993): 14.
[52] Amanda Holmes, 'That Which Cannot Be Shared: On the Politics of Shame', *Journal of Speculative Philosophy*, 29 (2015): 415–16.

9

The concept of 'Leidensdruck' in West German criminal therapy, 1960–85

Marcel Streng

In January 1983, thirty-year-old G., a prison inmate in the West German federal state of North Rhine-Westphalia, applied for admission to the Social Therapeutic Institution located in Gelsenkirchen. He had experienced 'various forms of imprisonment' since 1979 and had gone through 'an enormous amount of Leidensdruck', which he noted in a handwritten resume intended for the therapeutic director.[1] This experience, he said, made his future seem more hopeless than ever. In the social therapeutic institution, he wanted to 'quit his previous way of life' and 'start anew with all [his] strength'.[2] In the 1970s, it was not uncommon for inmates to apply for treatment in social therapeutic institutions in the Federal Republic. If they happened to address themselves to the Gelsenkirchen prison, they were sent an information sheet about the treatment program, which they could use to examine their motivation. The therapists then requested the applicant's prisoner file and the reports from the state's two 'diagnostic centers', through which male offenders passed after their conviction to prison sentences of more than one and a half years. Based on this documentation, the staff decided on the applicants' 'suitability' and their admission or rejection.

The wording of the quoted resume of prisoner G., however, makes one wonder. In what way might the expression 'enormous amount of Leidensdruck'

---

[1] Prisoner G., Handwritten resume, not dated [January 1983], Landesarchiv Nordrhein-Westfalen, Abteilung Westfalen, Münster, Q 918 Nr. 358. The names of all prisoners mentioned in this text are made anonymous. I wish to thank the editors as well as Alexa Geisthövel (Berlin) and Joachim Haeberlen (Warwick) who have read and commented on an earlier version of this paper.
[2] Prisoner G., letter to the therapeutic director, 24 January 1983, LAV NRW Abt. Westfalen Q 918 Nr. 358.

have made sense to the prisoner and his addressee? Did the prisoner mean to say that he had suffered enormously under the various conditions of confinement? Or was it a technical term that G. used to describe his feelings in prison, without knowing exactly its scholarly meaning? Both questions refer to the ways criminal psychologists, psychiatrists, and psychotherapists since the late 1950s to the mid-1980s transformed the discourse on the convict's personality and especially her/his emotional self. The rise of therapeutic penology after the Second World War, sustained by an alliance of various reform-oriented actors in the field of criminal policy, as well as the transfer of 'modern' rehabilitative concepts, strengthened a focus on new methods to treat convicts in order to reintegrate them into society. Addressing and reforming the convict's emotional self through psychotherapy and group dynamics, instructing her/him to work on negative feelings and affects judged detrimental to life in society, was at the centre of these rehabilitative strategies.[3]

One of the key concepts in the West German debate during this period was the enigmatic notion of 'Leidensdruck'. Literally meaning 'pressure of suffering', it signals heavy psychophysiological stress. Apart from the various contexts in which the concept was used, 'Leidensdruck' was ambivalent enough to combine several layers of meaning: it could evoke repentance; a soul-wrenching discomfort regarding the committed crime; a deep emotional distress that by its corporeal concomitants was close to the psychophysical pain a convict might (or should, according to the classic penal law theory) experience following his punishment.[4] However, crucially, the concept implied that the convicts also suffered from themselves, from certain personality patterns or disorders that caused or favoured criminal behaviour and against which they were powerless. In every sense, 'Leidensdruck' articulated the corporeal dimension of emotional suffering. As we will see, this was particularly difficult to imagine regarding notoriously 'callous' and 'incorrigible psychopaths'. Neuroticism, in contrast, offered a new psychodynamic way to think about criminal personalities, their emotionality and treatability.

Of course, the historical semantics of 'Leidensdruck' are far more complex. My aim here is to explore the genealogy of the term and to understand the emotionalizing strategies linked to it. As the aforementioned example of prisoner

---

[3] Annelie Ramsbrock, *Geschlossene Gesellschaft. Das Gefängnis als Sozialversuch – eine bundesdeutsche Geschichte* (Frankfurt a. M.: Fischer, 2020); Greg Eghigian, *The Corrigible and the Incorrigible: Science, Medicine, and the Convict in Twentieth-Century Germany* (Ann Arbor: University of Michigan Press, 2015); Imanuel Baumann, *Dem Verbrechen auf der Spur: eine Geschichte der Kriminologie und Kriminalpolitik in Deutschland 1880 bis 1980* (Göttingen: Wallstein, 2006).
[4] See Rob Boddice, *Pain: A Very Short Introduction* (Oxford: Oxford University Press, 2017), 22.

G. suggests, by the early 1980s, the term had made its way from the psy-experts' controversies into the prisoners' self-description. One way in which this transfer happened was through the practice of psychological diagnosis, which brought together psy-experts and convicts in the evaluation of the personality of the latter. My chapter is therefore based on an analysis of the general criminological discourse on 'Leidensdruck', as well as on psychological assessments carried out at the Gelsenkirchen institution between 1974 and early 1983.[5]

I use the example of facilities for male prisoners, for two reasons. On the one hand, male prisoners formed the overwhelming majority of the overall prison population. The assessment centres under scrutiny also admitted only male prisoners during the 1970s. On the other hand, 'Leidensdruck' was associated with qualities that used to be connotated as feminine, and the introduction of therapeutic categories and techniques into the masculine subcultures of the prison system was met with gendered reactions.

Healing criminal psychopaths? 'Leidensdruck' as an argument for social therapy in prison around 1960

Invented as part of the Criminal Law Reform in West Germany between the mid-1950s and the late 1960s, the social therapeutic institution was meant to solve a problem that had preoccupied prison officials and criminologists as well as psychiatrists and hospital staff since the 1920s. Prisoners who were significantly disruptive in jails were often transferred to psychiatric hospitals, from where they were soon sent back to prison. For institutional detention, 'psychopathic troublemakers' were considered insufficiently sane, while for psychiatry, not mentally ill enough. In the mid-1950s the Criminal Law Commission started to discuss the question of whether prisoners with 'psychopathic personalities' and reduced legal responsibility should be kept in special institutions.[6]

The canonical definition of psychopathic personalities developed by psychiatrist Kurt Schneider in the 1920s as 'people who suffer from their abnormality or whose abnormality makes society suffer' was a central reference

---

[5] The text is based on the evaluation of a sample taken at three points in time (all documented applications received from December 1974 to August 1975, from January to April 1979 and from October 1982 to January 1983, a total of 148 procedures).
[6] Baumann, *Dem Verbrechen*, 291–8; Eghigian, *Corrigible*, 183–8.

in these discussions.[7] Schneider, still an influential figure in post-war West German criminal psychiatry, advised the law commission on the problem of legal responsibility and its limitations. His expert opinion that all of these limitations should be based on some 'biological' element (e.g. neurophysiological impairments) prevailed in the debate, much to the dismay of many psychologists who argued that psychological disorders could have 'pathological value' as well.[8] In the ensuing controversy about appropriate forms of treatment for psychopathic delinquents, a shift in emphasis soon became apparent: in contrast to the pain and distress that psychopaths inflicted on society, the suffering of the psychopath from himself – his 'Leidensdruck' – came more and more to the fore.

A July 1956 meeting of the reform commission attested to this shift, which had been prompted by developments abroad. The commission heard two experts with irreconcilable positions. The first to speak was the Danish physician Georg Stürup, who headed the Herstedvester care facility for 'psychopaths'. His lecture was a demonstration of what an empathic attitude and psychotherapeutic treatment could achieve. To 'cure' criminal psychopaths, he argued, one had to address their emotional selves. The perception of psychopathic 'callousness' or 'lack of emotionality' in courtrooms was not wrong, he explained, but often it was 'a defence reaction for over-sensitivity'. Such a person was not necessarily also 'numb'. Moreover, the 'appearance of numbness could change in most cases'.[9] Cologne physician and criminal psychiatrist Paul Würfler, a former National Socialist, spoke next. He argued against the establishment of special institutions and referred to the deterministic assumption that hereditary 'deviant dispositions' predominated in criminal psychopaths. He believed the 'essence of the psychopath' could already be recognized in infants. The only treatment he recommended consisted of harshness and denial. Psychotherapy was baseless.[10]

As historian Imanuel Baumann has convincingly argued, the 'deconstruction of the psychopath' began in West German criminal science around 1960.[11] In the

---

[7] Kurt Schneider, 'Die psychopathischen Persönlichkeiten', Handbuch der Psychiatrie, ed. Gustav Aschaffenburg, Spezieller Teil, IV 2 und VII 1–3 (Leipzig: Deuticke, 1923); quoted after the English edition of Kurt Schneider, Clinical Psychopathology (New York: Grune & Stratton, 1959), 15.

[8] Eghigian, Corrigible, 141–53.

[9] Georg Stürup, Niederschriften über die Sitzungen der Großen Strafrechtskommission, vol. 4 (Bonn: Bundesdruckerei, 1958), 181–6, 199, and general discussion, 195–200. Some German prison doctors, however, would not subscribe to the conviction that psychopaths were not necessarily untreatable; see Johannes Hirschmann, 'Psychotherapie von Sittlichkeitsverbrechern im ausgesetzten Strafvollzug', Mitteilungen der Kriminalbiologischen Gesellschaft, 6 (1951): 81–8.

[10] Paul Würfler, Niederschriften über die Sitzungen der Großen Strafrechtskommission, vol. 4 (Bonn: Bundesdruckerei 1958), 186–95, 192–3.

[11] Baumann, Dem Verbrechen, 273–9. This process continued beyond criminology; see Alexa Geisthövel, 'Die Reform der "Psychopathie": forensisch-psychiatrische Begutachtung im geteilten Berlin, 1960–1980', Gesnerus, 77 (2020): 2, 244–78.

broader debate about the appropriate placement and treatment of 'psychopathic criminals', the reception of psychoanalytic knowledge was the main contributor to this process. The term 'Leidensdruck' did in fact go back to the reasoning of Harald Schultz-Hencke, an important figure in German psychotherapy since the 1920s, when he had been involved in the development of 'neoanalysis', who then became a proponent of 'Deutsche Seelenheilkunde' (the German art of healing of the soul) during the 1930s and 1940s.[12] According to him, 'Leidensdruck' played a major role in beginning an analysis. In the mid-1950s, the Göttingen psychoanalyst Franz Heigl, trained at Schultz-Hencke's Institute in West Berlin, took up his position. Heigl decided around 1960 to accept the patient's 'Leidensdruck' as an 'important motor for analysis, perhaps the most important one. Therapeutic successes diminish proportionately as Leidensdruck diminishes.'[13]

The designation of 'Leidensdruck' as the 'motor of therapy' points to the difficulties of an appropriate translation: the English word 'suffering' does not reflect the element of physical pressure that is linked to the term. However, for understanding the 'energetic self' conceived in early psychoanalytic discourse in general, this level of meaning is important.[14] This becomes clear in Heigl's definition of 'genuine Leidensdruck' as a kind of hydraulic system: if a person suffers from her/his inhibitions and symptoms, this suffering increases her/his 'capacity for suffering' and makes her/him overcome her/his 'pain barrier' instead of seeking substitute satisfaction; only if the suffering from the symptomatology is greater than the 'gain of illness' will the patient feel compelled to cooperate sufficiently in psychoanalysis.[15]

In this psycho- or post-neoanalytic understanding, 'Leidensdruck' was closely linked to neuroticism (and thus to psychotherapy), which began to override

---

[12] Wilhelm Blankenburg, 'Der "Leidensdruck" des Patienten in seiner Bedeutung für Psychotherapie und Psychopathologie', *Der Nervenarzt*, 52 (1981): 635–42, 636; Max Steller, *Sozialtherapie statt Strafvollzug* (Köln: Kiepenheuer und Witsch, 1977), 65 6.
[13] Franz Heigl, 'Vergleichende Betrachtung der prognostischen Faktoren bei Schultz-Hencke und Alexander', *Zeitschrift für psychosomatische Medizin*, 4 (1958): 2, 108–14, 109; Franz Heigl, 'Persönlichkeitsstruktur und Prognose', *Zeitschrift für psychosomatische Medizin*, 10 (1964): 2, 108–14, 109; see also Franz Heigl, 'Was ist wirksam in der psychoanalytischen Therapie?', *Zeitschrift für psychosomatische Medizin* 12 (1966): 4, 282–92.
[14] Uffa Jensen, *Wie die Couch nach Kalkutta kam. Eine Globalgeschichte der frühen Psychoanalyse* (Berlin: Suhrkamp, 2019), 270–9.
[15] Heigl, 'Persönlichkeitsstruktur', 109. 'Functional Leidensdruck' is caused by an 'attitude structure' in which 'the indirect consequences of inhibition in the form of error expectations, substitute satisfactions and overcompensation' predominate. Such a person suffers 'less from his inhibitions and his symptomatology than from the fact that he does not succeed in life with his attitudes, i.e. with his neurotic system of coping with the world'. Heigl, 'Persönlichkeitsstruktur', 108.

the concept of psychopathy in the discussion.[16] Around 1960, 'Leidensdruck' and neuroticism increasingly served to differentiate the treatability of delinquents. In 1963, physician Gerhard Mauch, who had been experimenting with psychoanalytic methods in offender treatment since 1954, assumed that most of his patients incessantly sought 'substitute pleasure', which he thought was an 'evasive reaction' that relieved the 'tension accumulated as a result of inhibition'. Because of this 'waywardness' as he wrote, citing psychoanalyst Annemarie Dührssen, another Schultz-Hencke adept, they could not feel emotionally distressed [Leidensgefühl] at all.[17] Likewise, in 1966, German-British psychoanalyst Melitta Schmideberg wrote that 'most delinquents ... rarely feel emotional distress [inneres Leiden]'.[18] Karl Pietsch, another physician turned prison psychoanalyst, took a nuanced position. Writing in 1957 and 1964, he distinguished delinquents on the basis of their psychological reaction to punishment and incarceration. Most prisoners, he noted, adapted rather well to the prison community. The psychotherapist rarely encountered them because they usually were of 'robust health' and did not feel emotional distress. Among those who did, Pietsch identified prisoners 'who suffer from the prison situation, but who are not able to take on this suffering manfully ... because of inner weakness, [and] who avoid this task by neurotic reactions' as the actual target group of the psychotherapist.[19]

The last statement points to the limits of psychoanalytical reasoning in these debates. While some considered at least some psychopathic inmates to have developed enough superego and inner complexity to react neurotically, others interpreted this reaction in gendered terms as a lack of self-control, a 'capitulation of rationality', and not as a consequence of pre-criminal inner conflicts.[20] However, the psychodynamic concept of neuroticism did alter the

---

[16] In 1971, Gerhard Mauch argued in favour of abandoning the distinction between psychopaths and 'neurotically wayward criminals' altogether, because it did not help to clarify whether delinquents could be treated or not. In order to assess their personalities, one had to start from the 'nature and extent of the disorder'; Gerhard Mauch and Roland Mauch, *Sozialtherapie und die sozialtherapeutische Anstalt: Erfahrungen in der Behandlung Chronisch-Krimineller. Voraussetzungen, Durchführung und Möglichkeiten* (Stuttgart: Enke, 1971), 15; Karl Pietsch, 'Der Psychopath in der Strafanstalt I', *Zeitschrift für Strafvollzug*, 7 (1957): 2, 102–16, 104. It was not far at this point from neurosis to 'criminosis'. See 'Engel in grau', *Der Spiegel*, 3, no. 10 (1966): 168.

[17] Gerhard Mauch, 'Psychotherapie Krimineller im Vollzug als Resozialisierungsmaßnahme', *Der Krankenhausarzt*, 36 (1963): 3, 74–9, 76. He later revised himself.

[18] Melitta Schmideberg, 'Prinzipien der Kriminalpsychotherapie', *Monatsschrift für Kriminologie und Strafrechtsreform*, 49 (1966): 4, 146–51, 150.

[19] Karl Pietsch, 'Der Psychopath in der Strafanstalt II', *Zeitschrift für Strafvollzug*, 7 (1957): 3, 143–55, 148.

[20] Karl Pietsch, 'Psychotherapeutische Bildungsarbeit an Strafgefangenen (I)', *Zeitschrift für Strafvollzug*, 13 (1964): 5, 224–33, 227.

ways criminologists around 1960 thought about the chances of treating and even healing notoriously incorrigible criminal psychopaths.

Distress of the disordered or the deviant personality? The delinquent's 'Leidensdruck' in criminological discourse, between generalization and differentiation in the 1970s

With the establishment and commissioning of the first social therapeutic institutions in the years 1969 to 1971 in the federal states of Baden-Württemberg, North Rhine-Westphalia and West Berlin, therapeutic penology in West Germany became increasingly differentiated, as these 'model institutions' also had a scientific mission. The teams implemented treatment programs and at the same time evaluated them scientifically. This gave the professional discourse on 'Leidensdruck' a new, institutional basis.

In this context, the psychoanalytic foundations of social therapy were quickly eroding. Criminologist and social pedagogue Stephan Quensel, who had taken part in group therapy experiments with inmates and was involved in training prison officers, conceded that the 'psychoanalytic model' had opened 'a broader field of selection and treatment compared to the classical psychiatric direction'. This opening, though, had not been wide enough, because 'the criteria for the treatability assessment, which all originate from classical psychoanalysis', restricted the circle of addressees too much.[21] Together with his wife Edelgard, a psychologist, Stefan Quensel introduced an alternative understanding of 'Leidensdruck' in 1971 that was based on the *labeling approach* borrowed from American criminal sociology. 'Leidensdruck', they argued, arose when someone adopted society's perception of the delinquent into his or her self-perception. The image of the 'self-confident gangster' was produced by the 'punitive organs of this society' and disregarded the social stresses that occurred 'repeatedly at a very early stage' in offenders' life histories. Since delinquents cherished the same 'ideals and dreams' as the rest of society, but were largely denied their realization, they began to see themselves as 'not quite normal' and suffered as a result: 'A "Leidensdruck", a depressive-hopeless feeling of being outcast, and an intense desire to get out of this role of delinquent, was present in these persons at least to the same degree as in the neurotics who sought out painful-expensive

---

[21] Stephan Quensel, 'Buchbesprechung', *Monatsschrift für Kriminologie und Strafrechtsreform*, 55 (1972): 4, 201–3, 201.

psychoanalysis or in the sick who, by necessity, endured surgery.'[22] The 'problem of treatment' therefore did not 'lie in the lack of emotional distress [Leiden]' but in the 'firmly ingrained behavioural and mistrust techniques' that the delinquent developed in order to not give himself up.

Forensic psychiatrist Wilfried Rasch, who in 1971 helped establish the much publicized first social therapy institution for convicts in North Rhine-Westphalia, in Düren near Cologne, problematized three other aspects of the psychoanalytic approach. First, Rasch rejected the notion of creating distress in delinquents who did not suffer in the first place by imposing infinite punishments, as had been envisioned by Stürup as well as Mauch and which had found its way into one of the first draft laws.[23] 'Therapy finds its meaning in providing help where it is requested. The dimension of subjective suffering offers itself as a criterion that can legitimize social therapeutic efforts. It is a prerequisite under which social therapy can also count on approval by its addressees.'[24] If 'Leidensdruck' did not arise spontaneously within the first weeks of imprisonment, there was no point in psychotherapy.[25] But Mauch had postulated that treatment would be given 'to anyone who wanted it.'[26] Since only those who felt 'Leidensdruck' were willing to undergo therapy voluntarily 'as, for example, the neurotically disturbed patient does',[27] there was no contradiction between coercion and voluntariness, but rather an almost productive relationship. Echoing critics in the left spectrum who suspected 'brainwashing'[28] here, Rasch demanded that the state's 'claim to re-education by means of medical-psychological methods should not be allowed to get out of hand' and that narrow limits should be set to the pathologization of deviant behaviour. The therapist's task could neither be to 'force adaptation to state norms' nor to 'try with humanitarian élan to undermine a system of sanctions that has been recognized as harmful'.[29]

---

[22] Edelgard Quensel and Stephan Quensel, 'Probleme der Behandlung im geschlossenen Vollzug', *Die Strafvollzugsreform: eine kritische Bestandsaufnahme*, ed. Arthur Kaufmann and Thomas Würtenberger (Karlsruhe: Müller, 1973), 159–73, 162.

[23] Stürup, *Niederschriften*, 199; Gerhard Mauch, 'Psychotherapie Krimineller im Vollzug als Resozialisierungsmaßnahme', *Der Krankenhausarzt*, 36 (1963): 3, 74–9, 76; Gerhard Mauch, 'Psychotherapie im Strafvollzug', *Monatsschrift für Kriminologie und Strafreform*, 47 (1964): 3, 108–21, 114; Bundestags-Drucksache V/4095, 31.

[24] Wilfried Rasch and Klaus-Peter Kühl, 'Subjektives Leiden als sozialtherapeutisches Behandlungskriterium – FPI-Ergebnisse bei Tätergruppen des §65 Abs. 1 2. StrRG', *Monatsschrift für Kriminologie und Strafrechtsreform*, 56 (1973): 237–45, 239.

[25] Wilfried Rasch, 'Unterbringung und Behandlung psychopathischer Rechtsbrecher', *Kriminalistik*, 23 (1969): 181–86, 184

[26] Mauch, 'Psychotherapie im Strafvollzug', 114.

[27] Mauch and Mauch, 'Sozialtherapie', 17.

[28] Dorothee Peters and Helge Peters, 'Therapie ohne Diagnose. Zur soziologischen Kritik am kriminologischen Konzept sozialtherapeutischer Anstalten', *Kriminologisches Journal*, 2 (1970): 114–20, 117.

[29] Rasch and Kühl, 'Subjektives Leiden', 239.

Second, while Gerhard Mauch saw 'chronic criminality' (recidivism) as the surest indication of a 'severe personality disorder' in a delinquent, which, according to § 65 2nd Criminal Reform Law, ought to have indicated admission to a social therapy institution, Rasch in 1973 saw this proposition as mainly 'the result of years of unsystematic procedure'.[30] A large part of his contribution to the social therapy discussion of the 1970s and 1980s consisted of empirical studies with the aim of developing more precise criteria for the diagnosis of personality disorders. The extensive selection of the first occupancy of the Düren institution underlined this claim.[31]

Third, Rasch came down hard on the assumption that delinquents felt no 'Leidensdruck'. In this supposition, advocates of psychoanalytic treatment methods met with staunch opponents of criminal therapy such as the Cologne psychiatrist Paul Bresser.[32] In 1973, Rasch stated that the 'complaint about the lack of Leidensdruck of criminals ... runs as a red thread through the criminal therapy literature'. The 'persistence of such stereotypes' was even more astonishing, he argued, because there was already a 'wealth of evidence' pointing in the opposite direction. The results of the extensive study that he himself had conducted with a team in 1970/71 as part of the preparations for the Düren experiment supported this finding.[33] The psychological testing of recidivists and sex offenders in the selection process had 'to a larger extent recorded persons who experienced themselves as disturbed and suffering'.[34] According to Rasch and his collaborator, psychologist Klaus-Peter Kühl:

> They most resembled neurotics or the psychosomatic patient of rehabilitation clinics. Neurotics, however, are more reserved and more self-contained than the delinquents and tend to be hesitant and wait-and-see. They do not possess the impulsivity and excitability of the criminals. Accordingly, the Freiburg Personality Inventory profile found in the present study shows strong correspondence with the neurotic character first described by [Franz] Alexander,

---

[30] Rasch and Kühl, 'Subjektives Leiden', 237.
[31] See Wilfried Rasch, 'Behandlungsbereitschaft und Behandlungsbedürftigkeit bei Probanden der Bewährungshilfe', *Bewährungshilfe*, 21 (1974): 1, 28–37, 31–6; Wilfried Rasch and Monika Stemmer-Lück, 'Diagnostik in der Sozialtherapie', *Diagnostik in der Psychotherapie*, ed. Manfred Zielke (Stuttgart: Enke, 1982), 179–202, see 182–99.
[32] Paul H. Bresser, 'Ziele und Grenzen der Sozialtherapie – Eine Diskussionsbemerkung', *Zeitschrift für Strafvollzug und Straffälligenhilfe*, 24 (1975): 1, 34–7, 35.
[33] In 1970/71, as director of the Department of Criminal Biology of the Institute of Forensic Medicine at the University of Cologne, Rasch advised the North Rhine-Westphalian Ministry of Justice on the establishment of the state's first model social therapeutic institution in Düren; see Wilfried Rasch, 'Grundsätze des Dürener Behandlungsprogramms', *Justizverwaltungsblatt*, 108 (1971): 6, 124–5.
[34] Rasch and Kühl, 'Subjektives Leiden', 242.

to which importance is attached in the Anglo-American criminal psychology literature for the development of deviant behavior.[35]

While Rasch and Kühl in 1973 condensed the results of their study to improve the diagnostics of personality disorders and help guide the selection of appropriate treatment methods, criminal psychologist Max Steller took a different path. In his 1974 PhD thesis at the University of Kiel, he observed that while the 'suitability criterion of Leidensdruck' was 'unanimously granted outstanding importance' in therapeutic penology it was nowhere 'sufficiently defined' or theoretically developed.[36] Based on a detailed critique of the German-language social therapy literature on the matter, Steller analysed the suitability of the concept for the selection of social therapy clients, then disassembled 'Leidensdruck' into five different 'variables of therapy motivation' ('Leidensdruck', dissatisfaction, desire for change, desire for help, expectation of success) and subjected these to empirical testing.[37]

Steller initially separated the term 'Leidensdruck' from 'desire for change'. Although the two had always been closely linked in psychoanalytic literature, Steller, who was trained in behavioural therapy, did not consider a 'close relationship between a negative emotional state and the desire to change one's personality' to be 'compelling'. He initially reserved the term 'Leidensdruck' for 'an emotional state of self-dissatisfaction, of being "depressed" by one's own suffering'.[38] However, for Steller this was not yet precise enough. In the literature, he argued, a distinction was made 'between suffering due to experiences of insufficiency related to one's own person', on the one hand, and, on the other hand, a 'suffering that has its origin in external conditions (for example, confinement, social position, etc.)'.[39] Therefore, he refined his definition of 'Leidensdruck' to an 'emotional state of (self-)dissatisfaction, of being depressed due to experiences of insufficiency, the source of which is seen in one's own personality'. The second dimension of its former meaning was not lost, however. Steller included it in the motivational variable 'dissatisfaction'. This could also consist in the 'refusal

---

[35] Rasch and Kühl, 'Subjektives Leiden', 242.
[36] Max Steller, '"Leidensdruck" als Indikation für Sozialtherapie? Eine Analyse motivationaler Klienten-Variablen und ihres Einflusses auf die Wirksamkeit von Psychotherapie bei Delinquenten', dissertation, Kiel University, 1974. See Steller, *Sozialtherapie*, 65–108.
[37] Max Steller and Wilfried Hommers, 'Zur Diagnose der Therapiemotivation durch konfigurale Klassifikation', *Diagnostica*, 13 (1977): 266–80.
[38] Steller, *Sozialtherapie*, 75.
[39] Steller, *Sozialtherapie*, 75. In a lecture that was only indirectly documented, psychiatrist Hans-Jürgen Horn had distinguished between 'primary', 'secondary' and 'tertiary Leidensdruck'; see Heike Jung and Heinz Müller-Dietz, '8. Kolloquium der südwestdeutschen kriminologischen Institute', *Monatsschrift für Kriminologie und Strafrechtsreform*, 56 (1976): 128–34.

to think about oneself and one's problems' while 'Leidensdruck presupposes a certain degree of self-observation and self-reflection'.[40]

Steller's semantic tweaking clarified and relativized the importance of the concept of 'Leidensdruck', which then had to be weighted and interpreted in terms of the overall therapy motivation of the delinquent client. In a revision of the various techniques used to enhance therapy motivation, Steller argued that coercive measures 'are likely to produce "dissatisfaction" rather than "Leidensdruck" because, although they produce a negative emotional state in the delinquent, this can be attributed by the delinquent to external conditions independent of himself'.[41] However, this relative decline in importance also resulted from Steller's behaviouristic approach to the problem. Negative stimuli caused dissatisfaction with one's situation but did not make the delinquent suffer from himself. With therapeutic measures, 'Leidensdruck' could actually be produced, Steller explained, because 'talk therapy techniques and selective reinforcement of certain client expressions increased the extent of self-exploration'.[42]

In other respects, Steller anticipated criticism of social therapeutic institutions raised around 1980. While in the 1950s and 1960s the primary question had been what characteristics clients had to have to be suitable for social therapy ('Leidensdruck', for example), the problem was then turned the other way around: what therapeutic methods were suitable for which clients? While in the first case – the psychoanalytic way – those prisoners were excluded who did not show any 'Leidensdruck' (meaning willingness to commit to the exertions of analytic treatment), in the second case prisoners could be admitted who were differently motivated and if suitable therapy offers were at hand.

During the 1970s, the psychoanalytic concept of 'Leidensdruck' was gradually decontextualized and transferred into the general debate on therapeutic penology. Assumptions about the psychophysical constitution of mentally disordered delinquents became less important, while the role of sociological factors of delinquency such as conditions of upbringing and socialization increased. This new epistemological context favoured the generalization of 'Leidensdruck', since it was increasingly incomprehensible why not every delinquent should be able to feel distressed by her/his incarceration, mental disorder, or stigma. Yet it was this very process of generalization that blurred the meaning of the concept

---

[40] Jung and Müller-Dietz, '8. Kolloquium'. See also Rasch and Stemmer-Lück, 'Diagnostik', 182–3.
[41] Steller, *Sozialtherapie*, 96.
[42] Steller, *Sozialtherapie*, 98.

of 'Leidensdruck' and stimulated semantic differentiation to save the term's usability in diagnostic practice.

Diagnosing 'Leidensdruck': Expert statements on male prisoners (North-Rhine Westphalia, 1974–83)

Starting in 1971, psychologists, sociologists, educators, social workers, employment counsellors, correctional officers and jurists collaborated in two assessment facilities in North Rhine-Westphalia.[43] The selection process, which all male offenders had to undergo following their conviction, lasted four to six weeks. [44] Based on the results of a series of personality and performance tests at the beginning of the process, it was decided which experts would interview the subject to complete the 'personality picture'. These interviews, as well as the study of the prisoner's personal file, and more or less elaborate research in the social environment and at public offices served to complete the 'social anamnesis'.[45] At the end of the procedure, a 'judicial panel' (Spruchkörper) issued the 'committal order', which classified the prisoner and – accompanied by 'treatment recommendations' – directed him to one of the state's correctional facilities.

Commissions as well as voluntary applications by inmates received by the Gelsenkirchen Social Therapeutic Institution, from its opening in January 1975 to the beginning of 1983, provide a suitable basis for examining the use of the concept of 'Leidensdruck' in expert practice.[46] The basis for the admission decision of the Gelsenkirchen prison was the prisoner's personal file (with verdict and, if applicable, psychiatric report) as well as the 'committal order' with psychological report and social anamnesis. Letters from the prisoners as well as from relatives and lawyers were also included in the files. Only exceptionally did members of the therapeutic team conduct their own diagnostics with the applicant prior to admission.

From a formal point of view, two correlations stand out in the analysis of the psychological reports and social anamneses. First, the psychological reports were divided into two parts, first briefly presenting the results of the

---

[43] LAV NRW Abt. Rheinland NW 460 Nr. 62, 1–2; Nr. 65, S. 1–2, 5–6, 15/16; Nr. 69 II, 1–4.
[44] LAV NRW Abt. Rheinland NW 460 Nr. 62, 1–2; NW 460 Nr. 65, 13, 14–15, 17–18.
[45] LAV NRW Abt. Rheinland NW 460 Nr. 66 II, 12–14.
[46] Since the legal basis (§ 65 StrRG) for admission to social-therapeutic institutions did not come into force during this period, the institutions had the opportunity to select and also reject applicants according to their own criteria.

intelligence, performance and personality tests and then those of the interviews. Without being able to assess this connection conclusively, an analysis of the reports suggests that the evaluators' attitudes towards the subjects during the exploration interview were strongly influenced by the test results. For example, they recommended inmates for social therapy when the tests showed relatively good intellectual ability on the one hand but hardly any motivation for therapy on the other. Conversely, if the intelligence quotient was relatively low, it was seemingly more difficult to work out aspects of the convict's personality in the interview that could be followed up therapeutically.

The word 'Leidensdruck' by no means appeared in all expert reports sent to Gelsenkirchen. Moreover, its use was limited to the psychological reports, while it hardly ever appeared in the social anamneses. In most cases, the reports mentioned 'Leidensdruck' at the end, when the question of whether therapeutic treatment of the patient was necessary, appropriate and promising was clarified. The term was not synonymous with the motivation for therapy; rather, it apparently served as a cipher for an ensemble of diagnostic findings concerning the subject's emotionality: to have feelings, to allow feelings, not to appear emotionally cold or uninvolved in personal contact, but to be 'able to resonate', to be 'responsive' in the 'emotional realm', 'accessible', 'not yet fixed'; to be able to speak more or less eloquently about oneself, to show in this way the ability to verbalize and be self-reflexive, to have insight into one's own guilt, 'awareness of problems' and 'personal difficulties', 'feelings of inferiority' and 'emotional lability'. Such findings seem to have been circumscribed and summed up by the term 'Leidensdruck'.

Second, the anamneses elaborated by sociologists, social workers, teachers and psychologists tended to follow a certain narrative scheme in terms of content. Special attention was paid to the conditions of upbringing from early childhood; to the parental home and family; to stays in institutional care; to school attendance, grades and the course of training; to professional career; to former and current love relationships as well as relationships within the parental family, to siblings; to the time of the first delinquency; to previous convictions and prison stays; and to the social situation at the time of the assessment. In this way, the biographical depth of the personal conflicts and tensions, 'breaks' and 'undesirable developments' were worked out.

Two different paths to 'waywardness' were identified in the anamneses. In some cases, an overpampering parental home or educational milieu had hampered the subject's development of 'realistic ideas about himself and his possibilities'. In the case of a 21-year-old prisoner, a 'personality with clear symptoms of waywardness', it was stated that 'the focus of his upbringing' had been his 'strong material pampering by his parents'. Their 'obviously only preconsciously applied unfortunate upbringing and affirmation methods' still strongly influenced the prisoner's behaviour at the time of the assessment, especially since the parents continued to be present as 'caregivers' of their imprisoned son. Although they only meant well, according to the expert opinion they 'objectively further strengthened the [prisoner's] lack of independence'. The well-meaning motivation was to be interpreted 'even as a special form of aggressiveness towards the prisoner'.[47]

In most cases, however, not too much but too little parental attention in childhood and adolescence was found. A 25-year-old sex offender assessed in the Duisburg centre in November 1982 was the 'third in a row of 15 siblings', the father an alcoholic, the mother 'not very affectionate'. Due to 'cramped quarters', the children had to sleep in twos or threes in one bed, which had 'encouraged sexual contact with some of the brothers'. One of the older brothers had introduced him to the 'hustler milieu', while with another he had committed the crimes.[48] Considering this dark misery, the psychologist was 'surprised' to discover an almost ideal client:

> His lack of ability to differentiate and his considerable self-uncertainty, combined with his sensitivity, frequently cause him to experience feelings of powerlessness and feelings of being dominated by alien forces. It is astonishing how sensitively and, in part, self-critically Mr. L. argues. He has dealt intensively with his social relationships and his personality disorders during his time in prison so far. In the interview he shows his high openness and a great degree of trust. Again and again he asked for the opinions and attitudes of his interlocutor and asked for advice. This demonstrated his strong effort to clarify his problems. Considering his background and his way of life, his fine sense of language and his good verbalization ability are surprising. Mr. L. is thus able to look at himself critically and in a distanced way. At the moment, the focus of his problems are his obsessive-compulsive symptoms, his self-doubt and his identity problems. Mr. L. clearly experiences his own inner ambivalence, an insecurity and his fears in contact with others. He cannot properly assess the effects of his behaviour on others and does not know how to clearly define his sexual position. His conflicts

---

[47] Psychological expert statement, Hagen, 16 July 1975, LAV NRW Abt. Westfalen NW Q918 Nr. 163. For a similar case see Committal order of Hagen, 6 September 1979, LAV NRW Abt. Westfalen NW Q918 Nr. 153.
[48] Psychological expert statement, Hagen, 16 July 1975.

create an intense Leidensdruck, which he does not try to escape by avoidance and flight behaviour.[49]

Initially, before the number of applications and the therapeutic work increasingly tied up the forces of the therapeutic team, some of them seem to have been prepared to question the psychological reports of the two assessment facilities. Regarding one of the first inmates, whose admission to the Gelsenkirchen correctional facility was examined in early 1975, the committal order of the Hagen selection facility stated: 'His comments on his crime (murder) at the time indicate a diminished affective and emotional capacity for sympathy, which is presumably constitutional. In his external behaviour, his uncontrolled urge to talk and his social lack of inhibition are impressive.'[50] The conference of the institution rejected his admission due to lack of motivation for therapy. The social worker in charge of processing and presenting the case previously had conceded that the report showed 'virtually no motivation and no Leidensdruck'. But because he had already been rejected twice by the state's second social therapeutic institution in Düren, and the admission in Gelsenkirchen being his last chance, she suggested that the prisoner at least 'be interviewed ... to convince me whether there really is no Leidensdruck, or at least to provoke it'.[51]

The prison's therapeutic director, psychologist Günter Romkopf, on the other hand, found even 'great Leidensdruck' in a prisoner serving time in the Cologne prison, who had described his situation to him in a letter of several pages in March 1979. This prisoner gave a vivid and eloquent account of his life, of his efforts on the second educational path, of his drug problems, of his participation in a self-awareness group and of the adoption of therapy-related practices in his everyday life (Zen meditation). He gave a sophisticated description of his feelings in custody and expressed regret for his wife, who was overburdened with the organic greengrocery and their baby child and who was herself undergoing psychotherapeutic treatment for depression. All in all, it was a life story that was shaped by the urban 'alternative' milieu in the 1970s.[52] Since the prisoner had been convicted of a drug offence and since social therapy institutions generally did not accept such convicts, Romkopf wanted nonetheless to do something for him. He contacted his wife, Ute Romkopf, a doctor who ran the drug programme at Münster Prison, via the short official channels (to probably no avail).[53]

---

[49] Psychological expert statement, 3 December 1982, LAV NRW Abt. Westfalen NW Q918 Nr. 358.
[50] Committal order Hagen, 24 January 1975, LAV NRW Abt. Westfalen NW Q918 Nr. 163.
[51] Handwritten note, not dated [before 29 January 1975], LAV NRW Abt. Westfalen NW Q918 Nr. 163.
[52] Letter to Romkopf, 14 March 1979, LAV NRW Abt. Westfalen NW Q918 Nr. 153.
[53] Günter Romkopf, letter to Ute Romkopf, 12 April 1979, LAV NRW Abt. Westfalen NW Q918 Nr. 153.

If prisoners were not recommended for social therapy by the assessment institutions or by the therapists working in the respective correctional facilities, but rather applied for admission themselves, this circumstance, from the therapists' point of view, at least spoke in favour of their mustering a certain amount of initiative, as in the case of the prisoner from Cologne. It seems misleading to regard the twisted and sometimes absurd use of psychological and therapeutic notions in such letters exclusively as an attempt to get into the supposedly easier-to-tolerate social therapeutic institutions.[54] Applications were basically characterized by their attempt to use the language of the person who would judge its merits. Romkopf, for example, almost always answered such inquiries in a friendly manner and sent a leaflet that the prison had prepared for this purpose in 1976.[55] When the prisoners wrote about themselves with the help of the technical terms contained in this leaflet or included elsewhere, they subjected themselves – just as prisoner G., quoted in the introduction, did – to the therapeutic discourse and thus contributed to its reproduction and distribution in the everyday life of penal institutions. Even if they often could hardly or only imprecisely formulate what they understood by 'therapy', the letters and the completed personality questionnaires at least show that they expected something else – more help! – from the social therapeutic institution than was offered by the prisons in which they served their sentence. And was this not precisely the claim of the prison reform in general?

The persistent attempt of a sex offender in 1975 and 1976 to be admitted to the Gelsenkirchen prison is a telling example in this regard. The therapists' conference turned him down three times. In several letters written by prisoner K. to the various institutions and offices implicated in his case, he insisted that only the social therapeutic institutions of the Federal Republic – if it was not 'all lies' – could help him not to relapse. Finally, the case found its way to a medical officer in the Ministry of Justice, who finally recognized the prisoner's efforts: his repeated attempts to be admitted to social therapy 'at least [show] … a clear initiative on his own part'. Moreover, at least one letter 'clearly unmistakably reveals a Leidensdruck', which is why 'really more needs to be done for the prisoner. … he will relapse again after his release, unless a "therapy" has been carried out in time beforehand'.[56]

---

[54] Eghigian, *Corrigible*, 193.
[55] Information sheet, Annex 1 to Annual Report for 1976, LAV NRW Abt. Rheinland NW 460 Nr. 81 II. It did not mention 'Leidensdruck' as motivation, though.
[56] Medical officer, report, not dated [January 1976], LAV NRW Abt. Westfalen NW Q918 Nr. 163.

When criminal psychologist Rüdiger Ortmann evaluated the recommendations for social therapy made by the expert panels at the Hagen and Duisburg assessment facilities in the mid-1980s, he emphasized the importance of the concept of 'Leidensdruck'. He himself differentiated 'prison-related' from 'personality-related' suffering. In almost five hundred assessment procedures of each of the two institutions examined, he found that the specialists diagnosed 'strong or very strong' prison-related 'Leidensdruck' in 37 per cent and 'strong or very strong personality-related Leidensdruck' in 18 per cent of the cases.[57] At the same time, the author stated that the number of recommendations for social therapy increased with the identification of 'Leidensdruck' (whether prison-related or personality-related).[58] One might conclude from Ortmann's findings that 'Leidensdruck' correlated highly with treatability in the assessment practice of the specialist teams at both institutions. Around 1980, the concept clearly had a regulating function in the selection of offenders for social therapeutic institutions.

Conclusion

The psychoanalytic term 'Leidensdruck' has been emblematic for the emergence of therapeutic penology, social-therapeutic facilities and specialized treatment techniques in the West German prison system since the late 1950s. When it first appeared in the debate, it indicated a shift in perspective. According to criminal psychiatrists, it was a waste of time to treat 'psychopathic criminals' who they deemed psychopathic by nature. As psychodynamic assumptions on personality disorders gained more and more ground in the discussion, 'Leidensdruck' was one of the key terms suggesting neuroticism, emotional accessibility and therefore treatability of the delinquent.

'Leidensdruck' played an important role in both the general criminological discussion and the statements of psy-experts on individual delinquents. The diagnostic processes in North Rhine-Westphalia around 1980 attest to that double aspect. Moreover, the emphasis placed on emotions in the therapeutic departments of the prison system suggested to some delinquents to 'stage'

---

[57] Rüdiger Ortmann, 'Resozialisierung im Strafvollzug. Eine vergleichende Längsschnittstudie zu Regelvollzugs- und sozialtherapeutischen Modellanstalten. Ein Beitrag zur Präzisierung von Grundbegriffen der sozialtherapeutischen Anstalt', *Zwanzig Jahre südwestdeutsche kriminologische Kolloquien*, ed. Hans-Jörg Albrecht (Freiburg im Breisgau: Max-Planck-Institut für Ausländisches und Internationales Strafrecht, 1986), 239–78, 244.

[58] Ortmann, 'Resozialisierung', 249.

emotions and present themselves as feeling, suffering beings, regardless of their actual diagnosis.

In the mid-1980s, however, the interest in the 'Leidensdruck' of delinquents and inmates declined very quickly among criminologists as well as in the general public.[59] One explanation for this decline might be found in yet another fundamental shift of criminal policy. During the 1980s, a 'punitive turn' in society favoured the re-emergence of conservative penal theories that vaunted deterrence and security over therapy and rehabilitation. Meanwhile, the influence of crime victims and their organizations like 'Weißer Ring' (White Ring) became more and more palpable in criminal policy. In 1987, the first victim protection law came into force in West Germany. From then on, it was the pain and distress of the victims that were in the spotlight; the 'Leidensdruck' of offenders, in contrast, was met with indifference.[60]

Nowadays, the 'White Ring', as well as police in larger cities, offers advice and information on local self-help groups and psychotherapists specializing in trauma therapy. The therapeutic impetus of these processes of victimization on the individual, as well as the societal, level has been such that, for instance in 2008, an initiative in the state of Baden-Württemberg, founded to promote offender therapy once again, argued that victim protection was most likely achieved through (preventive) therapeutic treatment of offenders. Not surprisingly, then, the selves of victims, as well as of offenders, are now both part of one and the same therapeutic regime.[61]

---

[59] Apart from psychologist Klaus-Peter Dahle, there was hardly any interest in 'Leidensdruck' as motivation to engage in therapy during the 1990s and early 2000s. See his *Therapiemotivation hinter Gittern: zielgruppenorientierte Entwicklung und Erprobung eines Motivationskonstrukts für die therapeutische Arbeit im Strafvollzug* (Regensburg: Roderer, 1995); since the Federal Constitutional Court in 2007 ruled unconstitutional the common practice to let convicts serve preventive custody under the same conditions as their sentence, the interest in therapy and the motivation of inmates is increasing again. See Melanie Spöhr, *Sozialtherapie von Sexualstraftätern im Justizvollzug: Praxis und Evaluation*, ed. the Federal Department of Justice (Mönchengladbach: Verlag Godesberg, 2009), 85; Lena C. Carl, Maike M. Breuer and Johann Endres, 'Leidensdruck und Behandlungsmotivation bei Gewaltstraftätern', *Forensische Psychiatrie und Psychotherapie*, 23 (2016): 1, 8–36.

[60] See Florian Schwanengel and Johann Endres, 'Kriminaltherapeutische Straftäterbehandlung. Theoretische Modelle und praktische Umsetzungen', *Forum Strafvollzug*, 65 (2016): 3, 158–62, 160, note 3: 'Nowadays criminal therapy is mainly about "protecting the public" and not, as in "general psychotherapy," about "curing or alleviating suffering".'

[61] Jens Elberfeld, *Anleitung zur Selbstregulation: Eine Wissensgeschichte der Therapeutisierung im 20. Jahrhundert* (Frankfurt: Campus, 2020); Maik Tändler, *Das therapeutische Jahrzehnt. Der Psychoboom in den siebziger Jahren* (Göttingen: Wallstein, 2016).

Construction and contingency of experience

Commentary

Diseases come and go, few remain. This is not only the case in the individual biography of each person. History also knows a number of diseases that were diagnosed only for a certain time and then disappeared from the repertoire of medicine: hysteria, neurasthenia and shell shock are among the best-known diseases of this kind. Therapies are at least as volatile. Something that was recognized as effective for a while, and possibly experienced as beneficial by patients, is at some point considered ineffective. This observation can be understood within the frame of reference of a history of medical progress, which hardly anyone dares to write so unambiguously anymore. Especially with regard to the affective experience of patients, the coming and going of disease diagnoses and therapies raises the question of the construction and possible contingency of experience. The following two chapters trace how profoundly the lived experience of dis-ease is shaped by the ever-changing relationship between medical theories, cultural beliefs and social framings.

The time, place and perspective of both chapters are vastly different. Brenda Lynn Edgar takes a look at American and European pain research and management in the second half of the twentieth century. She is interested in the use of landscape images as a means to increase pain tolerance. She makes clear that notions of pain and notions of 'nature' virtually converged during this period, until the moment when a conception prevailed according to which looking at or visualizing a simulated landscape in image or language was recognized as a means to reduce feelings of anxiety and stress. Thus, such images entered clinics and were simultaneously discovered as 'emotional commodities' that could be commercially exploited in the wellness industry.

James Kennaway's gaze, on the other hand, travels to Georgian England. He traces the career of 'fashionable' diseases, which were not 'fashionable' because they were only diagnosed in the eighteenth century, but because they were considered typical diseases of the successful, rich and clever. Gout or digestion problems were attributed to the luxurious lifestyles and mental exertion of this privileged class but were also seen as evidence of their more delicate bodies. Even if the public debate sometimes met these disease conditions with scepticism or moralizing undertones, turning them into a critique of expanding mercantile societies, the diagnosis of a 'fashionable' disease could be understood as proof of belonging to a social elite and paved the way to the exclusive spas of the Georgian period. Kennaway uses personal letters to show vividly how this added prestige had a consoling effect on the sufferers, which, however, failed in the case of serious pain.

Pain, then, is a relative limit for Kennaway to the soothing effects of a 'fashionable' disease, whereas the simulated 'landscapes' in Edgar's story can have their soothing effect precisely when pain is present. In medical history and the present, such effects have been explained by different concepts: from the gain of illness to placebo effects. Edgar and Kennaway, though, emphasize the dynamic interrelationship between medical and cultural concepts, social frames and affective lived experience. According to them, the experience of illness is neither a construction nor exclusively tied to an essentialized body. Here, too, the history of experience and emotions points to the fact that human beings are to be understood as biocultural beings.

10

The efficacy of Arcadia: Constructing emotions of nature in the pained body through landscape imagery, c.1945–present

Brenda Lynn Edgar

This essay examines the use of landscape imagery in clinical practices to elicit specific emotional responses in patients experiencing pain. One of the many different distraction techniques developed in the 1960s and 1970s to increase pain tolerance, landscape images are believed to lower patient stress and anxiety by inducing an emotional state of relaxation, ease and comfort. They can be verbally suggested in audio recordings or pictured in mediums such as photography, slide photography, films and more recently virtual environments. More generally, in the form of photographs or photomurals, landscape imagery has been integrated into the decorative schemes of medical environments where the image of 'nature' is thought to create relaxing atmospheres conducive to healing (Figure 10.1). Escalating with digital technology, this Arcadian imagery has become embedded in today's material culture and can be found on everything from computer screens, train bathrooms and shower curtains to building façades.

Simon Schama has argued that 'landscapes are culture before they are nature, constructs of the imagination projected onto wood, water and rock' intimately bound up in individual memories of places and collective nature myths.[1] Here I examine the emotions that attend these constructs of the imagination from the second half of the twentieth century, how they shaped and were shaped by notions of landscape and how they were bound up in the experience and treatment of pain. Through a selection of sources taken from North American and European medical reviews dating from 1962 to 2021, I will examine the evolving notions of

---

[1] Simon Schama, *Landscape and Memory* (London: HarperCollins, 1995), 61, 14.

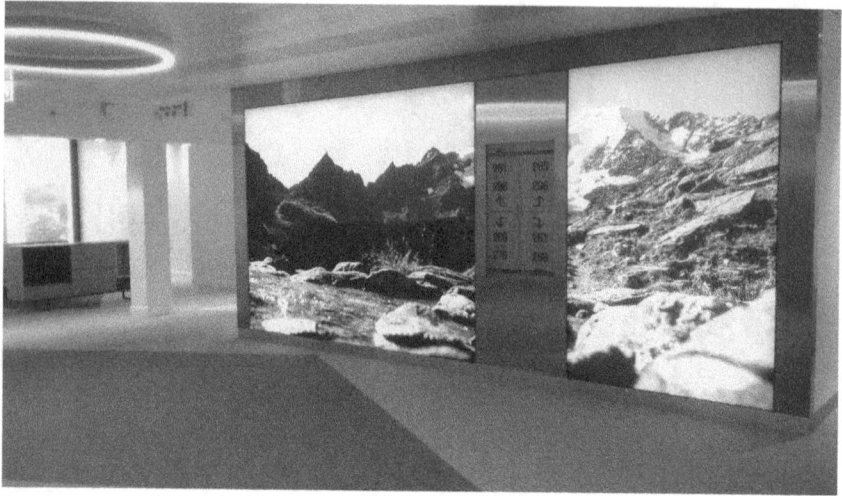

Figure 10.1 Photographic installations by David Carlier and Studiobivouac, La Tour Hospital, Geneva, Switzerland, 2017. Photo by Brenda Lynn Edgar.

pain and how landscape has been perceived as an agent of relaxation capable of altering patients' experience of pain by increasing their tolerance of it. I will then discuss this practice of landscape in clinical environments in relation to evolving emotions attending 'nature' from 1945 to the present.

Changing understandings of pain

Writing on hospital gardens in the nineteenth and twentieth centuries, Clare Hickman maintains that 'the explanations for the mechanisms by which the environment might affect patient recovery have changed over time, but the notion that the landscape can act as a therapeutic agent is as valid now as it was in previous centuries'.[2] Yet, the meaning and affective value of landscape are also historically contingent and condition its performative qualities (the 'mechanisms'). Likewise, how emotions shape and are shaped by landscape changes over time, as do the illnesses on which they are believed to act. The therapeutic value of nineteenth-century asylum gardens was largely normative; they were believed to restore a moral order thought to be inherent in 'nature' and missing in the mentally ill.[3] Asylums were also designed to resemble the

---

[2] Clare Hickman, *Therapeutic Landscapes: A History of English Hospital Gardens since 1800* (Manchester: Manchester University Press, 2013), 2.
[3] Hickman, *Therapeutic Landscapes*, 76.

large country homes of the wealthy, which were regarded as environments conducive to good health and moral development.[4] Views of cultivated gardens or 'tamed nature' as well as the 'wholesome occupation' of gardening activities were thought to promote 'a tranquil and cheerful tone of thought' in patients.[5] While mid- and late-twentieth-century sources also contain similar references to tranquillity and cheerfulness, landscape in the nineteenth century was not seen in the context of pain per se. Exposure to landscape was widely regarded as a curative practice for the psychiatrically ill (which would have included the intellectually disabled or deaf), who it was believed did not feel pain.[6] With the expansion of open-air hospitals and sanatoria in the late nineteenth and early twentieth centuries, the therapeutic value of walking and gardening activities became more important than viewing landscape. Likewise, long-standing medical beliefs in the curative and prophylactic qualities of 'nature' pertained to specific elements such as the air quality or altitude of a specific landscape or the sunlight it provided, and how these elements were believed to act directly on bodies suffering specific afflictions such as tuberculosis, or on healthy bodies as a reinforcing or prophylactic agent. These beliefs shaped a new architectural vocabulary for what was considered a healthy environment: roof terraces for sunbathing, large plate glass windows and even rotating garden pavilions that optimized exposure to the sun, fresh air or pinewood forests.[7]

While many of these notions still hold for what is deemed a healthy environment today, changing notions of pain that emerged in the mid-twentieth century conferred a new performative quality upon landscape and the emotions it is thought to evoke. Already in the late nineteenth century it was believed that 'emotional and psychological states dramatically affected levels of pain awareness and tolerance', but the physiological processes by which pain was transmitted to the brain, as well as questions of sensibility to pain, were debated up until the mid-twentieth century.[8] In the 1940s and 1950s, neurologists began

---

[4] Hickman, *Therapeutic Landscapes*, 76.
[5] Hickman, *Therapeutic Landscapes*, 91.
[6] Joanna Bourke, *The Story of Pain: From Prayer to Painkillers* (Oxford: Oxford University Press, 2014), 204.
[7] Philip L. Gallos, *Cure Cottages of Saranac Lake: Architecture and History of a Pioneer Health Resort* (New York: Historic Saranac Lake, 1985); M. Campbell, 'What Tuberculosis Did for Modernism: The Influence of a Curative Environment on Modernist Design and Architecture', *Medical History*, 49 (2005): 463–88; Richard Hobday, *The Light Revolution: Health, Architecture and the Sun* (Forres: Findhorn Press, 2007); Eva Eylers, 'Planning the Nation: The Sanatorium Movement in Germany', *Journal of Architecture*, 19 (2014): 667–92; Paul V. Stock and Chris Brickell, 'Nature's Good for You: Sir Truby King, Seacliff Asylum, and the Greening of Health Care in New Zealand, 1889–1922', *Health & Place* 22 (2013): 107–14.
[8] Bourke, *Story of Pain*, 203, 222.

to question the Cartesian concept of pain as a 'straight-through transmission system' by which pain was transmitted directly to the brain from an injured part of the body.[9] In the 1960s, Canadian pain psychologist Ronald Melzack and British neuroscientist Patrick David Wall would radically change this field of research with their Gate Control Theory of pain[10] whereby pain transmission to the brain is regulated by a gating mechanism located in the dorsal horns of the spinal column that 'modulates sensory input from the skin before it evokes pain perception and response'.[11] The possibility of modifying psychological perception of pain signified that 'mind and body were fully integrated'.[12] While racial, ethnic and gender biases would continue to influence beliefs about pain, the Gate Control Theory allowed research on pain perception and relief to focus on 'psychological variables such as past experience, attention and other cognitive processes'.[13] A new understanding of the effects of attention and anxiety on pain led to the development of cognitive strategies for coping with pain, such as distraction techniques.

'Emotive imagery'

The efficacy of distraction, or diverting the attention of a person away from their experiencing of pain, has been observed for centuries. However, in the 1970s there was a new focus on the use of cognitive techniques that would specifically induce relaxation and reduce anxiety in order to increase pain tolerance. Images deemed 'inherently relaxing' such as landscapes (either pictured or verbally suggested) were incorporated into these techniques. Relaxation techniques were already being developed at the time of Melzack and Wall's first study, and psychologists had experimented with visualization techniques to test the potential for positive emotions in reducing anxiety. In 1962, the term 'emotive imagery' was coined by psychologists Lazarus and Abramowitz to designate 'a method of engendering [positive] feelings through positive images vividly described by the therapist', referring to images 'which are assumed to arouse feelings of self-assertion,

---

[9] W. K. Livingston, *Pain Mechanisms* (New York: Macmillan, 1943); W. Noordenbos, *Pain* (Amsterdam: Elsevier, 1959).
[10] Ronald Melzack and Patrick D. Wall, 'Pain Mechanisms: A New Theory', *Science*, 150 (1965): 971–9.
[11] Melzack and Wall, 'Pain Mechanisms', 971.
[12] Bourke, *Story of Pain*, 229.
[13] R. Melzack, 'Pain: Past, Present and Future', *Canadian Journal of Experimental Psychology = Revue Canadienne De Psychologie Experimentale*, 47 (1993): 615.

pride, affection, mirth, and similar anxiety inhibiting responses'.[14] As their study involved children, they used guided imagery orientated towards wish fulfilment and hero identification that did not include landscapes.[15] A decade later, however, landscape imagery would be used by psychologists in pain tolerance experiments with adults using a method they called '*in vivo* emotive imagery'.[16] Subjects would remain alone in a room with one hand immersed in iced water – the pain stimulus – while listening to a guided imagery recording evoking landscapes in phrases such as 'walking through a lush meadow, looking at a clear blue lake' that, according to the authors, were 'assumed to arouse feelings of comfort and relaxation'.[17] In a prior, personal essay published in 1973, one of the authors, John Horan, claimed to have successfully distracted his wife from the pains of childbirth by 'verbally paint[ing] a picture of a clear blue sky, green grassy meadow, warm sun, gentle breeze, etc.', as well as images other than landscapes that seemed just as effective.[18] In a subsequent study comparing the in vivo emotive imagery method and the Lamaze Psychoprophylactic Method for childbirth (which uses focal point visualization and respiration techniques), Horan and his colleagues used a tape-recorded vignette that suggested subjects to picture themselves 'lying relaxed on a comfortable deserted lakeside'.[19]

Early experiments with guided imagery also used suggestions of sensorial experience of landscape that were intended to contrast the pain experienced by participants. A person with their hand immersed in ice water would be asked to imagine themselves in a desert on a very hot day, or a participant experiencing ischemic pain in their arm would be asked to imagine themselves going 'outside where it was a bright sun-shining day'.[20] Guided imagery recordings such as those made by Ohio-based company Health Journeys alternate between descriptions of visual aspects of landscape and the sensory experience of it (the smell of peat

---

[14] Thomas B. Westcott and John J. Horan, 'The Effects of Anger and Relaxation Forms of In Vivo Emotive Imagery on Pain Tolerance', *Canadian Journal of Behavioural Science/Revue Canadienne Des Sciences Du Comportement*, 9 (1977): 217; A. A. Lazarus and A. Abramowitz, 'The Use of "Emotive Imagery" in the Treatment of Children's Phobia', *Journal of Mental Science* 108 (1962): 191–5, at 191.
[15] Lazarus and Abramowitz, 'Use of "Emotive Imagery"', 192.
[16] John J. Horan and J. K. Dellinger, 'In Vivo Emotive Imagery: An Experimental Test', *Perceptual and Motor Skills*, 39 (1974): 359.
[17] Horan and Dellinger, 'In Vivo Emotive Imagery', 360.
[18] John J. Horan, '"In Vivo" Emotive Imagery: A Technique for Reducing Childbirth Anxiety and Discomfort', *Psychological Reports*, 32 (1973): 1328.
[19] Christopher I. Stone, Deborah A. Demchik-Stone and John J. Horan, 'Coping with Pain: A Component Analysis of Lamaze and Cognitive-Behavioral Procedures', *Journal of Psychosomatic Research*, 21 (1977): 453.
[20] Matt E. Jaremko, 'Cognitive Strategies in the Control of Pain Tolerance', *Journal of Behavioral Therapy & Experimental Psychiatry*, 9 (1978): 240–1; George A. Clum, R. L. Luscomb and L. Scott, 'Relaxation Training and Cognitive Redirection Strategies in the Treatment of Acute Pain', *Pain*, 12 (1982): 178.

moss, sea air, pine forests, etc.). In their recording 'Ease Pain' describing a 'special retreat' by the sea, listeners are guided through a series of suggested sensations and feelings provoked by the landscape. A dulcet-toned narrator encourages listeners to feel the 'healing presence' of the landscape [21] and imagine it relieving their pain:

> feel ... the healing vibrance of the place penetrate all the way into you, soaking into you, all the way through layers of tissue and muscle, all the way to the bone, down into each and every cell, softly seeping into the places that are tight, or tense, or sore, gently entering the places where pain is stored, and feeling the beginnings of a subtle shift deep inside, a softness, a gentle release.[22]

Health Journeys' additional guided imagery transitions from a description of an exterior landscape to a microscopic cellular landscape within the body, conflating a sensorial experience of the landscape with the experience of the body in pain. The recording *Overcoming Viral Infection* invites listeners to picture themselves atop a podium sitting in 'a great green field' and looking out on a mass of white blood cells that will marshal an inflammatory response to their pain.[23] More recently, the immersive environments of virtual reality (VR) have been observed to divert a greater part of a patient's conscious attention away from their pain.[24] SnowWorld, a VR game made specifically for burn victims during treatment sessions in water tanks, was designed to distract patients not only through gaming but also through pictured landscapes of icy canyons and rivers, igloos, penguins and exploding snowballs that are meant to counter the intense burning sensations felt by patients.[25]

In contrast to the constructionist approach to pain taken by doctors and psychologists since the 1960s and 1970s, medical literature reveals the persistence of an essentialist view of 'nature' (the term 'landscape' is rarely used) and the emotions it is thought to elicit. Recurrent descriptions such as 'pleasant images', 'pleasant scenery' and 'natural scenery' reflect the assumption that 'nature' is universally perceived as agreeable to behold (and a fortiori by people in pain)

---

[21] Belleruth Naparstek, *A Guided Meditation for Relaxation & Wellness*, mp3, accessed 25 June 2021, https://www.healthjourneys.com/AudioSamples/HJRelaxWellness.mp3.
[22] Belleruth Neparstek, *A Guided Meditation to Help Ease Pain*, mp3, n.d., https://www.healthjourneys.com/AudioSamples/HJ%20SMPL%20CID18%20Ease%20Pain.mp3.
[23] Emmett Miller, *Overcoming Viral Infection*, mp3, accessed 25 June 2021, https://www.healthjourneys.com/AudioSamples/Overcoming%20Viral%20Infection%20Sample.mp3.
[24] Hunter G. Hoffman et al., 'Water-Friendly Virtual Reality Pain Control during Wound Care', *Journal of Clinical Psychology*, 60 (2004): 190.
[25] UW Video, *Snow World*, accessed 24 June 2021, https://www.youtube.com/watch?v=Nh4K_dZ7LvQ.

and that its role is that of a spectacle or a background view. A study from the late 1980s describes 'natural' images used in distraction therapy as 'incompatible sensory imagery', so called because of the contrast between the distress of pain and the 'pleasant images of "blue skies", "grassy meadows", and "gentle warmth"' or 'images of "pure" visual, auditory or other sensations incompatible with pain but with no link to particular emotions'.[26] In a 1992 study on pain relief during treatment of severe burns, seventeen patients 'viewed video programs that were composed of scenic beauty with music'.[27] Others refer simply to 'relaxation-producing images' or 'scenic slides'.[28] In 2016, a research team at Imperial College used a panoramic photomural of a forest (Figure 10.2) to create a 'cosy and aesthetically pleasing' setting for trials of psychedelic substances which, according to them, 'increase feelings of nature connectedness'.[29] One study on stress recovery in what the authors call 'green' environments claims that the 'inherent quality of nature, such as noise reduction and spontaneous inductions of positive emotions', is effective in stress reduction.[30] Similarly, in literature from other fields such as environmental design, landscape is assumed to be 'enjoyable scenery' comparable to 'other pleasant distractions'.[31] Conversely, certain images are considered emotionally neutral. Westcott and Horan expressed surprise that images they considered 'devoid of affect', such as an orange, also proved effective in enhancing pain tolerance.[32]

In the 1970s, American psychologists Rachel and Stephen Kaplan conducted a series of studies on the psychological effects of 'nature' and its potential for generating positive emotions. Concomitant with the development of guided imagery in distraction techniques, their research also reflects certain assumptions about nature, such as the existence of 'wilderness' and the opposition of nature and culture. From 1972 to 1981, the Kaplans ran a 'Wilderness Laboratory' which involved taking groups of participants hiking through large 'wilderness'

---

[26] Ephrem Fernandez, 'A Classification System of Cognitive Coping Strategies for Pain', *Pain*, 26 (1986): 145.
[27] A. C. Miller, L. C. Hickman and G. K. Lemasters, 'A Distraction Technique for Control of Burn Pain', *Journal of Burn Care*, 13, no. 5 (1992): 577.
[28] Westcott and Horan, 'The Effects of Anger', 217; Fernandez, 'A Classification System', 147.
[29] Sam Gandy to Ros Watts and Brenda Lynn Edgar, 'Re: Psilocybin, 2016 Feasibility Study', 5 September 2020.
[30] Matilda Annerstedt et al., 'Inducing Physiological Stress Recovery with Sounds of Nature in a Virtual Reality Forest – Results from a Pilot Study', *Physiology & Behavior*, 118 (2013): 240.
[31] Roger S. Ulrich, 'Evidence-Based Health-Care Architecture', *Lancet*, 368 (2006): 39.
[32] Westcott and Horan, 'The Effects of Anger', 217. Another study featured a test group that used what was called 'neutral imagery' such as imagining 'activities of a routine nature, such as those activities done daily', to increase pain tolerance. See Everett L. Worthington, 'The Effects of Imagery Content, Choice of Imagery Content, and Self-Verbalization on the Self-Control of Pain', *Cognitive Therapy and Research*, 2 (1978): 230.

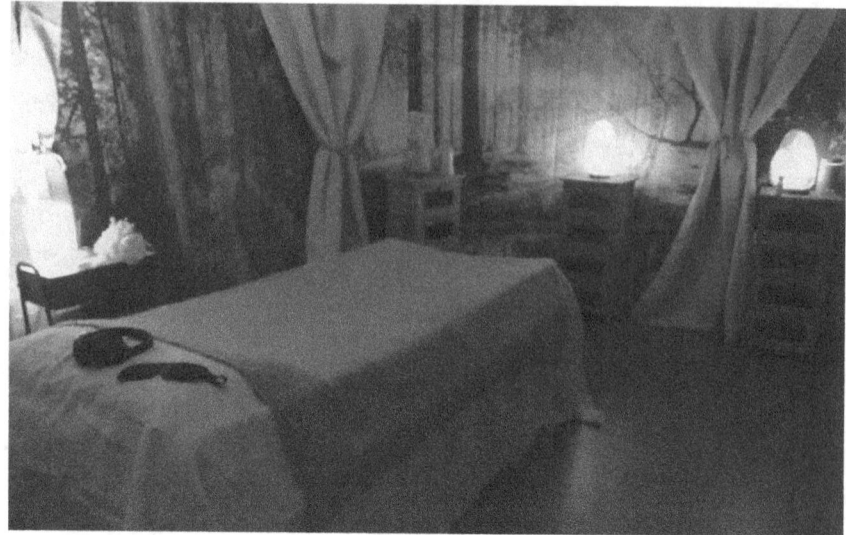

Figure 10.2 Room at Hammersmith Hospital, London, used for psilocybin trials, 2016. Photo: Rosalind Watts, Centre for Psychedelic Research, Imperial College London, UK.

areas of Michigan's Upper Peninsula for two-week periods of time, during forty-eight hours of which each participant would remain alone.[33] Certain features of the 'wilderness' were highly rated by participants as sources of comfort, such as 'the peace and quiet of the woods', the feeling that 'nothing is in a big hurry', the use of a compass, observation of surroundings and 'the sounds of nature'.[34] According to Kaplan and Kaplan, for the vast majority of participants 'the existence of the wilderness became a comforting thought' and their immersion in the 'wilderness' improved self-confidence and esteem and procured a sense of peace and tranquillity.[35] In their 1989 book *The Experience of Nature: A Psychological Study*, Kaplan and Kaplan also found that two key factors in restorative experiences were 'being away' from one's daily environment and being in a 'natural environment', which 'is universally preferred over many other environments'.[36]

---

[33] Rachel Kaplan and Stephen Kaplan, *The Experience of Nature: A Psychological Perspective* (Cambridge: Cambridge University Press, 1989), 122–3.
[34] Kaplan and Kaplan, *Experience*, 134.
[35] Kaplan and Kaplan, *Experience*, 146.
[36] Kaplan and Kaplan, *Experience*, 195.

Changing notions of landscape

The persistent belief that 'nature' exists somewhere in a prelapsarian state of 'purity' or 'wilderness', untouched by humans, and the desire for 'connectivity' with this landscape recalls ideas cast in the Romantic period when 'nature's' restorative powers became a remedy for nascent industrialization, 'a way of healing what modern society has damaged'.[37] The Romantic view of 'nature' as a state from which man was alienated by industrial society also gave rise to ecology. Scientists such as Alexander von Humboldt sought to demonstrate the interconnectivity of life systems on earth. The 'naturalized ecopoetics' of Romantic-period writers such as Coleridge and Wordsworth that created an 'embodied, heightened atmosphere' still forms the basis of how 'nature' is aestheticized.[38] In the United States, figures such as Henry David Thoreau (1817–1862) and Walt Whitman (1819–1892) still populate the American imagination of landscape. Nineteenth-century American landscape painting also played an important role in shaping cultural identities and notions of 'nature'.[39] Painters such as Thomas Cole (1801–1848), Asher Brown Durand (1796–1886) and Frederic Edwin Church (1826–1900) interpreted the American landscape in the European tradition of historical painting and Arcadian iconography.[40] Cole was influenced by Burkean notions of the sublime and his allegorical paintings of Arcadian themes express the tension between his nostalgia for a 'pastoral refuge' and the threat to this refuge posed by massive clearing for farming and industry, encouraged by national settlement policies.[41] Along with his contemporary, Charles Dickens, Cole lamented the environmental destruction caused by intensive deforestation, soil erosion and mining already in the first decades of the nineteenth century.[42] His most famous allegorical series *The Course of Empire* (1833–6) 'tells a prophetic tale of environmental destruction'.[43] According to

---

[37] Timothy Morton, *Ecology without Nature: Rethinking Environmental Aesthetics* (Cambridge, MA: Harvard University Press, 2007), 22. Morton is paraphrasing the ideas of Raymond Williams in *Culture and Society: Coleridge to Orwell* (London: Chatto and Windus, 1958).
[38] Morton, *Ecology*, 93.
[39] Angela Miller, *The Empire of the Eye: Landscape Representation and American Cultural Politics, 1825–1875* (Ithaca, NY: Cornell University Press, 1996).
[40] Van Wyck Brooks, *The Dream of Arcadia: American Writers and Artists in Italy, 1760–1915* (London: Dent, 1959), 90–1; Arne Neset, *Arcadian Waters and Wanton Seas: The Iconology of Waterscapes in Nineteenth-Century Transatlantic Culture* (New York: Lang, 2009), 21.
[41] Rebecca Bailey Bedell, *The Anatomy of Nature: Geology and American Landscape Painting, 1825–1875* (Princeton, NJ: Princeton University Press, 2002), 22–3; Miller, *Empire of the Eye*, 51.
[42] Angela Miller, 'Nature's History: The Changing Cultural Image of Nature, from Romantic Nationalism to Land Art', *Kunsttexte.De*, no. 1 (2015): 2.
[43] Miller, 'Nature's History', 3.

Rebecca Bedell, Durand believed his landscape paintings were imbued with the same restorative powers as 'nature' itself.[44] Durand was heavily influenced by John Ruskin's theory that scientific knowledge of 'nature' and its accurate representation in painting were key to spiritual enlightenment, bringing both painter and viewer closer to God's genius.[45] Equally important for Durand was Scottish geologist Hugh Miller (1802–1856), who believed that the awe and wonder inspired by 'nature's riddles' enabled man to transcend the trials and tribulations of mortal life.[46]

Yet however much Romantic and nineteenth-century sentiments of refuge, awe, wonder, restoration, nostalgia and even distress in relation to 'nature' and landscape might still resonate in the twentieth and early twenty-first centuries, they would be shaped in an entirely different ecosystem that included post-war technology and science, Cold War tensions, late capitalism, the Great Acceleration and the concept of the Anthropocene. Beginning with the dropping of the first atomic bombs in 1945, the Great Acceleration ushered in another complex entanglement of emotions related to 'nature' that were tainted by the existential threat posed by unprecedented levels of environmental destruction. According to Charles-François Mathis, emerging concepts such as James Lovelock and Lynn Margulis's Gaia theory would shape a new 'emotional relationship to nature' in which humans saw themselves as 'children lost to their "Mother Earth" whom they brutalize'.[47] Earth came to be understood as an auto-regulating biosphere: a sentient being whose welfare was in the hands of the human race. Interconnectivity with 'nature' in the 1970s took on a radically new meaning for certain movements, such as deep ecology's rejection of 'the human-in-environment image in favour of the relational, total-field image: organisms as knots in the biosphere net or field of intrinsic relations'.[48]

Environmental disasters with global repercussions such as Chernobyl, oil spills and ozone depletion created 'an anxiety ridden climate of insecurity', compounding that of the Cold War.[49] Rachel Carson's immensely popular 1962 *Silent Spring*, denouncing the effects of the pesticide DDT, indicates the sense of menacing fear and guilt that could be associated with landscape at this time. The

---

[44] Bedell, *Anatomy of Nature*, 58.
[45] Bedell, *Anatomy of Nature*, 50.
[46] Bedell, *Anatomy of Nature*, 51–2.
[47] Charles-François Mathis, 'La Terre Vaine: Mutations Du Sentiment de La Nature', *Histoire Des Émotions*, Points, 3. De la fin du XIXe siècle à nos jours (Paris: Seuil, 2016), 264.
[48] ArneNæss, 'The Shallow and the Deep, Long Range Ecology Movement: A Summary', *The Selected Works of Arne Naess Volumes 1–10*, vol. 10 (Dordrecht: Springer Netherlands, 2005), 2263.
[49] Mathis, 'La Terre Vaine', 265.

first chapter describes the idyllic landscape of 'a town in the heart of America where all life seemed to live in harmony with its surroundings' until blight, illness and death are suddenly brought on by a mysterious 'white granular powder' that readers recognize as DDT.[50] Carson concludes with an ominous accusation: 'No witchcraft, no enemy action had silenced the rebirth of new life in this stricken world. The people had done it themselves.'[51] Since 2002, the emotional regime of nature has become bound up in the notion of the Anthropocene, with the introduction of Glenn Albrecht's neologism *solastalgia* to describe the complex distress caused by ecological destruction.[52] Considered in the context of the latter twentieth century's landscapes-in-pain, emotions thought to be solicited by 'nature' such as appeasement, reassurance, comfort and bodily ease could also be rooted in myth-building, anxiety, denial, escapism or guilt attending the ecological catastrophes of the Great Acceleration. Picturing an unpolluted, intact landscape reminiscent of a familiar Arcadian or wilderness iconography is reassuring, just as tending to landscape also mitigates ecological anxiety. In their study on the psychological benefits of gardening, Kaplan and Kaplan found that participants who did not rely on chemicals 'found greater satisfaction in all phases of gardening, suggest[ing] a larger parallel feeling of partnership with the larger forces of nature'.[53]

Additionally, as Joanna Bourke has stressed, science and medicine in and of themselves became sources of anxiety and apprehension for patients, and the fear of pain itself was a major preoccupation in mid-twentieth-century medicine.[54] Many distraction techniques are aimed at diverting patients' attention away from particularly painful medical procedures where anaesthesia is not possible, such as bronchoscopy, recovery from colorectal surgery and burn treatment.[55] One study of audio and visual distraction techniques sought to improve pain tolerance during flexible sigmoidoscopy screenings for colorectal cancer because 'the discomfort associated with the procedure is one of the many

---

[50] Rachel L Carson, *Silent Spring* (London: Penguin, 1999), 21.
[51] Carson, *Silent Spring*, 22.
[52] Glenn Albrecht et al., 'Solastalgia: The Distress Caused by Environmental Change', *Australasian Psychiatry*, 15 (2007): S95–S98.
[53] Kaplan and Kaplan, *Experience*, 195.
[54] Joanna Bourke, 'Fear and Anxiety: Writing about Emotion in Modern History', *History Workshop Journal*, 55 (2003): 118.
[55] Gregory B. Diette et al., 'Distraction Therapy with Nature Sights and Sounds Reduces Pain during Flexible Bronchoscopy: A Complementary Approach to Routine Analgesia', *Chest*, 123 (2003): 941–8; Diane L. R. N. Tusek et al., 'Guided Imagery: A Significant Advance in the Care of Patients Undergoing Elective Colorectal Surgery', *Diseases of the Colon & Rectum*, 40 (1997): 172–8; Miller, Hickman and Lemasters, 'A Distraction Technique'; Hoffman et al., 'Water-Friendly Virtual Reality'.

possible explanations for [the] low participation rate'.[56] The dramatic contrast between idealized landscape imagery and standard hospital settings and machinery could also add to their efficacy, as it distracts people in pain from an environment that is readily associated with pain and death, as well as from more mundane anxieties such as the financial consequences of medical interventions. The forest photomural used in Imperial College's psilocybin study was intended in part to counter the sterility of the hospital room.[57]

Emotions such as relaxation, comfort and ease have also shaped and been shaped by the performance of landscape in transnational popular culture and mass media of the late twentieth century. The notion that landscape painting and its practice could be relaxing and even procure 'happiness' was widely disseminated by the American television artists Bill Alexander (1915–1997) and his famous disciple Bob Ross (1942–1995). Ross's television series *The Joy of Painting* aired weekly from 1983 to 1994 in Europe, North and South America and Asia (especially Japan) and is still rebroadcast today all over the world via YouTube. Each thirty-minute instructional episode features Ross executing an eye-catching technicolour landscape painting from start to finish. Over three hundred paintings were produced for the show, with compositions dominated by trees, mountains, clouds and various water elements with very little or no human presence.[58] Ross's soft voice and calm narration of landscape elements that he anthropomorphized as he painted (his most famous were 'happy clouds') is said to have a soothing effect on audiences and to 'put people at ease'.[59] According to Ross himself, audiences were more interested in his program for the relaxation it procured than they were in actually learning to paint.[60] Part of Ross's global posthumous fame is amongst adepts of autonomous sensory meridian response (ASMR).[61] In 2020, the BBC rebroadcast *The Joy of Painting* as a means of alleviating anxieties in viewers brought on by the Covid-19 pandemic and lockdown.[62] Both Ross and his mentor Alexander believed

---

[56] Tony Lembo et al., 'Audio and Visual Stimulation Reduces Patient Discomfort during Screening Flexible Sigmoidoscopy', *American Journal of Gastroenterology*, 93 (1998): 1113.

[57] Gandy to Watts and Edgar, 'Re: Psilocybin, 2016 Feasibility Study', 5 September 2020.

[58] Walt Hickey, 'A Statistical Analysis of the Work of Bob Ross', *FiveThirtyEight* (blog), 14 April 2014, https://fivethirtyeight.com/features/a-statistical-analysis-of-the-work-of-bob-ross/.

[59] Alexxa Gotthardt, 'Bob Ross Owes His "Happy Little Trees" to This Forgotten Painter', *Artsy*, 26 June 2018, https://www.artsy.net/article/artsy-editorial-bob-ross-owes-happy-trees-forgotten-painter.

[60] Joe Kloc, 'The Soothing Sounds of Bob Ross', *Newsweek*, 1 October 2014, https://www.newsweek.com/2014/10/10/soothing-sounds-bob-ross-274466.html.

[61] Zach Schonfeld, 'Inside the Whispery, Wonderful, Inexplicably Relaxing Golden Age of ASMR', *Newsweek*, 30 August 2018, https://www.newsweek.com/2018/09/07/asmr-whisper-videos-tingles-craig-richard-whisperlodge-1096749.html.

[62] Hannah Dean, 'Happy Little Trees – BBC Sounds', *BBC Radio 4*, 11 May 2020, https://www.bbc.co.uk/sounds/play/m000j1z2.

deeply in the therapeutic quality of landscape painting and its capacity to make people 'happy'.[63] Alexander even claimed he was 'in the happiness business'.[64] The kitsch quality of Ross's painting and television shows is what made their specific emotional appeal, according to C. E. Emmer, who further points out that the 'sense of release, relaxation, comfort and sweetness', which is the 'emotional core of Burkean beauty', is also that 'at the heart of traditional kitsch'.[65] Ross's paintings circulate not as physical oeuvres in galleries and museums but rather as performances via television and a now web-based franchise selling bespoke art supplies and instruction manuals.[66] Ross also carefully constructed these performances, making three versions of each painting: one kept off camera from which he painted, another that was produced during the show and a third, more detailed version which featured in the manuals.

'Biophilic' imagery

From the early 2000s onwards references to E. O. Wilson's *biophilia* hypothesis can be found in literature on guided imagery as an explanation for the efficacy of landscape images. Coined by Erich Fromm in 1964 to designate the love of life or living systems, *biophilia* is redefined by Wilson as 'the innate tendency' in humans 'to focus on life and lifelike processes'.[67] Authors of a randomized clinical trial at Johns Hopkins using landscape photomurals to distract patients undergoing bronchoscopy argued, 'The *biophilia* hypothesis suggests that humans are genetically predisposed to respond positively to nature. This can result in positive adaptive responses.'[68] Even if some authors admit that a deeper understanding is needed of 'the physiological pathway of action' between nature contact and health, they still evoke the possibility that 'these pathways may have an evolutionary origin, as proposed by the *biophilia* hypothesis'.[69]

A renowned entomologist, E. O. Wilson is better known as a proponent of controversial theories based on evolutionary biology, which he introduced in

---

[63] Gotthardt, 'Bob Ross'; Kloc, 'Soothing Sounds of Bob Ross'.
[64] Kloc, 'Soothing Sounds of Bob Ross'.
[65] C. E. Emmer, 'The Flower and the Breaking Wheel: Burkean Beauty and Political Kitsch', *International Journal of the Arts in Society*, 2 (2007): 156–7.
[66] https://www.bobross.com/.
[67] Erich Fromm, *The Heart of Man: Its Genius for Good and Evil* (New York: Harper & Row, 1964); Edward O. Wilson, *Biophilia* (Cambridge, MA: Harvard University Press, 1984), 1.
[68] Diette et al., 'Distraction Therapy', 946–7.
[69] Howard Frumkin et al., 'Nature Contact and Human Health: A Research Agenda', *Environmental Health Perspectives*, 125 (2017): 3.

his 1975 treatise *Sociobiology: The New Synthesis*, in which he argued that society and the human condition in general are genetically determined.[70] While popular with biologists and even anthropologists, critics of sociobiology were numerous, decrying the 'substantive flaws in its methods, science, logic and use of facts'.[71] Philosopher Mary Midgley called it 'biological Thatcherism' and described Wilson's language as 'crude', 'provocative' and 'ideologically loaded'.[72] In their 1984 book *Not in Our Genes: Biology, Ideology and Human Nature*, which largely opposed the tenets of sociobiology, evolutionary geneticist Steven Rose, neurobiologist Richard Lewontin and psychologist Leon J. Kamin attributed the popular success of Wilson's thesis to the simplistic nature of its 'reductionist, biological determinist explanation of human existence'.[73] As the influence of 'nature' and landscape imagery on emotions and mental states began to gain the attention of psychologists in the following years, Wilson attempted 'to apply the ideas of sociobiology to the environmental ethic' with his *biophilia* hypothesis, which also sparked controversy and criticism.[74] Jared Diamond contests Wilson's thesis that savannah environments inhabited by the first humans could still influence an 'innate' response to nature, especially given the wide range of habitats that could have equally influenced human responses to 'nature' since leaving the savannah over a million years ago.[75] Sociologist Claude Fisher criticized Wilson for 'notic[ing] commonalities across societies and historical eras and then leap[ing] to genetic explanations', further arguing that social learning and not innate tendencies explains 'the widespread liking of nature scenes'.[76] Fisher also criticized Wilson's conservationist agenda: 'Loving nature is in our genes ... justifies doing nothing. The real leverage for environmental activists lies in understanding the culture of nature-loving – the history of conservation, the social structure of environmentalism, nature ideologies – not biology'.[77] Indeed, conservationists have insisted that while *biophilia* is a useful ethical concept, the assumption by Wilson and his followers that it is innate

---

[70] Edward O. Wilson, *Sociobiology: The New Synthesis* (Cambridge, MA: Belknap Press, 1975).
[71] Peter Kahn, *The Human Relationship with Nature: Development and Culture* (Cambridge, MA: MIT Press, 1999), 27.
[72] Mary Midgley, *Beast and Man: The Roots of Human Nature* (London: Routledge, 2002), xiv.
[73] Steven P. R Rose, Richard C. Lewontin and Leon J. Kamin, *Not in Our Genes: Biology, Ideology, and Human Nature* (New York: Pantheon Books, 1984), 235–6.
[74] Kaplan and Kaplan, *Experience*; Stephen R. Kellert and Edward O. Wilson, eds, *The Biophilia Hypothesis* (Washington, DC: Shearwater Books, 1993), 55; Wilson, *Biophilia*.
[75] Jared Diamond, 'New Guineans and Their Natural World', *Biophilia Hypothesis*, ed. Kellert and Wilson, 347–8.
[76] Claude S. Fischer, 'Widespread Likings', *Science*, 263 (1994): 1162.
[77] Fischer, 'Widespread Likings', 1162.

is 'beyond scientific reason'.[78] Art historian Malcolm Andrews argues that the aesthetic codes of landscape painting have been so widely diffused since the early eighteenth century that it is difficult to determine any 'innate' appreciation of it.[79] The aesthetic codes of photography have also shaped our appreciation of landscape since the mid-nineteenth century. As Susan Sontag famously observed six years before Wilson's *biophilia* hypothesis appeared, one can no longer consider a sunset without comparing it to a photograph of a sunset.[80] The idea that reactions to 'nature' are innate also challenges the fundamentals of developmental psychology and the changing perception of 'nature' from childhood to adulthood, which has long been observed.

Despite Wilson's revision of the definition of *biophilia* in 1993, it remains unclear. He described it as 'the innately emotional human affiliation to other living organisms', whereby 'innate means hereditary and hence part of ultimate human nature'. But it was also combined with instinct and a complex of learning rules that become 'woven into symbols composing a large part of culture'.[81] Described as 'slippery and difficult to understand except in metaphorical terms', *biophilia* is open to a wide variety of interpretations.[82] This is perhaps why, despite its numerous critics, the *biophilia* hypothesis has gained considerable currency even outside of biology and medicine. In the beginning of the twenty-first century, it was taken up by designers as a scientific argument in favour of an 'evidence-based' approach to architecture that aims to create environments conducive not only to health but also to productivity and creativity.[83] A recent article in *Global Environmental Change* interprets *biophilia* as 'direct pathways by which experiences [of natural environments] affect the nervous system, bringing about stress reduction and restoration of attention', and as 'an adaptation to our reliance on the natural environment throughout all but the past 10,000 years of our history'.[84] A *technobiophilia* hypothesis even proposes 'an innate tendency to

---

[78] John P. Simaika and Michael J. Samways, 'Biophilia as a Universal Ethic for Conserving Biodiversity', *Conservation Biology*, 24 (2010): 903–6.
[79] Malcolm Andrews, *Landscape and Western Art* (Oxford: Oxford University Press, 1999), 19–20.
[80] Susan Sontag, *On Photography*, 6th print (New York: Farrar, Straus and Giroux, 1978), 85.
[81] Kellert and Wilson, *Biophilia Hypothesis*, 42.
[82] Kahn, *Human Relationship with Nature*, 40.
[83] Ulrich, 'Evidence-Based Health-Care Architecture'; Roger S. Ulrich et al., 'A Review of the Research Literature on Evidence-Based Healthcare Design', *HERD*, 1 (2008): 61–125; Stephen R. Kellert, Judith Heerwagen and Martin Mador, *Biophilic Design: The Theory, Science and Practice of Bringing Buildings to Life* (Oxford: Wiley, 2013); Mohamed S. Abdelaal and Veronica Soebarto, 'Biophilia and Salutogenesis as Restorative Design Approaches in Healthcare Architecture', *Architectural Science Review*, 62 (2019): 195–205; Mohamed S. Abdelaal, 'Biophilic Campus: An Emerging Planning Approach for a Sustainable Innovation-Conducive University', *Journal of Cleaner Production*, 215 (2019): 1445–56.
[84] George MacKerron and Susana Mourato, 'Happiness Is Greater in Natural Environments', *Global Environmental Change*, 23 (2013): 992.

focus on life and lifelike processes as they appear in technology' promising that 'we will benefit from trusting our ancient instincts in cyberspace'.[85]

Biophilia is also used as a selling argument for landscape images made specifically for the medical industry. According to the owner of Bedscapes, a company producing bespoke photomurals printed on hospital bed curtains, landscape imagery for their products is selected according to specific *biophilic* criteria as defined not by Wilson but by the 'evidence-based design' architect Roger Ulrich.[86] Yet these criteria seem to pertain more to cultural metaphors and symbols than to an 'innate' *biophilic* sense. Autumnal images or sunsets, for instance, are not to be used as Besdcapes because of their association with the end of life. Sunrises are equally undesirable because they evoke coming events and could therefore generate anxiety. Additionally, images must not be too large in size; panoramic landscapes that surround the whole bed can be experienced as 'oppressive' by patients.[87] In other words, the view must be clearly delimited, like a painting, a carefully landscaped prospect or a picturesque view from a window. Part of the reassurance generated by such views would then come from the distance between the viewer and the landscape, or their exteriority to it, and not their immersion in or connection with 'nature'.

Landscape: An emotional commodity

That a certain image of 'nature' has become a valuable commodity in health and well-being can also be understood as what Eva Illouz has described as an increased interconnectivity of capitalism and emotions in consumer markets of the latter twentieth century and their 'entanglement ... in a continual process of coproduction of emotions and commodities'.[88] Since the eighteenth century, tourism has contributed to shaping the belief that the non-human world is a source of desirable, strong emotions, and especially 'undomesticated emotions' experienced in 'wild' settings or by engaging in activities such as alpinism or camping.[89] In the late twentieth and early twenty-first centuries, the emotional

---

[85] Sue Thomas, *Technobiophilia. Nature and Cyberspace* (London: Bloomsbury, 2013), 11.
[86] Interview with Josaif August, Bedscapes, by Brenda Lynn Edgar, Skype, 20 January 2020.
[87] Interview with Josaif August.
[88] Eva Illouz and Yaara Benger Alaluf, 'Le Capitalisme Émotionnel', *Histoire Des Émotions*, Points, vol. 3. De la fin du XIXe siècle à nos jours (Paris: Seuil, 2016), 74; Illouz and Benger Alaluf, 'Le Capitalisme Émotionnel', 86; Eva Illouz, *Les sentiments du capitalisme* (Paris: Seuil, 2006).
[89] Sylvain Venayre, 'Transports Affectifs: Le Voyage, Entre Émerrvevillement et Déception', *Histoire Des Émotions*, Points, vol. 3. De la fin du XIXe siècle à nos jours (Paris: Seuil, 2016), 242, 253.

state of 'relaxation' is often procured by settings which might resemble 'wild' or 'primitive' nature, but are in reality highly manufactured and sanitized environments, such as those of Club Med. Designed to contrast with urban settings, these environments deploy sophisticated architectural and landscaping techniques that mask socio-economic signs and create the illusion of a place where 'money and work do not exist'.[90] They embody the paradox of idealizations of 'wild' natural settings which assuage anxieties related to survival.

Writing only a few years before the twenty-first-century world would conceive of itself as living in the Anthropocene, Malcolm Andrews noted that in light of looming environmental disaster, the growing awareness of the interdependency of man and 'nature' is incompatible with 'landscape as a way of seeing from a distance ... as a phase in the cultural way of life in the West'. Andrews writes, 'Landscape may already be over.'[91] If this is so, the idealized landscape imagery that has proliferated in both clinical and daily environments can be understood as what Sianne Ngai has called the 'entirely capitalist aesthetic' of the 'gimmick'.[92] Ngai's gimmick is a performative object that promises to save time and labour through technology that is either too sophisticated or not sophisticated enough for the essentially superfluous tasks it accomplishes.[93] Landscape imagery uses sophisticated technology such as HDR photography or virtual reality to produce an outdated, superfluous mode of viewing landscape under the pretext of procuring tranquillity and relaxation or of filling a putative biological need for an equally outmoded notion of 'nature'. In clinical practices, landscape imagery is perceived as a time-saving device that allays anxieties quickly and 'naturally', reducing patient recovery time in hospital and thus healthcare costs. Health Journeys advertises their guided imagery as 'cost effective, evidence-based meditation programs' capable of producing 'more contented, productive employees, stronger health outcomes for patients, and students who are less stressed, more resilient, and better able to learn'.[94] Landscape is a mere commodity exploited by late capitalist healthcare systems, shifting responsibility for psychological well-being onto individuals who, left to their own devices, increasingly rely on such 'gimmicks'.

---

[90] Illouz and Benger Alaluf, 'Le Capitalisme Émotionnel', 93.
[91] Andrews, *Landscape and Western Art*, 22.
[92] Sianne Ngai, *Theory of the Gimmick: Aesthetic Judgement and Capitalist Form* (Cambridge, MA: Belknap Press, 2020), 53.
[93] Ngai, *Theory of the Gimmick*, 2–3.
[94] Health Journeys, 'Partners | Health Journeys', accessed 27 June 2021, https://www.healthjourneys.com/partner-with-us.

There is a great deal of exchange between clinical practices of landscape imagery, commercial decoration and photography and recreational self-care practices such as *The Joy of Painting*, with each industry exploiting the other as validation for its respective 'gimmicks'. When guided imagery emerged in the 1970s, large-scale landscape photography had been a relatively popular product in interior decoration since the 1930s.[95] The wall size landscape photography from the 1940s to the 1960s promised to 'bring the world's loveliest scenic wonders right into your home or office' and 'create the illusion of rooms opening up onto utterly inspiring outdoor vistas', appealing to the suburban American ideal of living in 'nature'.[96] Documentation dating from the 1980s exists of decorative photomurals being used in medical environments, and the forest photomural used in Imperial College's psilocybin trials was purchased from a DIY online home decoration retailer.[97] Bespoke products made for clinical environments represent something of a niche market in the United States, for professionals from a variety of backgrounds. References can be found in medical studies to specific specialized companies such as the Oregon-based Muralvision, founded in 1978 by cinematographer Lee McCroury, which produced landscape films for in-channel diffusion in hospitals. Beginning with the three-volume series *Scenic America*, McCroury would make a total of five videos for hospitals between 1978 and 1988. The videos are cited in at least one study of distraction therapy with landscape imagery, which describe them as 'a composition of scenic beauty with music. Each program is a blend of scenes such as the ocean, desert, forest, flowers, waterfalls and wildlife.'[98] Another study mentions using guided imagery recordings by Health Journeys, founded in 1991 by Belleruth Naparstek, a clinical social worker and author in partnership with businessman George Klein.[99] At the beginning of the twenty-first century, medical or 'scientific' arguments were also used to promote decorative landscape views. In addition to its popularity in design industries, Wilson's *biophilia* hypothesis (and the medical research that refers to it) is widely quoted in the media by

---

[95] Brenda Lynn Edgar, 'L'invention Photographique et Le Paysage Mural: Le Photomural Décoratif Des Années 1930', *Les Inventions Photographiques Du Paysage*, ed. Pierre-Henry Frangne and Patricia Limodo, Art & Société (Rennes: Presses Universitaires de Rennes, 2016), 81–92.

[96] Foto Murals of California, 'Low Priced Foto Murals, Add Charm ... Depth ... Drama ... to Any Room for under $25', *Los Angeles Times*, 3 April 1955; Brenda Lynn Edgar, *Le Motif Éphémère: L'ornement Photographique et Architecture Au XXe Siècle*, Art & Société (Rennes: Presses Universitaires de Rennes, 2021), 222–6.

[97] Edgar, *Le Motif Éphémère*, 239; Robin L. Carhart-Harris et al., 'Psilocybin with Psychological Support for Treatment-Resistant Depression: An Open-Label Feasibility Study', *Lancet Psychiatry*, 3 (2016): 621; Gandy to Watts and Edgar, 'Re: Psilocybin, 2016 Feasibility Study', 5 September 2020.

[98] Miller, Hickman and Lemasters, 'Distraction Technique for Control of Burn Pain', 577.

[99] Tusek et al., 'Guided Imagery'.

journalists discussing the efficacy of 'nature' on health and well-being.[100] Some manufacturers market to healthcare institutions and to the greater public alike. While Health Journeys makes products specifically for medical institutions (endorsed by health insurance companies and hospitals alike), they also market to the higher education sector, boasting prestigious clients such as Duke University.[101] Also, their guided imagery recordings are sold online to the general public in a variety of different formats. Other actors of the 'happiness industry' such as self-help and meditation applications integrate HDR landscape photography and accompanying soundtracks (rain, ocean waves and forests) in their products.[102]

Conclusion

While the efficacy of landscape imagery in distraction techniques has been demonstrated in the medical literature examined here, these conclusions were reached within the controlled conditions of laboratory experiments and clinical trials. Viewing idealized landscapes might shape feelings and mental states, but how they are viewed also emotionally orientates: a doctor showing a patient an image might tell them it is supposed to relax or distract them. Given the aim of distraction therapy to increase tolerance for pain and anxiety, it is perhaps more appropriate to speak of placating patients rather than achieving a state of relaxation or ease. Why and how these images act on people (and vice versa) remains an area of speculation that can reveal deeply rooted cultural beliefs and the persistence of essentialist notions of 'nature' as a source of health and 'healing' emotions. Landscape in the past and present has been the locus of numerous and conflicting emotions: quietude, connectivity, wonder and awe but also anxiety, guilt, avoidance and passivity. However, the clinical practices of

---

[100] Sue Thomas, 'Can We Get All the Nature We Need from the Digital World?', *Aeon*, 24 September 2013, https://aeon.co/essays/can-we-get-all-the-nature-we-need-from-the-digital-world; James Hamblin, 'The Nature Cure: Why Some Doctors Are Writing Prescriptions for Time Outdoors', *The Atlantic*, 14 September 2015, https://www.theatlantic.com/magazine/archive/2015/10/the-nature-cure/403210/; Marc Jadoul, 'The Emotion of Nature and the Nature of Emotion', *Business Storytelling* (blog), 22 March 2017, https://b2bstorytelling.wordpress.com/2017/03/22/the-emotion-of-nature-and-the-nature-of-emotion/; Adrienne Matei, 'We're So Nature-Deprived That Even Footage of Wilderness Lifts Our Spirits | Adrienne Matei', *The Guardian*, 26 October 2020, https://www.theguardian.com/commentisfree/2020/oct/26/were-so-nature-deprived-that-even-footage-of-wilderness-lifts-our-spirits.

[101] Health Journeys, 'Partners | Health Journeys'.

[102] Edgar Cabanas and Eva Illouz, *Manufacturing Happy Citizens: How the Science and Industry of Happiness Control Our Lives* (Cambridge: Polity, 2019).

landscape examined here, as well as their reception in other disciplines, operate within a much more narrow and selective emotional spectrum which does not take into consideration the potential impact of the idealization of landscape itself.

The appropriation of 'efficacious' landscape images in other domains, such as 'evidence-based design' or the well-being industry, raises questions as to the reception of scientific research by a broader, non-specialist public and its exploitation for commercial gain. When the mass media diffuses the idea of the positive effects of 'nature' images on health, it only encourages consumption. The digital carbon footprint has yet to be calculated for the billions of idealized landscapes that decorate computer and telephone screens, illustrate meditation applications and crowd Instagram and Pinterest accounts. The enduring popularity of the *biophilia* hypothesis (and the biodeterministic reasoning behind it), despite the significant criticism it has received across the social and life sciences, is also disconcerting. Ambiguous concepts such as *biophilia* contribute to the commodification of landscape not only by conferring it with a 'scientifically proven' performative quality but also because the simplistic nature of its explanation makes it commercially exploitable as a slogan or meme.

The attempt to manufacture emotions through landscape imagery, either to control pain or to better live through a pandemic, raises certain ethical questions. While the moral agenda of nineteenth-century asylum gardens might be seen as coercive from today's perspective, one might consider it equally questionable to use landscape imagery to procure an emotional state that renders individuals more tolerant of pain, dis-ease and anxiety. Limited to specific invasive medical procedures such as bronchoscopy or the treatment of severe burns, the practice remains entirely justifiable. However, in the hands of healthcare providers eager to shift the costs of mental health onto individuals, people in pain with limited financial means might be left with only a guided imagery recording or a meditation app with bucolic visuals to deal with their dis-ease.

11

'Fashionable' diseases in Georgian Britain: Medical theory, cultural meanings and lived experience

James Kennaway

The whole idea of a 'fashionable disease' may seem perverse. After all, what is so enviable or fun about being ill? Nevertheless, there have been many examples of medical conditions being associated with the glamour of wealth, status, poetic sensitivity or genius. In particular, eighteenth-century Britain offers countless clichés of modish medical conditions, from gentlemen with gout and ladies with the vapours or weak nerves to consumptive poets, all reflecting what an anonymous author in *The Female Encyclopaedia* (1830) called 'the ridiculous mania of being fashionably ill'.[1] There was a range of complaints with strong connotations of elite standing, just as there were disorders linked to poverty, stigma, shame and exclusion. The period produced a rich medical, satirical and literary debate on fashionable maladies that drew on a perceived connection between beau-monde complaints and luxury, providing the basis for a medical-moral critique of the vices and excesses of modern urban life that proved enormously influential. At the same time, there was an extensive debate about faddish diagnoses that seemed to come rapidly into vogue before being replaced just as quickly, raising the spectre of 'imaginary' diseases, malingering and fakery.

These connections with glamour, depravity and inauthenticity help illuminate the relationship between medical theory, cultural and social framings and the lived experience of illness.[2] For in each of these one finds a complicated discourse

---

[1] Anon., 'Hints to the Domestic Practitioner', *The Female Encyclopaedia* (London: W. J. Sears, 1830), 208–12, here 208.
[2] For a discussion of the idea of experience in historiography, see Joan Scott, 'The Evidence of Experience,' *Critical Inquiry*, 17, no. 4 (1991): 773–97; Rob Boddice and Mark Smith, *Emotion, Sense, Experience* (Cambridge: Cambridge University Press, 2020), 18–29; Martin Jay, *Songs of*

about the paradoxical supposed positive side of illness and disease. Medical theory provided models of causation, combining long-standing theories with more recent ideas about nervous stimulation and novel diagnoses and terminology. These then were adapted for cultural use in endless forms, according to the moralizing, satirical, celebratory or ironical aims of commentators of many kinds. In turn, it is clear that medical theory and cultural framing mediated patient experience itself. Patients sometimes understood their own diagnoses as well as their symptoms and dis-ease in this context, as the price of luxury, whether associated with glamour or self-reproach. By avoiding a simplistic opposition between the 'real' somatic experiences of patients and cultural understandings of sickness, this chapter considers their dialectical relationship, showing the ways that sufferers' own subjective encounters with such maladies were themselves framed by medical thinking and broader cultural attitudes. The discourse among patients and physicians reflected shifting diagnoses as well as conceptions of physicians' authority, gender conventions and social hierarchies that arguably give it considerable relevance to wider methodological debates about the affective experience of patients, medical theory and the cultural meaning of disease.

Fashionable disease in Georgian medicine

The widespread discussion on fashionable disease had important roots in medical literature that went back centuries. For instance, since Antiquity there had been an intermittent discourse of the superior melancholic, notably in terms of (Pseudo-)Aristotle's *Problemata* and the Renaissance Humanism of Marsilio Ficino.[3] During the seventeenth century, much ink was spilled on the subject of the relationship between physical, mental and spiritual causation and symptoms of conditions like melancholy, often reflecting a certain kind of social prestige.[4] This long tradition provided some of the framework for Enlightenment

---

Experience: Modern American and European Variations on a Universal Theme (Berkeley: University of California Press, 2006).

[3] Marsilio Ficino, *De Vita libri tres* (Basel: Apud. Jo. Beb., 1529); Bernd Bösel, *Philosophie und Enthusiasmus* (Vienna: Passagen, 2008); Noel L. Brann, *The Debate over the Origin of Genius during the Italian Renaissance* (Leiden: Brill, 2002), 82–152.

[4] See Robert Burton, *Anatomy of Melancholy* (Oxford: John Lichfield and James Short, 1621); Erin Sullivan, *Beyond Melancholy* (Oxford: Oxford University Press, 2018); Michael Heyd, *Be Sober and Reasonable: The Critique of Enthusiasm in the Seventeenth and Early Eighteenth Centuries* (Leiden: Brill, 1995); Hannah Newton, *Misery to Mirth: Recovery from Illness in Early Modern England* (Oxford: Oxford University Press, 2018).

discussions of such conditions, but eighteenth-century commentators often added a clearer focus on luxury, a sharpened social critique and a medical terminology based on things such as nervous stimulation.

The period's most famous British book on nervous complaints, *The English Malady* (1733), by the Scottish physician George Cheyne, argued that the English elite were particularly apt to suffer from 'nervous distempers, spleen, vapours, and lowness of spirits' because of their luxurious lifestyles, and the consequent 'inactivity and sedentary occupations of the better sort' caused by the extraordinary 'wealth and abundance' created by the country's booming trade.[5] As he put it:

> Since our wealth has increase'd, and our navigation has been extended, we have ransack'd all the parts of the globe to bring together its whole stock of materials for riot, luxury, and to provoke excess. The tables of the rich and great (and indeed all ranks who can afford it) are furnish'd with provisions of delicacy, number and plenty, sufficient to provoke, and even gorge the most large and voluminous appetite.[6]

The maladies that Cheyne was referring to were chiefly 'nervous disorders', which he believed to account for 'almost one third' of those suffered in the country.[7] Although the book is sometimes thought of as being about nerves in a quasi-psychiatric sense, in fact its main focus was on diet and digestion, setting out an Enlightenment programme of 'plain Diet' in accordance with 'the Purity and Simplicity of uncorrupted Nature, and unconquer'd Reason', drawing on his own experience of dramatic weight loss.[8] Cheyne wrote that he looked with 'pity, compassion, and sorrow' on the suffering caused by excess among 'the Rich, the Lazy, the Luxurious, and the Unactive, those who fare daintily and live voluptuously'.[9] However, few readers can have really wished themselves instead members of the other part of society, 'the Poor, the Low, the meaner Sort', who were spared such complaints.[10]

A generation later, the Swiss physician Samuel Auguste Tissot also made an influential contribution to the British debate. His medical warnings in *L'Onanisme* (1760) about the dangers of masturbation have been the subject of

---

[5] George Cheyne, *The English Malady* (London: G. Strahan, 1733), i–ii.
[6] Cheyne, *English Malady*, 49–50.
[7] Cheyne, *English Malady*, ii.
[8] Cheyne, *English Malady*, 28.
[9] Cheyne, *English Malady*, 28. See Anita Guerrini, 'The Impossible Ideal of Moderation', *Lifestyle and Medicine in the Enlightenment*, ed. James Kennaway and Rina Knoeff (Abingdon: Routledge, 2020), 86–108.
[10] Cheyne, *English Malady*, 28–9.

a good deal of scholarship over the past few decades, but his advice books on regimen, notably his successful *Avis du peuple sur sa santé* (1761), were more famous in his lifetime. In his *Essai sur les maladies des gens du monde* (1770), translated into English as *Essay on the Disorders of People of Fashion* in 1771, as well as his 1768 *De la santé des gens de lettres* (in English as *An Essay on Diseases Incidental to Literary and Sedentary Persons* (1769)), he set out the links between sickness and the lifestyles of the rich, clever and idle. Although he insisted that 'none but a malicious satyrist can say that *it is not fashionable to be well*', his work did much to reinforce that very association.[11] 'The man of fashion', disturbed in mind, with 'trembled nerves' and an overstuffed stomach, was naturally vulnerable to sickness, he suggested.[12] In contrast, the 'labourer's morning briskness' was a source of health, and the obviously unglamorous peasant had nerves that 'are not agitated by any affection of the soul, or blood inflamed, or stomach labouring with the effects of an erroneous regime', and was able to breathe in salubrious country air and not the pestilential vapours of trendy metropolitan centres.[13]

In the work of Cheyne, Tissot and others, one thus sees a clear critique of expanding mercantile societies. Drawing on traditional medical notions of avoiding excess, as well as on humanist conceptions of corruption and luxury, it attacked modern urban sophistication as excessive and sickly, mirroring the contemporaneous moral critique of that society put forward by Jean-Jacques Rousseau and others. Behind much of the debate was a theory of decadence, the sense that individual moral failings, especially in relation to sexuality, were a threat to social order, echoing Roman and Greek texts, well known in the eighteenth century, that fretted about the impact of eastern luxury on manly character and military ethos.[14]

While doctors' lamentations about the evil consequences of the luxuries and excesses of beau-monde life were often highly moralistic, there was also an implicit positive note to these descriptions of the diseases of the fashionable.

---

[11] S. A. D. Tissot, *An Essay on the Disorders of People of Fashion* (London: Richardson and Urquhart, 1771), 162.

[12] Tissot, *Essay on the Disorders of People of Fashion*, 38.

[13] Tissot, *Essay on the Disorders of People of Fashion*, 37–8, 20–2. See James Kennaway and Rina Knoeff, '"For It Is the Debilitating Fibres That Exercise Restores": Movement, Morality and Moderation in Eighteenth-Century Medical Advice Literature', *Lifestyle and Medicine in the Enlightenment: The Six Non-Naturals in the Long Eighteenth Century*, ed. James Kennaway and Rina Knoeff (Abingdon: Routledge, 2020), 111–38.

[14] WalterRehm, *Der Untergang Roms in abendländischen Denken: Ein Beitrag zur Geschichte der Geschichtsschreibung und zum Dekadenz-Problem* (Darmstadt: Wissenschaftliche Buchgesellschaft, 1969).

Cheyne, Tissot and their ilk had no intention per se of praising the vices of the English upper classes or their medical conditions, but by linking them so overtly to success and status they inadvertently laid the foundation for both a medical assault on a rapidly developing commercial society and a culture that put a positive spin on the diseases in question. The tension between the moral-medical denunciations of the illnesses of the elite on the one hand and its glamour on the other provided enormous scope for the social and literary pleasures of irony, of ribbing others or mocking oneself, safe in the knowledge that benign connotations of such conditions meant that no stigma would necessarily accrue.

Physicians' descriptions of the character of the diseases in question provide countless instances of apparent social gains. For example, Cheyne linked phthisis (consumption) with nervousness, writing that it could 'afflict and destroy the noblest spirits and finest genius's [sic]'.[15] Another influential Scottish physician, William Buchan, made parallel arguments in his popular *Domestic Medicine* (1769). He was clear that intellectual work made men 'very subject to the gout ... stone and gravel' and 'consumptions of the lungs', weakening the 'functions of the heart' and 'the powers of digestion' and meaning that 'the whole constitution goes to ruin', with resulting 'grievous head-achs [sic], which bring on vertigoes, apoplexies, palsies, and other fatal disorders'. It was also likely to lead to 'disorders of the mind' and thus to 'delirium, melancholy, and even madness'.[16] That is to say, a great number of the diseases that afflicted the body were linked to the kind of mental exertion found among the clever, wise and industrious.

There was also an implicit degree of national narcissism involved, an implied bonus for sickness, as Britons could enjoy hearing that their bad health was the result of their glorious superiority over other countries. William Hogarth's *The Roast Beef of Old England* (1748) was typical in contrasting his well-fed countrymen with the starving French (fat and greedy Catholic priests aside). The high-flying physician James Johnston, originally from Ulster, was as fierce a critic as any of the luxury lifestyle and its medical implications, but his explanations for the ill health of his British clientele were a rhapsody of exuberant national self-confidence. Britain's sicknesses, he suggested in 1831, were in direct proportion to its prosperity, something reflected in the fact, as he saw it, that 'our fields [are] better cultivated, our houses better furnished, our villas more numerous, our

---

[15] George Cheyne, *The Natural Method of Cureing the Diseases of the Body* ((London: G. Strahan, 1742), 186. See Clark Lawlor, *Consumption and Literature: The Making of a Romantic Disease* (Houndmills: Palgrave Macmillan, 2007).
[16] William Buchan, *Domestic Medicine* (London: A. Strahan, T. Cadell, J. Balfour, W. Creech, 1815), 55–61.

cottons and our cutlery better manufactured, our machinery more effective, our merchants more rich'.[17] It surely took a sober-minded reader not to feel some satisfaction in the fact that these were the factors causing the country's maladies, even (and perhaps especially) if that involved symptoms for oneself.

A key sense in which a disease could be said to be fashionable was when a diagnosis, for various reasons, became *à la mode*. The period certainly produced a seemingly constant stream of new faddish diagnoses: Nervousness, spleen, hypochondria, biliousness, the vapours and indigestion, to name just a few, all had their advocates, adherents and their time in the sun. Since medicine is often dependent on the subjective observations of doctors, this has been a general tendency. As the English Tory critic and satirist William Gifford put it in 1816, looking back to the life of the Jacobean playwright Ben Jonson, 'This noble art has always had its jargon, and its fashionable diseases'.[18]

The Georgian period was perhaps especially liable to this phenomenon, given the combination of a booming and often unregulated medical marketplace, the rising influence of formal medical thinking and the continuing relative social and economic power of elite patients over physicians. To attract attention and to please their sometimes self-indulgent client base, there were many incentives for doctors to assert a novel terminology or model of causation for the symptoms they came across. Contacts among the elite and consequent financial success for a physician could result from his ability to link sickness, luxury and prestige in an appropriate manner. Thus, while many physicians were critical of the phenomenon of faddish diagnoses, they were often complicit in it. Mainstream practitioners, as well as so-called quacks and purveyors of proprietary medicines, were often happy to provide their patients with a curious social boon in the form of a novel diagnosis. In the words of a 1795 poem in *The European Magazine*, 'The art of physic with a license kills/And keeps its empire with our fancied ills.'[19]

Nervous complaints were at the centre of much of the Georgian debate on fashionable diseases. Discussion of the role of the nervous system in medicine was based on the anatomical and physiological work of scholars such as Thomas Willis, Robert Whytt and Albrecht von Haller. Rather than overturning older conceptions of the body, the nerves were incorporated into those models, with ideas of the 'nervous fluid' that exhibited a high level of continuity with

---

[17] James Johnson, *Change of Air, or the Diary of a Philosopher in Pursuit of Health and Recreation* (London: S. Highley, 1831), 3.
[18] William Gifford, ed., *The Works of Ben Jonson*, 9 vols (London: W. Bulmer, 1816), 1:126.
[19] Anon., 'Godeau', *European Magazine* (June 1795), 398.

humoural theory mixed up with theories of electric and elastic nerves.[20] The nerves offered an apparently clear explanation for the effects of emotional and mental distress and bad behaviour on health, which in turn helped explain why, in Tissot's words, 'nervous complaints are frequent with people of fashion'.[21] Overstimulation of the nerves joined older ideas of excess and imbalance in diet as a cause of sickness, well suited to medical fears about the dubious thrills of modern city life.

Nervous complaints offered particularly wide scope for paradoxical enjoyment of disease. The whole culture of 'sensibility', the cult of exquisite feeling, drew many of its key ideas from the medicine of nerves, as George Rousseau has long argued.[22] The Scottish naval surgeon and medical writer Thomas Trotter, a man with some stern views on the overstimulations of fashionable life, nevertheless echoed conventional wisdom when he wrote that 'all men who possess genius, and those mental qualifications which prompt them to literary attainments and pursuits, are endued by nature with more than usual sensibility of nervous system'.[23] To suffer from nervous complaints was to have an implicit claim to intelligence, refinement and status.

Gout can be an agonising chronic condition, but its connotations of excess and idleness gave it some cachet as a disease of gentlemen. Furthermore, the diagnosis of gout also included several other symptoms, especially in the guise of the 'flying gout' that linked it to a variety of other fashionable complaints. The suggestion from Thomas Sydenham ('The English Hippocrates') that gouty patients might find 'consolation' in the fact that so many 'kings, princes, generals, admirals, philosophers, and several other great men' were similarly afflicted, and 'that it destroys more rich than poor persons, and more wise men than fools', was often echoed in later years.[24] A. Rennie's *Treatise on Gout and Nervous Disorders* of 1828, which quoted Sydenham on this point, also mentioned the elite connotations of suffering from gout, saying that it was passed by heredity like an aristocratic heirloom, and that the lifestyles of the rich ('indolent and sedentary inactivity') and their supposed sexual excesses ('indiscreet excess in venery') were also to blame.[25]

---

[20] Jean Starobinski, 'Notes sur l'histoire des fluids imaginaries (des esprit animaux a la libido)', *Gesnerus*, 23 (1966): 176-87.
[21] Tissot, *Essay on the Disorders of People of Fashion*, 113.
[22] George S. Rousseau, *Nervous Acts: Essays on Literature, Culture and Sensibility* (Basingstoke: Palgrave, 2004).
[23] Thomas Trotter, *A View of the Nervous Temperament* (London: Longman, Hurst, Rees, and Orme, 1807), 39.
[24] Thomas Sydenham, *The Works of Thomas Sydenham MD on Acute and Chronic Diseases* (Philadelphia, PA: Benjamin and Thomas Kite, 1809), 312-13.
[25] A. Rennie, *A Treatise on Gout and Nervous Disorders* (London: Charles Wood and Son, 1828), 9-11.

The stomach and digestive system played a starring role in many of these debates on modish disease, due to the association of gluttony with wealth and social status, combined with medical theories that linked the guts directly with emotional and mental states. As Byron put it in *Don Juan* (1819–24), the mind depends 'so much upon the gastric juice'.[26] For instance, those fashionable complaints hypochondria and the vapours originally related to the supposed rising of gases ('vapours') from the guts to the brain, where they would supposedly lead to mental and physical symptoms. An entry in the 1830 *Female Encyclopaedia* drew on a wide consensus to suggest that 'flatulence is always the forerunner of approaching nervousness' and advised those wanting to avoid the 'bodily and mental horrors of nervousness' to 'change their mode of living on the very first approach of flatulency'.[27]

Despite such decidedly unglamorous symptoms, there were apparent social advantages to be found from having digestive conditions. An 1821 article on 'The Alimentary Function and its Disorders' in *The Edinburgh Medical and Surgical Journal* noted that stomach complaints were especially a problem in 'a refined and wealthy community', characterized by 'luxury'.[28] It admitted that digestive conditions were not 'exclusively' something for a 'fashionable gourmand or your turtle eating alderman' but asserted that 'affections of the alimentary canal, and derangement of its functions, are generally more frequent in such a state of society as the present, where the operation of habits of this description is favoured by the aversion to the laborious and manly exercises, which seldom fails to distinguish the more refined stages of society'.[29] With stomach complaints, nerves and gout, as well as in other conditions with positive connotations such as consumption, biliousness and so forth, one sees a mingling of medical thinking, social critique and class and gender ideologies that could console the sufferer with notions of individual excellence, social status and national pride.

---

[26] See James Kennaway and Jonathan Andrews, 'The Grand Organ of Sympathy: Fashionable Stomach Complaints and the Mind in Britain', *Social History of Medicine*, 32, no. 1 (2019): 57–79; Jonathan Andrews and James Kennaway, 'Experiencing, Exploiting and Evacuating Bile: Framing Fashionable Biliousness from the Sufferer's Perspective', *Literature and Medicine*, 35, no. 2 (2017): 292–333.

[27] Anon., 'Hints to the Domestic Practitioner', *The Female Encyclopaedia* (London: W.J. Sears, 1830), 208–12, here 209.

[28] Anon., 'The Alimentary Function and Its Disorders', *Edinburgh Medical and Surgical Journal*, LXIX (1821): 574–608, here 595.

[29] Anon., 'Alimentary Function and Its Disorders', 595.

Fashionable diseases in Georgian culture

A striking feature of the debate on fashionable disease among physicians was its wide resonance in lay culture. Medicine was gaining in prestige as an explanatory framework but individual doctors were often viewed with considerable scepticism. Lay people could therefore adapt both the medical critique of elite vice and the implied kudos of the consequent maladies for their own ends. The published writing of the period showed a range of responses, from moralism, mockery and invective to praise of nervous sensibility as a source of exquisite feeling and smug satisfaction in the symptoms of digestive and gouty complaints as evidence of wealth and status.

A medicalized critique of the whole world of fashionable elite society as wicked and sickly, which depicted fashionable diseases as a symptom of broader moral and physical malaise, was common. One consequence of the association between luxurious and even louche living and disease was that the phrase 'fashionable disease' was commonly understood to connote sexually transmitted conditions. As Noelle Gallagher notes, VD was in vogue because of its associations with sexual libertinism and a Francophile upper-class lifestyle.[30] For instance, in his 1825 novel of the Napoleonic Wars, *Ned Clinton; Or the Commissary*, Francis Glasse patriotically denounced Paris as so full of 'vice' and 'folly' that 'a poor youth' who ended up there would be destined for poverty and 'the cure of a fashionable disease' at the Hotel de Dieu hospital.[31] More broadly, medical attacks on the world of the elite often had a clear fixation on moral questions related to sexuality. The sense that disease was a just punishment for sin is sometimes close to the surface, but moralizing references were matched by others that gave the notion a knowing wink and an upbeat interpretation that gave scope for consolation for one's own sufferings, even in such inauspicious circumstances.[32]

The sensual indulgences that were supposedly bringing sickness to the elite also included such menaces as tea and coffee, dangerous exotic imports and symbols of decadence. The writer and philanthropist Jonas Hanway's *Essay on Tea* (1756) argued that that beverage 'hurts health and shortens life'. Tea was

---

[30] Noelle Gallagher, *Itch, Clap, Pox: Venereal Disease in the Eighteenth-Century Imagination* (New Haven, CT: Yale University Press, 2018).
[31] Francis Glasse, *Ned Clinton; or The Commissary*, 3 vols (London: W. March, 1825), 2: 134
[32] As Rob Boddice has observed, debates on vaccination from this period often involved parallel allusions to sin and civilization. Rob Boddice, 'Bestiality in a Time of Smallpox: Dr. Jenner and the "Modern Chimera"', *Exploring Animal Encounters*, ed. Dominic Ohrem and Matthew Calarco (London: Palgrave Macmillan, 2018), 155–78.

responsible, he suggested, for all those ladies who 'languish with weak digestion, low spirits, lassitudes, melancholy, and twenty disorders, which in spite of the faculty have yet no names, except the general one of nervous complaints'.[33] However, by linking such symptoms to consumerism and the opulent East, critics did little to diminish their glamorous associations.

The cultural habits of the elite were also thought to be a cause of overstimulation, leading to nervousness and other fashionable complaints, especially among the women of the elite.[34] Making and listening to music, dancing and reading and writing books were all subject to regular moral-medical attack.[35] Unitarian minister John Platt's collection *The Female Mentor* (1823) included a denunciation of the 'superfluous susceptibility' of the nerves and mind that he believed to be rife among modern young ladies. They were, he wrote, unconcerned by what they might see as the 'coarse and common' duty to address real suffering nearby, because the 'sensibility of the moral novel-reader is too deliciously delirious, and her nerves are too delicately strung'. Such sensitive beings were, he continued, made 'dizzy by the fume of this intoxicating sensibility', their nerves 'thrilling with the noxious effluvia of some inflammatory romance', that is, of an overexciting novel.[36]

While jeremiads of this kind were closely linked to implied positive aspects of modish complaints, other lay observers wrote more directly about their apparent positive side. The idea that health was something achieved by demeaning hard work outdoors and that sickness was often the result of the luxurious habits and heredity of the elite was widespread, even if it is often hard to tell where paradoxical admiration ends and critique and irony begin. For instance, Maria Edgeworth's novel *Harrington* (1817), which deals with the theme of anti-Semitism, describes a character exactly in terms of the classic sensitive and talented nervous case:

> My mother was a woman of weak health, delicate nerves, and a kind of morbid sensibility, which I often heard her deplore as a misfortune, but which I observed

---

[33] Jonas Hanway, 'An Essay on Tea', *A Journal of an Eight Days' Journey from Portsmouth to Kingston-Upon-Thames* (London: H. Woodfall, 1756), 201–353, here 215, 274, 220.

[34] James Kennaway, 'The Dietetics of the Soul in Britain in the Long Eighteenth Century', *Lifestyle and Medicine in the Enlightenment: The Six Non-Naturals in the Long Eighteenth Century*, ed. James Kennaway and Rina Knoeff (New York: Routledge, 2020); James Kennaway, 'From Sensibility to Pathology: The Origins of Nervous Music', *Journal for the History of Medicine and Allied Sciences*, 65, no. 3 (2010): 396–426.

[35] James Kennaway, 'The Diseases of the Learned and Morbid Novels: Reading as a Cause of Disease', *Literature and Medicine*, 34, no. 2 (2016): 252–77; James Kennaway and Anita O'Connell, 'Pathological Reading', *Literature and Medicine*, 34, no. 2 (2016): 242–51.

[36] John Platt, *The Female Mentor* (Derby: Henry Moseley, 1823), 137–8.

every body about her admired as a grace. She lamented that her dear Harrington, her only son, should so much resemble her in this exquisite sensibility of the nervous system. But her physician ... assured her, that this was indisputably 'the genuine temperament of genius'.[37]

Likewise, the image of a prosperous Georgian gentleman laid up with a case of fashionable gout after a lifetime of overindulging in claret, beef and cheese is a recurring one, often reflected in the period's culture. Some observers took this association between gout and high status as the starting point for elaborate satire, generally acknowledging the implicit social prestige as much as lamenting the real suffering involved. The poem *On the Gout* suggested that 'plenty, parent of excess and ease' were the 'fatal cause' that brought gout into the world, while it was a 'stranger to the lowly cells/Where health with poverty and labour dwells', found only 'where luxury swells the dome and bids the column rise'.[38] In such waggish verse, sufferers could perhaps find some positive meaning for their pain.

A significant connection between medicine and the public culture of the beau monde was the world of spa towns such as Bath, Tunbridge Wells, Islington, Buxton and Brighton, which reached the apogee of their social prominence in this period. While there are places in the world where patients still 'take the waters', today it can be hard to imagine the combination of alluring social scene and medical establishment found in such resorts. The reputation of places for fun lent an air of fascination to the conditions involved, a key positive side of illness for some. Bath was referred to as a 'Region of Pleasure' because of the 'plays, music, cards, balls, and so many different amusements' by the Irish writer Samuel Derrick, a friend of Johnson and Smollett, who was made the town's 'Master of Ceremonies'.[39] The fun involved had an aristocratic ambiance. At certain times of year spas could be so full of members of the elite as to leave other visitors feeling positively ostracized. A letter written in 1811 to Edward Turner, steward of the grand stately home Welbeck Abbey, contained the lament: 'The hotels are full of nobility and gentry; all people above my cut – therefore I had no society at all.'[40]

---

[37] Maria Edgeworth, *Harrington, A Tale, and Ormond, a Tale*, 3 vols (London: R. Hunter, 1817), 1:14–15.
[38] Anon., 'On the Gout', *London Magazine*, 3 (January 1734): 660.
[39] Samuel Derrick, *Letters*, 2 vols (London: L. Davis and C. Reymers, 1767), 2:83, 2:88.
[40] Letter from P. P. Merlin, Buxton, to Edward Turner, Welbeck Abbet, Notts, 6 October 1811 (Nottingham University Special Collections Pw H 2021).

Along with a positive depiction of the benefits of having a modish disease and a medical critique of the elite, Georgian Britain also included many observers who depicted the whole business as a sham, a mere pose. For instance, in June 1795 *The European Magazine* recounts: 'When Mr ------ was dismissed being Prime Minister, he became ill, and sent for Sir William Duncan, who asked the servant who came for him, what ailed his master? "He has a bilious complaint, Sir," was the answer, "I never in my life," replied he, "knew a Minister out of place without a bilious complaint."'[41]

In a similar vein, William Makepeace Thackeray's *Vanity Fair* (1847–8) looked back on the Georgian era and contains several allusions to the period's culture of fashionable complaints. For instance, the hapless Joseph Sedley, East India Company collector of Boggley Wollah, who poses as a 'man of fashion' but whose own father regards him as 'vain, selfish, lazy, and effeminate', is described as having 'Luckily' caught a 'liver complaint'.[42] This was a 'source of great comfort and amusement', which allowed him to return to England: 'Were it not for his doctor, and the society of his blue-pill, and his liver complaint, he must have died of loneliness.'[43] In this view, elite patients were likely cynically to exploit modish complaints, trying to reap the positives without ever experiencing anything like a symptom.

Georgian culture also included explicit rejections of the move to medicalize social and moral issues. In this regard, Protestant ideas of sin retained substantial influence. John Owen, Fellow of Corpus Christi, Cambridge and Secretary of the British and Foreign Bible Society, fulminated in his 1806 *The Fashionable World Displayed* that the real problem was not a 'disorder of the nerves' or a matter of the 'disarrangement of the animal economy', which, for Owen, explains why 'fashionable nostrums' at Bath, Weymouth or Tunbridge failed to effect a cure. Whatever 'these Medicins de la mode' might have said, a 'fashionable' lifestyle of excess and vice meant that the 'disease is altogether moral' and its seat 'is not in the nerves, but in the Conscience'.[44] Such an approach, by denying the medical basis of the 'symptoms' concerned, also undermined any claims to prestige, reflecting the ways that the nexus of medicine and social status were central to the whole discourse of fashionable disease.

[41] Anon., 'Godeau', *European Magazine*, 27 (June 1795): 398.
[42] William Makepeace Thackeray, *Vanity Fair* (London: Bradbury and Evans, 1853), 230, 40, 17.
[43] Thackeray, *Vanity Fair*, 17.
[44] John Owen, *The Fashionable World Displayed* (New York: Hopkins and Seymour, 1806), 94–5.

Lay perceptions of 'fashionable' disease in Georgian Britain

It would be easy for a study of fashionable diseases to be waylaid by droll cultural expressions, but an affective history of the topic should take into consideration the feelings of sufferers too. While we have, of course, no unmediated access to the lived experience of Georgian sufferers of supposedly fashionable complaints, it is important to be aware of the extent to which their own experiences (and ours) were themselves also profoundly mediated by cultural understandings.[45] For this reason, 'real' experience, medical theory, the culture of fashionable disease, the attitudes of lay observers and the understandings of such diagnoses by patients are impossible to separate. First-hand testimony from sufferers' diaries and letters may be marked by literary conventions of irony and moralism, and generally relate to a tiny proportion of the population, but they do offer insights into how patients experienced modish complaints. So, how did patients and other sufferers talk about putatively modish conditions when it was not just a matter of stylized posturing but of pain, disability and discomfort?

It is clear that medical thinking that associated the beau monde with disease found widespread resonance among lay observers. For example, the extensive correspondence between the 'bluestocking' circle of female intellectuals included many discussions of the links between the world of fashion and medical conditions such as headaches and nervousness. In a letter to Rev. Friend in 1749, Elizabeth Montagu, by her own account a martyr to nervous complaints, described Tunbridge Wells as being full of lords and ladies, 'the great and rich who have bad nerves', whom she juxtaposed to the 'healthful and laborious peasant' who was spared such elite maladies.[46] The fundamental link between status and sickness was summed up in a 1770 letter from Montagu's friend Elizabeth Carter to another one of the group, Catherine Talbot, suggesting that 'fashionable life is a hard service', and for the people 'engaged' in such service, health 'is not very easily procured'.[47]

---

[45] See Barbara Rosenwein, *Generations of Feeling: A History of Emotions, 600-1700* (Cambridge: Cambridge University Press, 2016); Barbara Rosenwein and Riccardo Cristiani, *What Is the History of Emotions?* (Cambridge: Polity, 2018); Boddice and Smith, *Emotion, Sense, Experience*, 9–17; Joanna Bourke, *The Story of Pain* (Oxford: Oxford University Press, 2014).
[46] Matthew Montagu, ed., *The Letters of Elizabeth Montagu*, 3 vols (Boston, MA: Wells and Lilley, 1825), 186.
[47] Montagu Pennington, ed., *A Series of Letters between Elizabeth Carter and Miss Catherine Talbot*, 4 vols (London: Rivington, 1809), 4:6.

It seems that while patients may not have 'enjoyed' their symptoms in general, some were able to internalize or sublimate their dis-ease to derive advantages from sickness in terms of prestige and self-satisfaction. In that sense, modish diseases were not just a matter of fanciful cultural 'superstructure' but also of lived experience, something that was always profoundly mediated. To give a famous instance, James Boswell, doyen of biographers and a self-proclaimed sufferer of nervous complaints, wrote in 1778 that '*We Hypochondriacks*' could 'console ourselves in the hour of gloomy distress, by thinking that our sufferings mark our superiority'.[48] A generation later, Thomas Carlyle drew similar consolation about his own condition. In a letter from Kirkcaldy in February 1821, he linked the 'disorder in the stomach' from which he was suffering to his own 'superior' nature, 'something different from the vulgar herd of mortals'.[49] And in another letter, from December of the same year, he wrote to complain about his insomnia: 'The feeling around one's heart is as if you had planted fifty daggers there all in a moment; and the burning tremor that ensues extends to every fibre of the body. I speak, of course, of nervous persons, poor hypochondriacs, with whose agonising sensations, a sound plump husbandman is happily secure from having the remotest sympathy.'[50]

However, perhaps more common among patients was scepticism about fashionable diagnoses and about physicians' opinions. Often this can be seen in the form of light irony on the subject. For example, in October 1770 Henry Mackenzie, the author of the epitome of the novel of sensibility, 1771's *The Man of Feeling*, wrote to his cousin Elizabeth Rose of Kilravock, near Inverness, 'We have at present an epidemical cold which nobody escapes; I am seldom violently in the fashion, & therefore have had only a gentle touch of it; but Hannah, who is, & should be more modish than me, has suffer'd pretty severely from it these eight or ten days past.'[51] Others expressed cynicism about modish or faddish diagnoses and the physicians who promoted them. The doctors involved were not the titans of the later nineteenth century. The elite patients concerned were often confident in their own ideas about their symptoms, based on their own observations, and, no doubt, second-hand medical theory and prevailing cultural assumptions.

---

[48] James Boswell, 'On Hypochondria', *Hypochondriack*, 5 (February 1778), 42–7, here 42–3.
[49] The Carlyle Letters Online, https://carlyleletters.dukeupress.edu/volume/01/lt-18210219-TC-AC-01, accessed 26 December 2020.
[50] The Caryle Letters Online, https://carlyleletters.dukeupress.edu/volume/01/lt-18211225-TC-AC-01?term=fifty%20daggers%20, accessed 26 December 2020.
[51] Horst W. Drescher, *Henry Mackenzie, Letters to Elizabeth Rose of Kilravock* (Edinburgh: Oliver and Boyd, 1967), 58.

A tone of ironic scepticism can already be found in the letters of the French aristocrat Madame de Sévigné to her daughter in the 1680s, translated and published in English in the eighteenth century. Writing about her son-in-law's illness, she alludes to what was already a cliché, that 'the gout is a sign of wealth', but argues that in reality 'gout or rheumatism' are 'twin brothers', the latter being lower of the aristocratic pecking order, but essentially 'the same stuff'.[52] She also gently mocks doctors for using trendier terms for well-known complaints, writing that 'the physicians with pomp of erudition, declare his disorder *arthritic*' when the 'plain and homely appellation of the *gout*' would do just as well.[53] In England, instances of similar attitudes were also common. For example, Lady Betty Germain, who had met her husband at Bristol's hot wells in 1706, alluded to the supposed 'virtues' of gout in letters to Jonathan Swift. In September 1731, she wrote of its putative hereditary character: 'I do derive it from my ancestors.'[54] Four years later she teasingly referred to the idea that gout could act against other medical complaints, calling it 'that infallible cure for all diseases, which all great fools and talkers wish joy of'.[55]

Others were dubious about parts of medical theory concerning the causes of fashionable diseases. The Anglo-Irish writer and landowner Richard Lovell Edgeworth (father to twenty-two children, including the novelist Maria Edgeworth, quoted above) wrote to Erasmus Darwin, a fellow member of the Lunar Society, in October 1786, querying some of the precepts of the physicians' critique of excess. Kept awake by pain caused by illness himself, despite only drinking a couple of glasses of wine a day (which made him 'notorious' for sobriety in Ireland, he said), he questioned the link between boozing and sickness.[56] He felt that while 'the lower class drink as much whiskey as they can get, and are, notwithstanding, strong and healthy!' 'the gentlemen who drink wine, and eat luxuriously, are, on the contrary, afflicted with all the demons of disease, and flock to Bath and Spa, like regular birds of passage, every autumn'.[57]

It must be noted, however, that the most widespread theme in first-hand testimony about modish complaints relates to feelings of physical pain, with little hint that fashion offered much by way of consolation. In his letters, the

---

[52] Madame de Sevigne, *Letters of Madame de Sevigne to Her Daughter and Her Friends*, 9 vols (London: J. Walker, 1811), 6:129.
[53] *Letters of Madame de Sevigne*, 6:146.
[54] John Hawkesworth, ed., *Letters Written by the Late Jonathan Swift DD, Dean of St. Patrick's, Dublin and Several of His Friends from the Year 1703 to 1740*, 2 vols (London: T. Davies, 1766), 2:142.
[55] Hawkesworth, *Letters*, 2:222.
[56] Richard Lovell Edgeworth and Maria Edgeworth, *Memoirs of Richard Lovell Edgeworth* (London: Richard Bentley, 1844), 300–1.
[57] Edgeworth, *Memoirs of Richard Lovell Edgeworth*, 300.

historian Edward Gibbon writes about the suffering caused by his gout, which, in a letter of 1787, he called 'the capricious tyrant'.[58] In a letter in 1777, he gave an account of his gout symptoms in stylish prose reminiscent of his *Decline and Fall of the Roman Empire* (1776–89):

> With regard to myself, the gout has behaved in a very honourable manner; after a complete conquest, and after making me feel his power for some days, the generous enemy has disdained to abuse his victor, or to torment any longer an unresisting victim. He has already ceased to torture the lower extremities of your humble servant; the swelling is so amazingly diminished, that they are no longer above twice their ordinary size. Yesterday I moved about the room with the laborious majesty of crutches; to-day I have exchanged them for a stick.[59]

The only solace on offer here is of an essentially literary and ironic kind.

The role of suffering in accounts of the afflicted is also related to a strong recurring religious element. The fundamental moral argument behind medical critiques of fashionable lifestyles, that excess led to sickness and death, had obvious religious overtones: there was an understandable urge to seek succour in faith when in suffering. It is perhaps not surprising that evangelical self-condemnation and a search for consolation were common. Willielma Campbell, Viscountess Glenorchy, was a prominent evangelical who understood her supposedly modish diseases in terms of Protestantism, having undergone a conversion experience in the 1760s while recovering from illness. Her usual doctor was the great Edinburgh physician William Cullen, but in London she saw Dr Fothergill. Her diaries reflect her sober and pious approach to putatively glamorous complaints. For instance, in May 1780 she wrote about the 'gout in the head and stomach' she had experienced before moving to Bridport in Dorset for her health, seeing in these changes evidence that 'God's path is in the deep, and his footsteps are not known'.[60] Other pious observers drew on their faith to consciously reject the whole idea of fashionable diseases. In a letter to his father in 1749, the Quaker Philip Eliot wrote about the 'great fitts of sickness' experienced by his sister, which he said bore no relation to what are 'vulgarly called Histericks in Women & Vapours in Men, names commonly given by Physicians when they can't comprehend the Disorder'. Instead, he argued that

---

[58] Edward Gibbon, *The Miscellaneous Works of Edward Gibbon*, 5 vols (London: John Murray, 1814), 2:401.
[59] Gibbon, *Miscellaneous Works*, 2:215.
[60] T. S. Jones, ed., *The Life of the Right Honourable Viscountess of Glenorchy* (Edinburgh: William Whyte, 1822), 471.

it was 'a visitation from the Almighty in order to rectify her Inside and so form both Soul and body for his peculiar use and service'.[61]

Medical thinking of these kinds provided the vocabulary needed to talk about symptoms and supplied models of the connection between lifestyle and disease, but the etiquette and power dynamics of medical practice also played a key role in the wider discourse of fashionable maladies. The Georgian period was arguably an era in which formal medical thinking was coming to have more widespread cultural impact than ever before, and medical theories were regularly used to make broader social arguments. However, it was not yet an age of the quasi-omnipotent 'medical gaze' of nineteenth-century anatomo-clinical medicine. The elite patients that formed the bulk of clients who have left us substantial written records were by no means passive recipients of the wisdom of their physicians. Rather, they were customers with considerable financial, social and cultural power that helped frame their symptoms and the diagnoses they were given: a key reason for the period's efflorescence of fashionable diseases.

A sense of the role of patients, or rather of the interaction between physicians and wealthy patients, in creating fashionable diagnoses, can be found in the mocking account given by the mischievous Scottish doctor James Makittrick Adair. Explaining how faddish diagnoses gained attention, he noted the regular shifts in modish diagnosis, arguing that it was driven by the social status of those involved more than by rigorous medical judgement.[62] In his *Essay on Regimen* (1799), he blamed a 'fashionable apothecary' for making nerves modish. Having read a serious book on the subject, the apothecary told the next fashionable patient who consulted him, '"Madam, you are nervous," ... nervous diseases became quite the *ton*, and spleen, vapours and hyp were kicked out of doors'.[63] Adair went as far as to suggest that some of the conditions concerned were merely 'imaginary', something echoed in modern suggestions that 'trendy' complaints are just the result of rich people malingering.

Conclusion

The lived experience of suffering was mediated by medical and cultural ideas, and the feelings of sufferers in turn played a significant role in the development

---

[61] Eliot Howard, ed., *Eliot Papers: John Eliot, of London, Merchant 1735-1785* (London: E. Hicks, 1895), 12-13.
[62] James Makittrick Adair, *An Essay on Diet and Regimen* (London: James Rideway, 1812), 122-3.
[63] James Makittrick Adair, *An Essay on Regimen* (London: J & P Wilson, 1799), 130.

of the discourse of fashionable complaints, feeding back into medical diagnostic discourse. The power of elite patients therefore meant that diagnosis retained an important element of negotiation between patients and physicians. Trendy medical thinking provided attractive new models of causation and a new vocabulary for symptoms, but the culture of the period and first-hand testimony reflected widespread scepticism about specific disorders and about the insights of individual physicians and of the profession as a whole. The elite Georgian patients who were chiefly involved in the debates on modish conditions thus often provide clear instances of the autonomy of the patient in the generations before the advent of any overweening medical gaze.

At the same time, physicians' ideas helped validate positive conceptions of certain maladies even if their arguments were framed in terms of moralizing social critique. Those ideas, made ironic or paradoxical, helped reinforce notions that the rich were almost biologically different from the lower orders, blessed with more delicate bodies and feelings: in David Hume's notorious words, 'the nerves of a day-labourer are different from those of a man of quality'.[64] In contrast to the cliché of the hypersensitive gentleman or lady weeping at the sight of the suffering of the poor, the sense that 'they don't feel it like we do' provided an alibi for a lack of pity for others.[65] James Johnston, for instance, wrote that 'factory girls' should be thankful that they did not have the fragile nerves of young ladies of the elite.[66] Even for those ladies, the prestige of being associated with modish conditions was at best a double-edged sword. Their supposed sensitive nervousness and vulnerability to beau-monde conditions may have lent them a certain Romantic air, but if their education or family life was influenced by the strictures of doctors in this regard it could have disempowered them, leading to a rather Spartan existence in which even reading and music were to be avoided.

As the Georgian era ended, there seems to have been a notable decline in interest in the subject. Rachael Johnson has noted that in the Victorian era images of vigorous healthy people rather than elite valetudinarians began to dominate depictions of spa towns.[67] More broadly, it seems that the class associations of

---

[64] David Hume, 'Of Liberty and Necessity', *The Philosophical Works of David Hume*, 4 vols (Boston, MA: Little, Brown, 1854), 2:148–57, here 151.

[65] See Jonathan Lamb, *The Evolution of Sympathy in the Long Eighteenth Century* (London: Routledge, 2009); Rob Boddice, *The Science of Sympathy: Morality, Evolution and Victorian Civilization* (Urbana: University of Illinois Press, 2017); Joanna Bourke, 'Pain Sensitivity: An Unnatural History from 1800 to 1965', *Journal of Medical Humanities*, 35 (2014): 301–19.

[66] James Johnson, *The Economy of Health, or the Stream of Human Life from the Cradle to the Grave, with Reflections Moral, Physical and Philosophical on the Successive Phases of Human Existence* (London: S. Highley, 1837), 32–4.

[67] Rachael Johnson, 'The Venus of Margate: Fashion and Disease at the Seaside', *Journal for Eighteenth Century Studies*, 40, no. 4 (2017): 571–86.

luxury were being undermined as a growing middle class sought to emulate their social superiors. Charles Scudamore, in his *Treatise on the Nature and Cure of Gout and Rheumatism* (1819), for example, argued that the associations with wealth that Sydenham had noted with gout no longer applied, since 'luxury has so much increased among the whole community' and that even 'butchers, innkeepers, butlers and porters in wealthy families' often suffered from it.[68] The term 'neurasthenia' was famously coined by the American George Miller Beard in 1869, but its fundamental argument about modernity, work and nervous disease can thus be found in British sources from decades earlier, linking formerly fashionable diseases not with the glamorous classes but with men in trade.[69] This shift in class associations created the basis for the Victorian debate on nervousness as a problem for an increasingly large part of the population, which obviously undermined its social cachet. By the end of the nineteenth century, the neurasthenia of the urban capitalist was matched by fears of the degeneration of the masses, radically challenging the whole notion of elegant sickliness for all except small numbers of self-conscious decadents.[70] However, in new permutations, the discourse of diseases of the rich, clever and stylish intermittently recurred throughout the twentieth century and in constantly shifting forms is thriving in our own time.

---

[68] Charles Scudamore, *A Treatise on the Nature and Cure of Gout and Rheumatism* (London: Charles Scudamore, 1819), 66–7.
[69] George Miller Beard, 'Neurasthenia or Nervous Exhaustion', *Boston Medical and Surgical Journal*, 80 (1869): 245–59; Roy Porter, 'Nervousness Eighteenth and Nineteenth Style: From Luxury to Labour', *Cultures of Neurasthenia*, ed. Roy Porter (Leiden: Brill, 2001), 31–49.
[70] See Daniel Pick, *Faces of Degeneration: A European Disorder* (Cambridge: Cambridge University Press, 1989); Jill Kirby, *Feeling the Strain: A Cultural History of Stress in Twentieth-Century Britain* (Oxford: Oxford University Press, 2019); Amelia Bonea, Melissa Dickson, Sally Shuttleworth and Jennifer Wallis, eds, *Anxious Times: Medicine and Modernity in Nineteenth-Century Britain* (Pittsburgh: University of Pittsburgh Press, 2019).

Material, objects, feelings

Commentary

The final section might just as easily have been titled 'Space and Place', for many of the theoretical considerations of the relation between spatiality and emotion/experience overlap with approaches to materiality and the relationship between actors and objects. Here we encounter two distinct forms of spatial planning and prescription, replete with detailed analysis of the design and arrangement of objects to which people 'stick'. From a design point of view, both the bed-treatment approach to early twentieth-century psychiatry and the realization of the Montreal Neurological Institute lobby in the 1930s were deterministic about the human experience they were to evoke. Yet both chapters discuss the vicissitudes of lived experience within and beyond the limits of such prescription. The two themes return us to the opening note of our introduction and the question of what the focus of the emotional and experiential history of medicine should be: patient/doctor; macro/micro. Both these chapters show the value of complicating the response to such a question, with Ankele juxtaposing experiences of doctors and patients in the encounter, and allowing for the divergence of expectation and experience, and with Adams situating the focus in the space itself, with its bespoke objects, and using these in turn to find Wilder Penfield's experience of neurosurgery and, perhaps, herself.

Monika Ankele's chapter discusses a fundamental shift in psychiatric treatment in which patients were compelled to lie prone in bed in a ward. The prescription was to inculcate an experience of sickness to psychiatric patients who might otherwise have rejected or resisted a diagnosis. Ankele shows how the deliberate narrowing of the sensory repertoire actually heightened certain sensory perceptions and evoked acute memories as patients strove to visualize wellness, the outside, the upright or just another place. She elegantly juxtaposes the felt dis-ease of patients that was experienced in a manner at odds with the prescription for the experience of sickness. Here, the orientation and arrangement of beds, the placement of windows and doors and proximity of other patients are key. In a space aimed ultimately at wellness, with an intention to induce a feeling of illness, the result was a complex third thing.

Annmarie Adams puts herself squarely in the frame of her own chapter on the MNI lobby, weaving a double-threaded narrative about the design of the space and its furnishings and her own encounter with it. The foremost aim is to demonstrate the design intentions of the lobby interior: to inspire a kind of compound awe, itself a form of dis-ease, at nature and at science's power of 'discovering' nature. Running alongside this is a narrative about Wilder Penfield's own emotional investment in the space, which transforms the MNI lobby from a space designed to inspire a certain experience to a space that reveals Penfield himself. Every piece of furniture, every design consideration, becomes a primary source for the emotional biography of Penfield. By recording her own thoughts and experience, *sotto voce*, Adams mirrors her own argument, artfully revealing the connections of academic positioning to personal reflection and reaction.

Thus, the book ends as it began, with an innovative first-person narrative account of the experience of medicine and illness. The two could not be farther apart in terms of their subject matter, but they share an impulse to find an understanding of past experience through the exercise of personal reflection, weighed against an array of other sources. Is this not a call to action in exploring the feeling of dis-ease in history? Do we not need to expose ourselves, as historians and scholars in adjacent fields, to our own feelings of dis-ease and, in accounting for them, to find a way to explore their relationship to the experiences of the past? Sometimes, as with the opening essay in this volume, the connection seems immutable. But at other times, as with the last essay here, we see the necessary work of disambiguation and disconnection. Making both visible is uncomfortable and delightful, an historiographical dis-ease. We should embrace it.

12

From a patient's point of view: A sensual-perceptual approach to bed treatment

Monika Ankele

Introduction

The State Archive Schaffhausen in Switzerland contains numerous works of art by patients who were treated at the now-defunct Breitenau psychiatric hospital between 1891 and 1930.[1] One is a drawing by Bernhard(t) B.,[2] which provides a helpful introduction to the topic of this chapter (Figure 12.1). Drawn with red and black pencil, the image renders the perspective of a patient lying in a sickbed and looking around. The lines on the paper are determined by the perspective disclosed by the artist's lying position, which in turn conditions his perception of the space. In a broad sense, Bernhard(t) B. represented the situation in which he found himself, as the style of the drawing suggests that he was depicting his own perspective. Thus, artist and patient are one here. The drawing's vanishing point is an open door with a massive frame. Everything is oriented around this central point: the walls on both sides of the room, the dark grey hatched flooring, the

---

[1] This article was composed as part of the project 'Bett und Bad. Räume und Objekte therapeutischen Handelns in der Psychiatrie des 19. und 20. Jahrhunderts' (SCHM1311–11/1 – Bed and Bath: Spaces and Objects of Therapeutic Practice in Psychiatry in the Nineteenth and Twentieth Century), funded by the German Research Foundation, at the Institute for History and Ethics of Medicine at the University Medical Center Hamburg-Eppendorf and at the Medical University of Vienna. Special thanks to Céline Kaiser, Heinz-Peter Schmiedebach and Kai Sammet for their many helpful suggestions and Adam Bresnahan for the translation.
On the history of the Breitenau psychiatric hospital see 'Psychiatrie-Zentrum/Klinik für Psychiatrie und Psychotherapie Breitenau. Sammlung Breitenau, Staatsarchiv des Kantons Schaffhausen', https://blog.zhdk.ch/bewahrenbesondererkulturgueter/schaffhausen/. The website contains a list of the patients' digitalized works.

[2] As a patient of the Breitenau hospital, Bernhard(t) B. produced a series of drawings with various subject matter. On Bernhard(t) B. see Katrin Luchsinger, '"Alles Ferne, Fremde, Ungewöhnliche". Kunst in der Klinik Breitenau, 1904–1935', *125 Jahre Psychiatrische Klinik Breitenau Schaffhausen, 1891–2016*, ed. Historischer Verein des Kantons Schaffhausen und den Spitälern Schaffhausen (Zurich: Chronos, 2018), 164–6.

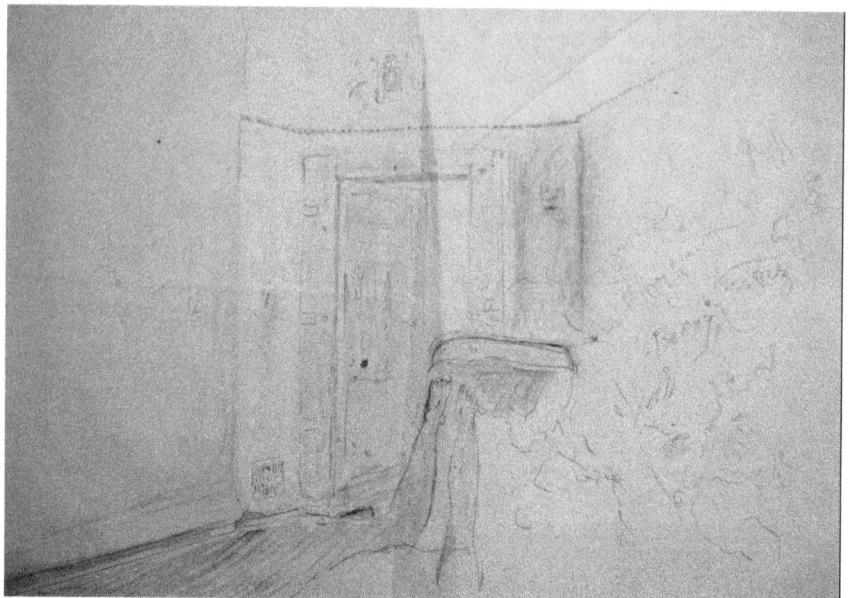

Figure 12.1 Room drawn from the perspective of a hospital bed by Bernhard(t) B., Breitenau psychiatric hospital, 1932. Staatsarchiv Schaffhausen, DI 39/639.

body lying in bed and, finally, the patient's perspective, which becomes our perspective, taking us along into the room and allowing us to see not only what the patient-artist sees but also how he sees it.

Another striking feature of the drawing are the two bare legs that lie stretched out on the sickbed. They, too, are pointed towards the open door. The drawing does not depict the patient-artist's head, arms and torso. Because the person drawing himself and his perspective is identical with the person lying in bed, we only see the body parts that the drawer can himself see from his lying position. The legs seem remarkably stiff. These are not legs that are about to get up, leave the bed and walk through the open door. The bed's footrest and the bedframe that supports it are clearly defined. They mark off the space to which the body is confined and thus delimit a space within a space. The patient is positioned so far to the left side of the bed that it seems like he could fall out at any minute. On the right side of the drawing, where the bed butts up against the wall, the scene is chaotic. The wall and the bed seem to merge into one another. The lack of colour gives the impression that something is forcing its way from the wall towards the bed. Pencil strokes break away from the wall and form rhythmic lines, curves and loops that have no apparent relation to anything else in the image. Letters and words flow towards the bed, proliferating above it and rambling into the room.

Wherever they appear, the clear, straight lines of bodies and objects break apart. Their dynamic movement infuses the image with restlessness and interrupts the order of the delicately compact composition. Do they symbolize noises that Bernhard(t) B. hears through the wall alongside his bed? What relation do they have to his supine body? And what do they say about the experience of space represented in the image?

The drawing suggests that Bernhard(t) B. was housed in a one-bed room and was required to stay in bed. German psychiatrist Wilhelm Weygandt (1870–1939) described this form of treating patients with mental illness as 'optical isolation'.[3] While bed treatment, which psychiatrists began using around 1900, was focused on reducing all sensory stimuli, optical isolation was primarily concerned with minimizing just visual stimuli. Might this medically prescribed sensory deprivation have sharpened Bernhard(t) B.'s receptiveness for other impressions? Might the signs on the right side of the image be a manifestation of this?

The drawing's gestural, expressive style informs the recipient not so much about the actual layout of the space, with its furniture, objects and walls, as about how Bernhard(t) B. perceived it and his own position within it: lying in bed, with stretched out legs, in a narrow, almost empty room with a door that, though open, provided no view to anything outside. By selecting elements and perspectives that he found relevant, Bernhard(t) B. established relations between the space and his body, his posture and his perception. By requiring him to remain in a lying position, the doctors put him into a particular relationship with this spatial constellation. However, he also drafted his own relationship to it. By enabling the recipient to experience the space through the eyes (and, in a sense, through the body) of the patient, the drawing reverses the power relation between the gaze of the doctor and that of the patient and places the patient as someone who sees – instead of as someone who is seen – front and centre. Thus, the drawing can be conceived of as an assertive gesture.

Problem and analysis

This chapter engages with questions on the relationship between space, body, posture and perception in psychiatric institutions, issues that Bernhard(t) B.'s drawing explores. I engage with these questions through an in-depth analysis of

---

[3] Wilhelm Weygandt, *Atlas und Grundriss der Psychiatrie* (Munich: Lehmann's, 1902).

doctors' and patients' varying perspectives on the introduction of bed treatment in psychiatric hospitals at the turn of the twentieth century. Bed treatment denotes the systematic use of bedrest for the mentally ill, which doctors could prescribe for days, weeks or months. The specially furnished room, the lying body and the intentional limitation of sensory perception were, together with the duration, the cornerstones of bed treatment. As the following demonstrates, they were closely connected and were intended to influence the patients in concert by calming them, making them pliable and pushing them to acknowledge that they were ill.

The first section focuses on the spatial and material dimensions of the sense regime that the implementation of bed treatment sought to influence. In this context, the concept of 'sense regime' signifies measures taken to exert power over patients by intentionally regulating their sensory perception. The term comes from an article by sociologist Andreas Reckwitz: 'Social macro-phenomena such as institutions, social fields, and classes cultivate within the totality of their practices their own sense regimes.'[4] This applies to the institution of the psychiatric hospital. As historian Madeline Bourque Kearin notes, 'The asylum was an institution primarily aimed at transforming the lunatic into a sane person by manipulating his senses.'[5] This claim might be slightly modified to describe the goal of bed treatment: to transform the 'lunatic' into a patient by manipulating his senses. I thus conceive of bed treatment as a complex of practices that, by arranging objects and bodies in space in a particular way, forged its own material environment and moulded sensory perception. 'Every practice and complex of practices', Reckwitz writes, 'is in its way perceptually organised, meaning that it mobilises, limits and structures the *what* and the *how* of sense perception in a specific way.'[6]

In the second section, I engage with the effects of doctors' intentional organization of patients' perception. To this end, I juxtapose the perspectives of doctors and patients, especially in regards to the spatial constellations in psychiatric hospitals. I also analyse the forms of perception and practices of perception that the patients developed in their interactions with the clinic's sense regime. Where the sources permit, I also explore what emotions the sense regime of bed treatment evoked in individual patients.

---

[4] Andreas Reckwitz, 'How the Senses Organise the Social', *Praxeological Political Analysis*, ed. Michael Jonas and Beate Littig (New York: Routledge, 2017), 63.
[5] Madeline Bourque Kearin, '"As Syllable from Sound": The Sonic Dimensions of Confinement at the State Hospital for the Insane at Worcester, Massachusetts', *History of Psychiatry*, 31, no. 1 (2020): 79.
[6] Reckwitz, 'How the Senses Organise the Social', 63.

I take a praxeological approach to picking apart the interdependencies of space, objects, bodies and sensory perception.[7] This approach holds that practices – and thus practices of perception – are 'materially anchored' in bodies and objects.[8] The analysis of perception is thus conditioned by an analysis of the physical environment, of the spatial and material constellations that are brought forth by specific practices and that influence how people perceive and what they perceive. This holds for the analysis of the historical sense regimes represented by institutions like psychiatric hospitals.[9] I will not dissect in detail the environment of one particular psychiatric hospital but will instead sketch out the defining features of the arrangement and sense regime of bed treatment by drawing on contemporaneous specialist literature. The analysis in the second section is based on patients' own accounts, such as written notes, letters and drawings, as well as on medical records from various psychiatric institutions. The sources used in the article are from Germanophone countries.

A sensorial shift: The implementation of bed treatment

A praxeological analysis of bed treatment will make visible how senses and emotions are interrelated, since the sense regime of bed treatment changed

---

[7] See Reckwitz, 'How the Senses Organise the Social'. On the relation between perception and material culture, see Hanna Katharina Göbel and Sophia Prinz, eds, *Die Sinnlichkeit des Sozialen: Wahrnehmung und materielle Kultur* (Bielefeld: Transcript, 2015). Researchers in disciplines from philosophy to the cognitive sciences have engaged with the question of what perception is. I dispense with a survey of the various theories here and limit my discussion to those approaches that are directly relevant to the article, while acknowledging that this unavoidably under-researched topic in the history of a lot.
[8] Andreas Reckwitz, 'Affective Spaces: A Praxeological Outlook', *Rethinking History*, 16 (2012): 241–58, at 248.
[9] In the history of psychiatry, therapeutic methods have often focused on patients' senses and emotions. For an example, see the analysis of Johann Christian Reil's 'psychic remedy doctrine' (Reil 1803/1818) in Céline Kaiser, *Szenographien des Subjekts. Eine Kulturmediengeschichte szenischer Therapieformen seit dem 18. Jahrhundert* (Bielefeld: Transcript, 2019), 127–38. The intertwining of power, agency and the senses is a key, though unfortunately under-researched topic in the history of psychiatry. There are only a few historical studies on the sense regimes of psychiatric hospitals and these regimes' effects on patients. See Kai Sammet, 'Silent "Night of Madness"? Light, Voice, Sounds, and Space in the Illenau Asylum in Baden between 1842–1910', *Material Cultures of Psychiatry*, ed. Monika Ankele and Benoît Majerus (Bielefeld: Transcript, 2020), 44–73; Kirsi Heimonen and Sari Kuuva, 'A Corridor That Moves: Corporeal Encounters with Materiality in a Mental Hospital', in Ankele and Majerus, *Material Cultures of Psychiatry*, 334–53; Madeline Bourque Kearin, ' "A State of Conscious and Permanent Visibility": Sight as an Instrument of Cure and Control at the Worcester State Hospital for the Insane, 1833–1900', *New England Quarterly*, 92, no. 3 (2019): 431–76; Kearin, 'As Syllable from Sound'; Monika Ankele, 'The Fabric of Seclusion: Textiles as Medias of (Spatial) Interaction in Mental Hospitals', in Ankele and Majerus, *Material Cultures of Psychiatry*, 140–56. For a 'sensual approach' to the history of hospitals see the UCRI project by Victoria Bates, University of Bristol, 'Sensing Spaces of Healthcare: Rethinking the NHS Hospital', https://hospitalsenses.co.uk/2019/11/15/ukri-future-leaders-fellowship/; however, up to this point (spring 2021), the project has not studied psychiatric institutions.

the emotional signature of the mental hospital.[10] In other words, it sought to transform the hospital into a place where patients would no longer feel as if they were being 'buried alive' and where they would no longer view doctors as their 'jailers' (*Kerkermeister*).[11] But how could the introduction of a rather simple form of treatment like bed rest achieve such fundamental change?

The senses and sensory perception of the space of the mental hospital played a significant role in German-speaking psychiatrists' view of what they considered to be the advantages (at the time, they identified practically no disadvantages) of bed rest as a new method of treatment at the end of the nineteenth century. While their reports published in scientific journals should be read with caution (medical records might reveal different insights into the everyday life of a ward), they are indicative of doctors' views on bed treatment. In their support of bed treatment, physicians tended to contrast two different sensory environments on the psychiatric ward: the first before the implementation of bed rest and the second after its implementation. Their message was clear: making bed rest a standard part of psychiatric treatment would not just promote patients' well-being but would also change the institution as such – its entire atmosphere – for the better.

One of the reasons they gave for these improvements was a shift in the way the space of the hospital was sensually experienced and how it affected patients' (self-)perception. As psychiatrists vividly illustrated, bed treatment changed the way the asylum space looked, smelled and sounded. There is hardly a report on the introduction of bed treatment that does not include a review of how things were at the hospital before it. In their reports, psychiatrists highlighted unpleasant smells, disturbing sounds and disgusting sights that had permeated and penetrated the hospital space before bed rest was applied. As they pointed out, these smells, sounds and sights had been frequently caused by the way that the sick had been treated (or, more likely, had not been treated at all) and how they reacted to this (lack of) treatment. In their accounts, doctors identified the spatial and material environment as a possible cause of certain patient behaviours,

---

[10] The concept 'emotional signature' is defined in Rob Boddice and Mark Smith, *Emotion, Sense, Experience* (Cambridge: Cambridge University Press, 2020), 4, 23.

[11] The expression 'buried alive' was used by proponents of the movement for the rights of people living with mental illness around 1900. See Heinz-Peter Schmiedebach, '"Zerquälte Ergebnisse einer Dichterseele" – Literarische Kritik, Psychiatrie und Öffentlichkeit um 1900', in *'Moderne' Anstaltspsychiatrie im 19. und 20. Jahrhundert*, ed. Heiner Fangerau and Karen Nolte (Stuttgart: Franz Steiner Verlag, 2006), 259–82. The term 'Kerkermeister' (jailer) appears in multiple contemporaneous texts by psychiatrists. See, for example, Adolf Gross, *Allgemeine Therapie der Psychosen* (Leipzig: Franz Deuticke, 1912), 133; Gustav Kolb, 'Reform der Irrenfürsorge', *Zeitschrift für die gesamte Neurologie und Psychiatrie*, 47 (1919): 142.

practices and even their alleged pathologies.[12] In particular, proponents of bed treatment criticized the clinics' isolation sections. They established a direct connection between the practice of segregating anxious patients in closed rooms, where they were left to themselves and shut off from sensory stimuli, and some of those patients' behavioural patterns, such as smearing the cell walls with faeces, pounding on the doors, screaming loudly and tearing up clothes. While the cells' thick walls did succeed in isolating the patients from the outside world, they could not necessarily shield the outside world from the sensory aspect of the patients' actions – the smells and noises emanating from the cells that shaped the sensory environment of the wards.[13]

Doctors also thematized patients' appearances. German psychiatrist Otto Klinke recalled with 'discontent' the era before bed treatment, homing in on the 'terrifying', 'oppressive' sight of agitated patients moving uncontrollably, screaming and lying on the floor or benches.[14] Jakob Salgó, a psychiatrist at the State Mental Hospital in Budapest, described the sight of patients in isolation cells – who were often naked or smearing excrement on the walls – as 'unspeakably dismal', and he found the long corridors 'swarming with patients aimlessly wandering and staggering around' to be 'depressing'.[15] In retrospect, Salgó remembered the 'horrid figures of slurping, tottering paralytics and epileptics', the 'dishevelled, poorly dressed, somewhat unclean terminal imbeciles' and the 'apathic, stuporous patients that cause shame and pain to all human sensibility'. He wrote that they all 'bleakly' gathered in the ward's halls, which took on a 'repulsive character' as a result.[16] But most important for him was that the sight of these patients, whom the psychiatrist described both vividly and disparagingly, almost entirely nullified the institution's 'curative purpose'.[17]

The advent of bed treatment was supposed to have relegated all this to the past. If one takes the psychiatrist at his word, prescribing patients to lie in bed largely put an end to the 'lethargic sitting around',[18] the

---

[12] See Clemens Neisser, 'Ueber die Bettbehandlung der akuten Psychosen und über die Veränderungen, welche ihre Einführung im Anstaltsorganismus mit sich bringt', *Zeitschrift für praktische Aerzte*, 18 (1900): 730; Gross, *Allgemeine Therapie*; Monika Ankele, 'Sich aufführen. Rauminterventionen und Wissenspraktiken in der Psychiatrie um 1900', *Aufführen, Anordnen, Aufzeichnen. Wissenspraktiken in Psychiatrie und Psychotherapie*, ed. Monika Ankele, Sophie Ledebur and Céline Kaiser (Wiesbaden: Springer, 2019), 71–89.
[13] Kearin, 'As Syllable from Sound'.
[14] Otto Klinke, 'Zur Geschichte der freien Behandlung und der Anwendung der Bettruhe bei Geisteskranken', *Allgemeine Zeitschrift für Psychiatrie und psychisch-gerichtliche Medizin*, 49 (1893): 680.
[15] [Jakob] Salgó, 'Die Bettbehandlung der Geisteskranken', *Psychiatrische Wochenschrift*, 4 (1899): 34.
[16] Salgó, 'Die Bettbehandlung', 34.
[17] Salgó, 'Die Bettbehandlung', 34.
[18] Neisser, 'Ueber die Bettbehandlung', 682.

'screaming',[19] the 'spinning around'[20] and the 'pointless wandering'[21] omnipresent in doctors' reports. Bed treatment gave the patient a clear place to be (a bed) in a common room (a sick ward); it specified the posture that the body was to assume (lying); it restricted patients' movements and actions to the micro-space of the bed; and it unified patients' external, visible appearance: 'They are all lying, ward upon ward, in clean beds.'[22] This was how Salgó summarized the transformation that bed treatment accomplished, or, more precisely, the transformation it was supposed to accomplish.

In many institutions, the implementation of bed treatment necessitated that the existing spatial layout be restructured. The isolation cells were combined into larger wards, and the benches and tables of the common rooms, which had been open to patients (walking, sitting, lying) during the day, were swapped out with rows of beds. This created rooms where patients could be housed together during treatment, which doctors viewed as particularly important for their acclimatization. They reasoned that seeing other patients lying in their beds would make patients more receptive to doctors' orders and stay in bed without complaint. Psychiatrist Clemens Neisser, who coined the term 'bed treatment', explained this phenomenon: 'Many patients who, in their own rooms, would flatly refuse to follow the doctor's orders, do not resist … when doing so would disturb the calm and order of many others. In other respects, the hospital-like character of the surroundings makes it easier for patients to become oriented and behave properly, and for many, the desire to imitate kicks in instinctively.'[23] In short, the configuration of perception through the spatial arrangement of bed treatment was intended to influence the behaviour of newly admitted patients in a specific way.

The bed became the definitive feature of treatment. It took on a structuring function within the hospital space, giving doctors orientation and creating a kind of visible classification of patients. Moreover, it facilitated surveillance, because doctors and nurses walking through the ward could see all of the patients lying in their beds, while patients in their lying position had no choice but to expose themselves to this gaze. Surveillance, in turn, enabled staff to intervene quickly if anything happened. For patients, the bed was the spot reserved for them, the place where they had to stay and could only leave with the doctor's permission.

---

[19] Gross, *Allgemeine Therapie*.
[20] Neisser, 'Ueber die Bettbehandlung', 682; Gross, *Allgemeine Therapie*, 134.
[21] See Salgó, 'Die Bettbehandlung', 34.
[22] Salgó, 'Die Bettbehandlung', 34.
[23] Neisser, 'Ueber die Bettbehandlung', 686.

It forced their body to assume a specific posture, regulated their contact with their environment and demarcated the space that they could perceive and inhabit. Patients could only touch the textile surfaces of the bed and their own body, though doing the latter could have consequences. They could only see the space around them, though sometimes this was expanded if they had a window view.[24] Lying in their beds, their blankets pulled up to their chins, every patient's external appearance was similar to that of the next.

The layout of the wards for bed treatment was modelled on the sick wards found in general hospitals. The purpose was to turn the 'insane asylum' into a hospital and the 'mad' into sick patients. Thus, psychiatrist Adolf Gross remarked that the 'large, bright, well-ventilated dayrooms' of bed treatment, 'where patients lie cleanly in beds with white sheets, looked happier and more like hospitals'.[25] The transformation from individual cells to the open sick ward also opened an opportunity to redefine the doctor–patient relationship. Gross wrote that bed treatment supported the doctor's attempt to make the patient view him as a 'helper'.[26] And for the patient, too, he claimed, it was 'more charitable and beneficial … to be in a bed rather than in a cell'.[27]

Bed treatment was intended primarily for new patients, who had to become accustomed to living in an institution, and patients with acute illness. Psychiatrists assessed one of the treatment's main effects to be the pacification of patients, which was achieved through a series of techniques, one of which was the reduction of sensory stimuli and the concomitant alteration of patients' field of perception. In contrast to isolation, the reduction of sensory stimuli in the context of bed treatment was spatially configured differently and the patients were permanently monitored so that negative effects did not unfold. The wards were supposed to contain as few stimuli as possible, while still being pleasing. As Neisser explained, patients entering the ward should encounter 'no kind of exciting, sudden, or indeed any strange impression'.[28] Neisser also recommended linoleum flooring in order to dampen 'acoustic stimuli'.[29] The beds were to be arranged such that the space between them made it impossible for patients to touch one another, even with outstretched arms. Neisser recommended that 'the

---

[24] See Monika Ankele, 'Sehen/Berühren. Das Bett als Beziehungsraum', *Unbehaust Wohnen. Konflikthafte Räume in Kunst – Architektur – Visueller Kultur*, ed. Irene Nierhaus and Kathrin Heinz (Bielefeld: Transcript, 2020), 325–42.
[25] Gross, *Allgemeine Therapie*, 200.
[26] Gross, *Allgemeine Therapie*, 200.
[27] Salgó, 'Die Bettbehandlung', 34.
[28] Neisser, 'Ueber die Bettbehandlung', 684.
[29] Clemens Neisser, 'Die Bettbehandlung der Irren', *Berliner Klinische Wochenschrift*, 27 (1890): 864.

cleanest white sheets' be used, and patients were compelled to wear nightgowns.[30] Psychiatrist Albrecht Paetz underscored the additional advantages of a 'friendly view into nature', because he thought this would make 'the impression on the mind all the more friendly and salutary'.[31] But the unassuming arrangement was not the only feature of the space intended to pacify patients. According to Salgó, another was the 'sleep-inducing effect of the lying position in bed'. Paetz admonished doctors to ensure that patients 'really lie in bed and do not sit', because, he asserted, pacification could only occur in a horizontal position.[32] Other calming aspects of the treatment included the 'comfortable, consistent bed warmth' and the 'freedom from tight clothing', which, according to Gross, could alter patients' perception of their bodies.[33] Moreover, minimal clothing like the nightgown was intended to make sure they stayed in bed, as psychiatrists speculated that patients' feelings of shame would hinder them from showing themselves to their fellow patients if they were dressed in nothing more than a nightgown.

Keeping patients lying horizontally in a room together was intended to have yet another effect. It was supposed to suggest to patients that they were sick. Bed treatment was built upon the association between being bedridden and being sick, thus encouraging patients to see themselves as such and doctors to treat them as such. As Neisser wrote, 'lying in bed and being sick' constitute 'an association that has been engraved in our minds through repeated experience'.[34] At the same time, the sight of the sick ward evoked memories and emotions that coloured the experience of the present moment. For instance, Adolf Gross thought that upon seeing the ward, patients would draw an association between the 'image of the sick ward familiar to them from previous experience' and the sick ward of the psychiatric institution they were entering.[35] Bed rest also suggested to patients they were sick, since 'spending time in bed' could show patients 'the sickness of mental disturbances' and thus cause them to acknowledge they were ill, which doctors considered a necessary condition for recovery.[36]

---

[30] Neisser, 'Die Bettbehandlung der Irren', 865.
[31] Albrecht Paetz, *Die Kolonisirung der Geisteskranken in Verbindung mit dem Offen-Thür-System: ihre historische Entwickelung und die Art ihrer Ausführung auf Rittergut Alt-Scherbitz* (Berlin: Julius Springer, 1893), 53.
[32] Paetz, *Die Kolonisirung*, 213.
[33] Gross, *Allgemeine Therapie*, 133.
[34] Neisser, 'Die Bettbehandlung der Irren', 864.
[35] Gross, *Allgemeine Therapie*, 133.
[36] On the distinctions between feeling ill, knowing one is ill and acknowledging one is ill, see Karl Heilbronner, 'Über Krankheitseinsicht', *Allgemeine Zeitschrift für Psychiatrie*, 58 (1901): 608–31.

Almost every textbook from the era worked with the concept of 'acknowledging one's own illness' (*Krankheitseinsicht*). It denoted the patient's capacity to make an objective judgement about their own state of health and to distinguish between their own self and the actions and thoughts produced by the illness.[37] Proponents of bed treatment argued that it helped patients arrive at a point where they acknowledged their own illness. In these discussions, psychiatrists often touted bed treatment's 'suggestive power' and its 'psychological dimension',[38] which were generated through the combination of its features: the sick ward, the sight of other patients lying in bed, the experience of staying in bed and remaining in a horizontal position. All these physical aspects of bed treatment coalesced into a sense regime that was supposed to convince patients that they were sick and to subjectivize them as sick persons.

In their reports on bed treatment, doctors compared how they themselves perceived the clinical space, their patients and the sensory environment (sight, smell, noise) before and after it had been implemented at their institutions. In doing so, they attributed significance to their own perceptions. By applying bed treatment, doctors sought to create a space that would enable them to perceive what they as doctors wanted or thought they were supposed to perceive. As Salgó pithily put it: 'They are all lying, ward upon ward, in clean beds.'

From the patient's view

The archive of Bern's psychiatric museum holds a drawing by Léon Alphonse Kropf that depicts a sick ward at the nearby Waldau psychiatric hospital (Figure 12.2). The drawing offers a patient's perspective on the treatment space. At the same time, the drawing is the expression of Kropf's detailed observations, which required – alongside his ability to put what he saw onto paper – time.

Kropf's drawing depicts a large, bright, open space. The middle ground of the page shows three beds, with a male patient lying down in each one. There is a bed abutting the wall and two beds in the middle of the room. A fourth bed is obscured by a patient in the foreground who, wearing a nightgown, walks through the room carrying a kind of laundry sack, perhaps his bedding, over

---

[37] Heilbronner, 'Über Krankheitseinsicht'.
[38] Psychiatrist Wilhelm Deiters also viewed bed rest as a powerful means of suggestion. He claimed that it could 'suggest to the patient, who often does not acknowledge that he is ill, that he is in fact so'. See Wilhelm Otto Deiters, 'Zweiter Bericht über die Fortschritte des Irrenwesens, nach den Anstaltsberichten erstattet', *Psychiatrisch-Neurologische Wochenschrift*, 12 (1903): 129–37.

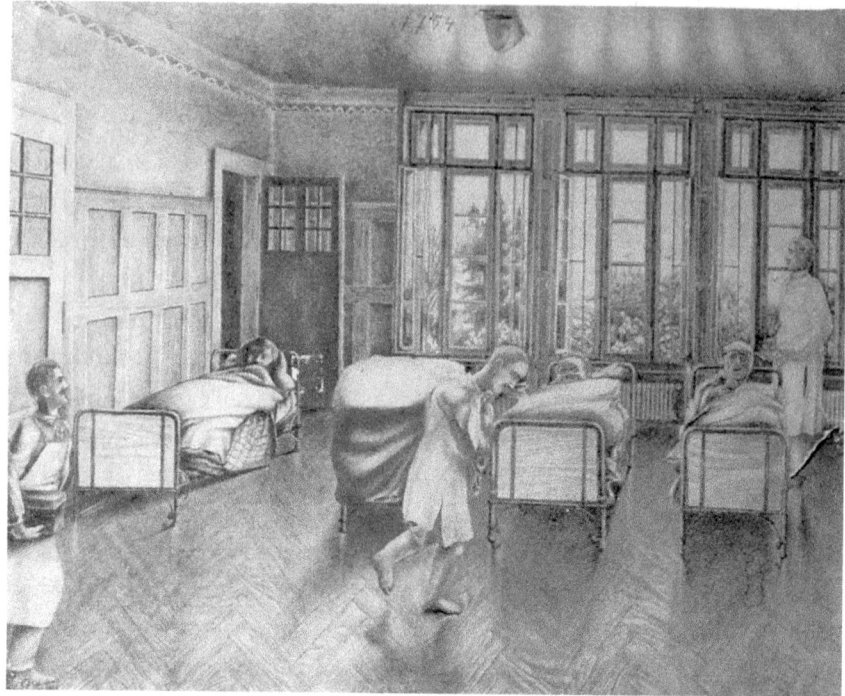

Figure 12.2 Sick ward using bed treatment at the Waldau psychiatric hospital near Bern, drawn by Léon Alphonse Kropf. Psychiatrie-Museum Bern, inventory number 1631.

his shoulder. While the patient on the right side of the drawing sits somewhat upright in his bed, the other two patients have their blankets pulled so far up that only their faces can be seen. Sunk into their blankets, they appear tired, weak, sickly. In the foreground on the left, a nurse enters the room. Diagonally across from him is a doctor who looks over at the opened door on the other side of the room. There are no other objects or furniture in the room aside from the beds. There are no pictures on the walls. The only decorative feature is some plaster around the ceiling, which must have been particularly visible for those lying down. Behind the row of beds, there is – at least from the artist's perspective – a view outside. In their letters, patients regularly wrote about how much they desired to be outdoors. The three large windows let daylight into the room, and Kropf also drew the bright squares of light that they cast onto the ceiling. The sides of the windows are open. They are not barred, but they are so thin that it would be impossible to slip through them. Still, they not only let sunlight into the room but also fresh air. Perhaps the patients in their beds are not positioned towards the windows because they do not want to be blinded by the sun. The windows open out onto a park with trees, bushes and flowers. The big, cloudless sky is not coloured in. The view out the window into the blossoming flora creates a stark contrast to the austerity, emptiness and sadness of the sick ward. Being able to look outside was likely of considerable significance for the patients relegated to long days in bed.

Kropf's drawing leads us to the next section of the chapter, which deals with how patients reacted to the sense regime of bed treatment and the prescription of bed rest. It also analyses the forms of perception that this regime produced, bolstered or re-evaluated. How did patients' place in space, their supine posture, the sense regime that confronted them and the time that they spent in bed alter what and how they perceived? And did the treatment evoke specific feelings?

Body posture and self-perception

Entries in patients' medical records and patients' own writings provide fruitful sources for studying the relation between body posture and self-perception. The supine position and the temporal dimension of bed rest impacted how patient Margaretha W. perceived herself. In a letter from the psychiatric clinic in Heidelberg from September 1895, Margaretha W. described how bed treatment affected her: 'I am currently back in the ward next to the dormitories, where the agitated sick people are, where I am almost always in bed, discouraged and made into a little child.'[39] The effects that she described were certainly intended by the doctors. As Salgó put it, bed treatment made the sick person 'helpless in a most beneficent way'.[40] Psychiatrist Ludwig Scholz also used the term 'helplessness' when discussing bed treatment. He noted that when the sick were put to bed, they calmed down 'as if a feeling of helplessness and neediness lay dormant in the depths of even the most confused mind'.[41] While psychiatrists conceived of patients' situation as a positive state of helplessness, Margaretha W. thought it made patients needy, compliant and docile, a condition, she explained, that increased their willingness to follow doctors' orders. Bed treatment was intended

---

[39] Universitätsarchiv Heidelberg, medical records of the Irrenklinik Heidelberg, L–III, medical records of Margaretha W., signature 01/1, letter from 16 September 1895, no pagination. Original text: 'so dass ich mich momentan wieder in der Abteilung neben den Schlafsälen, wo die aufgeregten Kranken sind, befinde, wo ich fast immer zu Bett bin mut+willenlos gemacht worden wie ein Kleinkind.'

[40] Salgó, 'Die Bettbehandlung', 35.

[41] Ludwig Scholz, *Leitfaden für Irrenpfleger* (Halle a. S.: C. Marhold, 1909), 238. Original: 'als ob ein Gefühl der Hülflosigkeit und Hülfsbedürftigkeit in der Tiefe auch des verworrensten Bewusstseins schlummere.'

to evoke this state of being. Margaretha W. experienced constantly lying down in bed as belittling and identified it as a cause of her feelings of resignation, loss of self-determination and loss of self.

Lying versus standing

Patients thematized the different corporeal feelings associated with both lying down and an upright posture, a discrepancy that grew starker the longer they remained in bed. These distinct feelings were not only connected to different modes of self-perception but could also signify different modes of being in the world. Marta K., a patient at the University of Tübingen's psychiatric clinic, remarked to doctors in June 1919 that 'in bed, she sometimes [has] the feeling as if somebody were draining her body's energy, and that when she stands up, she is herself again'.[42] It is likely that doctors interpreted this lack of energy as a desirable, pacifying effect of bed treatment, with the patient lying in bed as she was supposed to. However, Marta K. interpreted it as a loss of autonomy, as if her actions were being dictated by others ('she sometimes [has] the feeling as if somebody …'). Only after getting out of bed and standing upright did she feel as if she were 'herself'. In a letter from July 1919, Marta K. wrote that she had been in bed for months, while asserting that the 'working life' was more in line with her wishes. She contrasted the active life with 'compulsory lying in bed', which she called the 'heaviest burden'. Thus, in her mind, an upright posture and lying down were associated with distinct forms of self-perception and differences in her (in)ability to participate, to determine her own life and to act.

Gerda L., a patient at the psychiatric clinic in Heidelberg, also reflected on the differences between upright and lying postures. She observed a connection between how her body felt when she was upright and when she was reposed and the clothing that patients wore during the day and at night. She associated lying with night-time and rest and standing upright with daytime and work. Her account expounds 'that one, as long as one is up and dressed, has a completely different feeling of activity and exertion than when one has completed the day's work, put on one's nightgown, and laid down in bed'.[43] Bed treatment intended to blur the lines between these familiar associations by forcing patients to wear a

---

[42] Universitätsarchiv Tübingen, medical records of the Universitätsklinik für Gemüts- und Nervenkrankheiten Tübingen, signature 669/1537 (copy of the medical records held in the Sammlung Prinzhorn, Universitätsklinikum Heidelberg), medical records of Marta K., entry from 23 June 1919.
[43] Universitätsarchiv Heidelberg, medical records of the Irrenklinik Heidelberg, L–III, medical records of Gerda L., signature 00/151, 20/272, undated report, no pagination.

nightgown and remain in bed during the day. The corporeal and mental effects of lying in bed, which Gerda L. contrasted with 'exertion' and Marta K. described as 'energy draining', were simply parts of the treatment itself. It was intended to pacify and tire the awake, energetic body.

Bed rest affected Siegfried L. in a way wholly divergent from doctors' intentions. His medical records from the psychiatric clinic in Heidelberg note that every day, he asked to be released, requested his clothes and told the doctors he would no longer remain in bed because it was 'making him crazy'.[44] He did not see the sickbed as a site of healing, and he did not acknowledge he was sick in the way that doctors wanted. Instead, he felt that the bed itself was what was making him sick in the first place.

Helene K. also expressed the feelings that constantly being in bed evoked in her. Her medical records from February 1899 note that her mood had been good when she was outdoors and that it changed suddenly when she entered the ward, where she seemed depressed. She told the doctors: 'I am so unhappy that I always have to lie here.'[45] Helene K. traced her changed mood back to the medically prescribed bed rest and the experience of perpetually lying in bed (indeed, patients often used the word 'perpetually' in their accounts of bed treatment). In doing so, she attributed her unhappiness not to an 'inner' state or to something wrong with herself but, like Siegfried L., to an external cause. Helene K.'s explanation could also have had the intention of getting permission to stand and go outside, where she, according to the doctors, was not unhappy.

Rest and movement

During bed treatment, most patients were immobilized, their world limited to the small space around their beds. This could amplify their need for movement and contact with an outside world that seemed out of reach. Permanently lying in bed certainly increased Marta K.'s desire to go outside and breathe the fresh air. In a letter to her grandmother dated 1 January 1920, she wrote: 'Unfortunately, I am always lying in bed and waiting every day for my release, as my stay here has no point any longer. The wish for fresh air and movement, to go home and be in a familiar place is often almost unbearable.' At the end of the letter, she

---

[44] Universitätsarchiv Heidelberg, medical records of the Irrenklinik Heidelberg, L–III, medical records of Siegfried L., signature 00/43, entry from 23 September 1900.
[45] Original medical records held in the Sammlung Prinzhorn, Universitätsklinikum Heidelberg, without signature, Heil- und Pflegeanstalt Illenau, medical records of Helene K., entry from 18 February 1899, no pagination.

repeated that she was in the hospital 'without movement' and that she had to live 'in a stench'. In an undated letter to her mother that was probably penned in December 1919 or January 1920, she again expressed her strong desire to go outside and again establish a connection between this need and her current situation of lying in bed all day. She related that she had not been outdoors for a long time and then, in the same sentence, complained that she felt 'the constant lying down in all my limbs'. She also gave voice to the joy she experienced at the prospect of taking a walk with her mother. Marta K. wanted to go outside to inhabit a different space, to move her body, to inhale fresh air, to be together with loved ones and to take in the world with all her senses again. Thus, in a comprehensive sense, being outdoors constituted the opposite of lying in bed and being closed off mentally, spatially and sensorily.

The reduction of sensory stimuli that doctors sought to achieve through bed treatment could remind patients of familiar experiences that were part of a life that seemed far removed from the isolated one they were leading at the hospital. Memories of life outside the institution were filled with a variety of sensory impressions that represented that life and its experiences in the minds of patients. In contrast to the positions of patients in Kropf's drawing, Metta W. described her view out the window in a letter to her mother. She reported that 'the yard here is so sad and the vegetation so lean; one sees just a few flowers from the window and they stir up melancholic thoughts inside of me. Do the magnolias and acacias still smell so sweet like they did back then?'[46] Metta W. articulated the loss of a world, painfully recalled. Instead of experiencing these sights and memories as salubrious, as the doctors intended, they saddened her by reminding her that she was not allowed to touch, smell and see them directly.

In a letter from 15 December 1919, Marta K. also recalled a sensory experience: 'Movement in my mind without moving my limbs is all that I have for recreation here; I hardly remember anymore how snow crunches when one rolls it into a ball.' At the end of her letter, she voiced little hope for recovery, writing, 'The only solid thing here are castles in the air.' In this sense, the world of imagination and ideas represented the world in which she could (still) move without leaving the bed and thus while at least superficially following the doctors' orders.

---

[46] Universitätsarchiv Heidelberg, medical records of the Irrenklinik Heidelberg, L–III, medical records of Metta W., signature 03/25, letter from 17 March 1903 (copy).

Conclusion

'There is nothing intrinsically meaningful in any object, but the way in which an object is constructed in a space, placed into a narrative, associated with something beyond itself, and with past experiences, all endow said object with meaning,'[47] writes Rob Boddice on how many entangled factors have to come together to make an object significant. This holds for the bed and its place in the context of bed treatment. I have grappled with two 'perceptual' perspectives on bed treatment. First, the perspective of doctors who employed bed treatment to create a space that was fundamentally different from the sensory environment of the individual cells that had been customary in psychiatric institutions. The space of bed treatment was intended to evoke forms of spatial perception different from those evoked by the cell. Its material, spatial and sensual layout was supposed to shape patients' perceptions in a specific way. Succinctly put, the space's visual appearance and the bodily experience of constantly lying down in bed were supposed to generate both the feeling that one was ill and the feeling that one could recover. Bed treatment worked with associations (lying down in bed and being sick) and memories (hospitals as such) to affect patients' perception and suggest to them that they were sick. Second, the perspective of patients, who reacted to the experience of always lying down in bed with particular emotional responses, whether it be feelings of unhappiness or feelings that they would soon go crazy. The lying position also impacted patients' perceptions of themselves, as they distinguished between what it meant to lie down and what it meant to be upright. Stuck in bed, the need to move around, change surroundings and do different things weighed heavily on them, because the bed limited their ability to participate in social situations and have contact with others. The reduction of sensory stimuli during treatment could turn the sense of sight and the view out the window into a channel for other senses, stirring up memories and exciting the senses of smell, touch and hearing. Patients' accounts articulate thoughts, explanations, reflections and experiences. They give the impression that patients, at least to outward appearances, followed doctors' orders and remained in bed. However, they offer little insight into the concrete practices that patients developed to deal with the bed, into how they resisted, subverted or challenged bed treatment and its sense regime. After all, patients did not always lie 'ward upon ward, in clean beds' as the doctors wished.

---

[47] Rob Boddice, *The History of Emotions* (Manchester: Manchester University Press, 2018), 345.

The patients' perspectives, revealed in ego documents and medical records, can rarely be situated in a broader context. It is difficult to draw nuanced conclusions about differences in perception on the basis of gender or class; about how patients' perception was impacted by the duration of bed treatment, the actual appearance of the rooms and the presence or absence of a view out the window; and about how past life experiences, diagnoses and opinions influenced how and what patients perceived.[48] But even though these questions might go unanswered and the patients' statements thus remain fragmentary and detached, taking them into account opens up important insights into bed treatment and its sense regime, which sets the stage for further comparison and deeper analysis. Thus, I offer an initial exploration of the connections between bed treatment and perception and of some of the source material that might aid further research.[49]

---

[48] See Victoria Bates, 'Sensing Space and Making Place: The Hospital and Therapeutic Landscapes in Two Cancer Narratives', *Medical Humanities*, 45 (2019): 10–20, http://dx.doi.org/10.1136/medhum-2017-011347.

[49] When criticisms of bed treatment gained in volume after the First World War, they often remonstrated that it only furthered patients' solipsistic tendencies because the constant bed rest and lack of activity made patients focus their attention on themselves too much. Work therapy, which became increasingly popular after the war, was supposed to distract patients from their own thoughts by making them focus on their work and engagement with concrete objects. Indeed, this type of treatment was sometimes also called 'distraction therapy'.

13

Feeling Penfield

Annmarie Adams

Neurosurgeon Wilder Penfield commissioned New York decorator Barnet Phillips to curate a particular atmosphere for the Art Deco hospital lobby of the Montreal Neurological Institute (MNI), often called The Neuro. It is highly significant that Phillips was not the architect of the building – Montreal architect Robert Macdonald (of Ross & Macdonald) designed the overall hospital – but was hired to design this particular space. *Funny that Penfield misspells Macdonald in his autobiography. How could he get that wrong?* Phillips was well known as a designer of stunning interiors, including at least five hospitals or related medical buildings: the New York Academy of Medicine, Fifth Avenue Hospital, Lenox Hill hospital, St Luke's Hospital Nurses Home and the Allegheny General Hospital of Pittsburgh.[1] Penfield may have (*would have*) known the buildings from his time in New York from 1921 to 1928.[2] As a special interior commission, part of the lobby's visual power derives from its distinctiveness from the rest of the building – it is the only space like it and demanded a specialized design and designer. Phillips designed the lobby in a style that art and architectural historians would describe as Art Deco, but the hospital is not an Art Deco building. Our information about the design intentions of the lobby mostly comes from Penfield's copious correspondence with the decorator and other stakeholders. Since the lobby and its striking furniture are extant, however, personal *observation and life experience also inform this chapter. My private thoughts are in italics. I quote here from one of our daughter's favourite books, the 1973 romance novel* The Princess Bride, *written in two voices: 'This is me. All abridging remarks and other comments will be in this fancy italic type so you'll*

---

[1] 'Barnet Phillips, Designer, 65, Dies: Interior Decorator Worked on Federal Reserve Bank, Club and Hospital Buildings', *New York Times (1923–Current File)*, 2 August 1942.
[2] 'W.G. Penfield, Neurologist Dies: Refined Techniques to Treat Epilepsy – Founded an Institute in Montreal', *New York Times (1923–Current File)*, 6 April 1976.

*know.*³ Conceptually I move back and forth from the lobby to the archives to the lobby, looking for how Penfield expressed his intentions to professional designers. What does one see and from where? How does neurology *feel* through architecture? *And how can I communicate that in words? Can architectural experience be transcribed? Music and architecture are often compared, since they both occupy time. Architectural drawings are like musical notation. Architectural experiences are like performances. Can a building be a notation of a feeling?*

Writing in two or more voices serves several purposes. Needless to say, it shows that different individuals experience architecture and art differently. *I am a subject in this text. I use the sense of my own body, my age, my gender, my education to experience the space. My positionality as an architectural historian and even my role as a mother have shaped it. I am aware of my biases. I think about my feelings. I try to record them in writing.*⁴ *I choose to share them with readers.* Additionally, the approach simulates the mental and written notes many of us take as researchers while producing research papers. In this case, it allows me to make unorthodox associations to seemingly unrelated architectures such as a Baroque urban space, the traditional Japanese tea garden, a rural Catholic church and the generic fenced schoolyard. It also captures some of my personal feelings about Penfield, judgements I could not draw from sources and that I would otherwise not dare to write in an academic text.⁵ As academic authors we rarely reveal our feelings about our subjects or our writing process. That is one reason why this approach may be illuminating, especially in a book about feeling, sensing and experiencing disease. It exposes/reveals the author, me, as a feeling, sensing, experiencing subject. What might we lose from this approach? Certainly we sacrifice some coherence. The text flickers between past and present; between Penfield, others and me. This chapter may become outdated quickly. It is a snapshot of what I feel about one place at one time. We also lose some things we need to lose, such as the presumption that any one body – Penfield's, mine, yours – should serve as a universal instrument to experience and assess architecture. Penfield co-designed the lobby with a particular user in mind: male, tall, with perfect eyesight and a familiarity with other famous medical institutions.

---

³ William Goldman, *The Princess Bride* (New York: Ballantine, 1973), 38.
⁴ On other historians who have tried this, see Emily Robinson, 'Touching the Void: Affective History and the Impossible', *Rethinking History*, 14 (2010): 503–20; and the collection *Emotion and the Researcher: Sites, Subjectivities and Relationships*, ed. Tracey Loughran and Dawn Mannay (London: Emerald, 2018). Thanks to Agnes Arnold-Forster for these recommendations.
⁵ 'An older commitment to objectivity looked in askance at such feeling.' See Katie Barclay, 'The Practice and Ethics of the History of Emotions', *Sources for the History of Emotions: A Guide*, ed. Katie Barclay, Sharon Crozier-De Rosa and Peter N. Stearns (Abingdon: Routledge, 2021), 33.

Approaching the Neuro

The street leading up to the neurological hospital is wide and steep, framed on the west by the greystone campus of McGill University and on the east by a charming residential neighbourhood, known as the McGill Ghetto. In the Ghetto, a grid of streets comprised of rundown and 'earlied-up'[6] triplexes is peppered with 1960s high-rise towers and corner dépanneurs. The sounds are of students, walking and talking, and of cars, forced to stop and start at every block. Cyclists ignore the stop signs, darting brazenly among the moving cars. An ambulance siren blares from a distance. The northward slope of University Street marks the base of Mount Royal, the gentle, picturesque mountain that gives the island and the city its name.

The Neuro sits above busy Pine Avenue, something of a northern boundary to the campus and a traffic speedway, and just eastward of the now-empty Royal Victoria Hospital, a stunning Victorian, pavilion-plan hospital with a dozen or so layered additions (Figure 13.1).[7] At the moment, the massive, empty hospital awaits reuse by the adjacent university, which will refashion it into a site to accommodate interdisciplinary, student-centred learning and other yet-to-be named reuses. Falling into disrepair from six years of emptiness, the RVH is currently serving as a shelter for refugees and homeless Montrealers with pets.[8] The main entry to the MNI, a relief after the climb, comes mid-block on the east side and without much notice. Just before an overhead footbridge, a two-storey section of the castle-like hospital projects slightly towards the street, signalling the location of the door. Just south of the machicolated footbridge, one takes a sharp right inside, ascending a short flight of stairs into a modest vestibule, opens double doors and *enters into another world. By its scale and elegance, it feels like a New York apartment building. The warmth and peaceful quiet are welcome.* Across a busy, north-south running corridor, echoing the street outside, the lobby of the MNI is a glowing, Art Deco, windowless cave (Figure 13.2).

I enter the short end of its rectangular shape and spot a shallow, fluted apse at the far end, framing a white statue. I settle on one of two wooden settees that face each other on the long walls, resting from the climb, and take in the yellowish

---

[6] This is a colloquial term used by conservation architects that suggests making a place seem older than it is.
[7] The layering concept is the central argument of Annmarie Adams, David Theodore and Don Toromanoff, *Royal Victoria Hospital: A Layered History* (Montreal: Ville de Montreal, 2012).
[8] Teddy Elliot, 'Montreal's Royal Victoria Hospital Will Become a Pet-Friendly Homeless Shelter This Winter', *MTL Blog*, 12 November 2019, https://www.mtlblog.com/en-ca/news/montreal/montreals-royal-victoria-hospital-will-become-a-pet-friendly-homeless-shelter-this-winter.

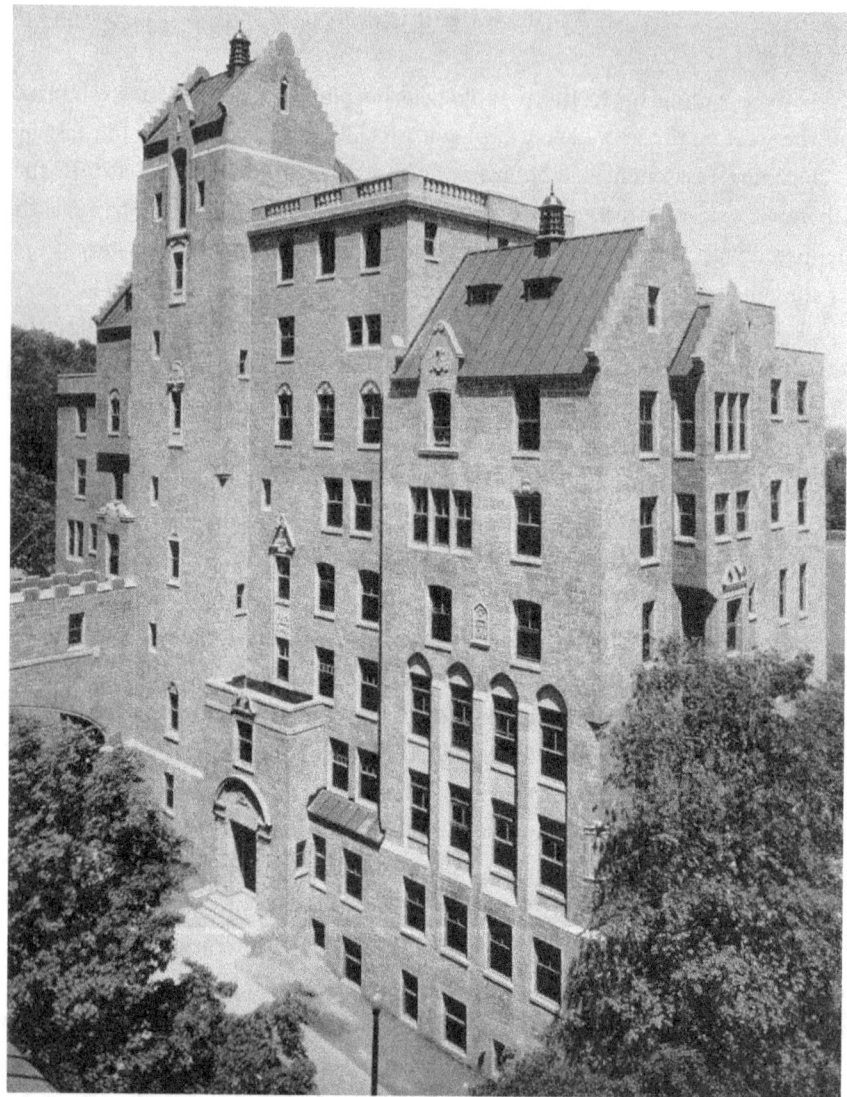

Figure 13.1 Exterior view of the MNI, from 'The Montreal Neurological Institute', *Royal Architectural Institute of Canada*, 11 (1934): 143.

veneer walls and unusual ceiling decoration. An image of a large ram's head peers down from the centre of the ceiling. Beside the settees are four floor lamps and in front is a round table, ornamented on top with a map-like feature. *Some pamphlets about epilepsy are strewn on it, as well as a Montreal Gazette – 'Quebec surpasses total of 200,000 COVID-19 cases on New Year's Eve' – my hearts sinks – and an empty, disposable coffee cup from Timmy's. Vive le Tim des fêtes, the cup*

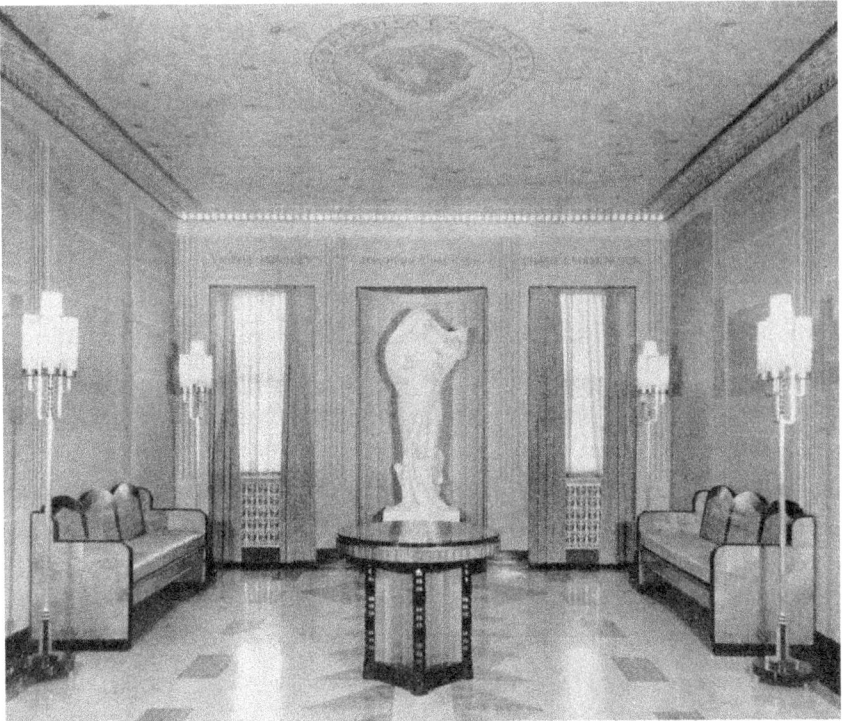

Figure 13.2 MNI lobby view, from 'The Montreal Neurological Institute', *Royal Architectural Institute of Canada*, 11 (1934): 144.

says, in red and green lettering with mistletoe shaped like a maple leaf. The table is a messy spot in an otherwise immaculate hospital lobby. Hospital cleaners are doing an especially thorough job during the pandemic. I feel grateful for that. To the east, towards the statue in her apse, are boarded-up windows over massive radiator grills, blasting heat my way. These windows must have looked out on the site of the McGill stadium. *Hochelaga would be under us now, I think, remembering François Girard's extraordinary film,* Hochelaga Land of Souls. Early floor plans in the Canadian Centre for Architecture (CCA), dated 22 July 1932, show doors where these ghosted windows are today, leading outside to a modest terrace.[9] The design of the entry sequence, with its expensive materials and existential glow, suggests a special place. *It feels a bit like a church, with pews and apse, or maybe a museum, with its hushed atmosphere and carefully placed art. Furniture must be felt.*

---

[9] A 'plot plan' of 25 November 1932, also in the CCA, shows a wide, sweeping driveway with banked edges leading to this terrace.

Intentions

The scholarly mission of this chapter is to explore the potential of interior design to generate feelings and shape experience of a public space designed for neurology; its experiential mission explores how it actually feels to move through that same public space today,[10] *capturing my own thoughts and feelings as I write.* In particular, I consider the prescribed movement, the seat I occupy, the round table, the radiator grills and floor lamps mentioned above, in their purpose-built architectural context (*an understatement*), to understand how material culture shapes architectural meaning for medicine. Archival sources reveal what Penfield wanted the space and objects to say, but how were they understood and experienced? During the nearly ninety years since the building officially opened, subsequent cultural references have shaped the experience of medical architecture. Additionally, non-traditional sources (such as a menu, for example) illuminate ways Penfield thought about the institute. Can a menu reveal architectural intentions? *Yes!*

Movement inside a building is also significant, both actual and prescribed. *Architecture doesn't just illustrate the history of medicine; it is evidence of intentions and aspirations. Also note that users don't always move as prescribed.* Pedestrian and car movement in a city are almost entirely shaped by design. Cars drive on roads. The linearity of a sidewalk impels us forward. A crosswalk indicates a safe place to cross. A lobby, on the other hand, is a resting or pausing space. It receives visitors to a building, invites us to pause by its widened shape and furniture designed for seating and then spatially and visually reorientates us towards whatever might come next: a work shift, a visit, a meeting, an appointment, a delivery. Historians rarely acknowledge that patients are a small percentage of users of hospitals. Lobbies address this wide array of users.[11] *Nowadays it is a place people talk on their phones. Nobody anticipated that. Just like when smoking indoors was suddenly unacceptable, the entries of public buildings became places*

---

[10] I have written two architectural histories of the MNI. See 'Designing Penfield: Inside the Montreal Neurological Institute', *Bulletin of the History of Medicine*, 93 (2019): 207–40; Annmarie Adams and William Feindel, 'Building the Institute', *The Wounded Brain Healed: The Golden Age of the Montreal Neurological Institute, 1934–1984*, ed. William Feindel and Richard Leblanc (Montreal: McGill-Queens University Press, 2016), 441–58. The lobby is included in my 'Art Deco Medicine', *The Routledge Companion to Art Deco*, ed. Bridget Elliott and Michael Windover (London: Routledge, 2019): 160–75.

[11] *Hospital lobbies are understudied. The type I have written most about is the post-1980 atrium.* See Annmarie Adams, David Theodore, Ellie Goldenberg, Coralee McLaren and Patricia McKeever, 'Kids in the Atrium: Comparing Architectural Intentions and Children's Experiences in a Pediatric Hospital Lobby', *Social Science & Medicine*, 70, no. 5 (March 2010): 658–67.

to gather and smoke. Note that the space isn't called a Lobby in the architectural documents. On some drawings architects Ross & Macdonald call it an entrance hall or a 'reception hall'. *Time spent in a lobby can feel like the architectural equivalent of being 'on hold' on a phone call – or in an unmoving/immobile queue. A lobby is a hiatus that invariably anticipates something happening next. In grammar, it might be a colon: the link that anticipates the completion of the sentence.*

Visitors receive mixed spatial messages as they enter the MNI lobby (Figure 13.3). The rather small, rectangular space is axial. Axiality means that users are compelled to move forward in a straight line, towards a destination, like in a church procession towards the altar. In the case of the MNI lobby, this directionality is signalled by the niche form behind the statue, which functions like arms reaching out to us as I enter. The most famous example of this type of 'reception' is the design of St Peter's Square in the Vatican City, whose Baroque shape emits an almost magnetic pull of visitors towards the church. This design was key to the Counter Reformation in which it played a part, by literally bringing Catholics back to the church. At the Neuro, additionally, a pattern in the darker-coloured tiles on the floor leads from the entry to the location of the mid-space, round table. *Following the pattern of the tiles, subconsciously or not, I stop at the table. I look up and I see the statue.* Such a sequence of movement is akin to the design of the classical Japanese tea garden, where visitors might cross streams of water on stepping stones. When a line-up of stepping stones ends, pedestrians instinctively look up and are then confronted by a carefully calculated view. The end of the stones determines when and where users look up. *It is 100 per cent controlled.* Design historian Marc Treib refers to this as 'restriction and then release', noting how it heightens the impact of whatever comes into focus.[12]

Note that unlike most hospital lobbies, the MNI lobby has no admissions desk. *In hospitals today the check-in is the threshold, even in the emergency room. You're admitted when you're admitted. Here the architecture of the lobby admits.* The design was all about education and orientation to neurology, more than enrolment in the hospital. Working closely with Phillips, Penfield ensured that the entrance lobby familiarized staff, patients and visitors to the unique work being done there and particularly to the 'place' of the MNI in history. *The names high up on the walls do this most explicitly.* With relation to 'feeling', it demonstrates what architectural historians might call architecture's 'world-making capacity'.

---

[12] Marc Treib, 'Lessons from the Japanese Garden', *Pacific Horticulture Society* (Winter 1991), https://www.pacifichorticulture.org/articles/lessons-from-the-japanese-garden.

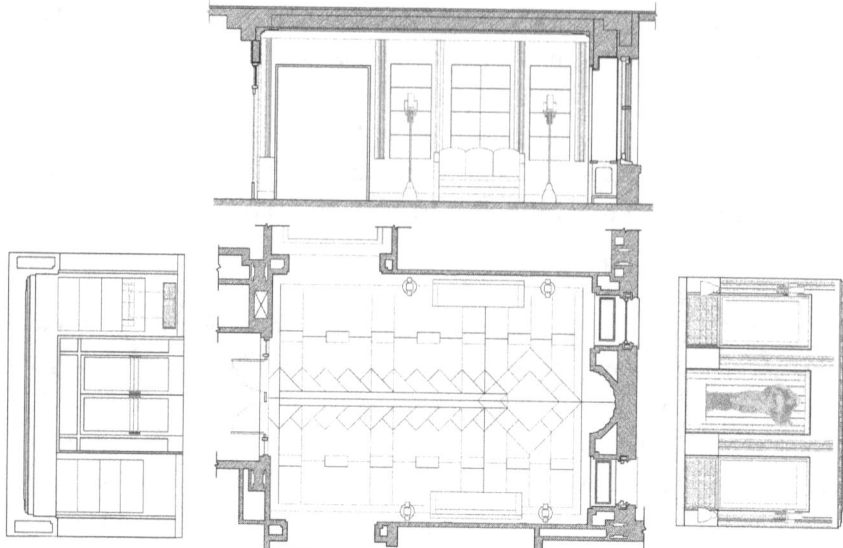

Figure 13.3 Fold-out diagram of the MNI lobby, Jennifer Phan.

Architecture can create a momentary state that suspends its occupants in a particular belief system. Churches are the most obvious example, but many secular spaces function like this too. Like music, architecture can whisk us away to another time and place, allowing us to momentarily escape the present. In his collaborative work on Quebec rural churches, architectural historian Martin Bressani explains, 'An architectural setting is the creation of an alternative universe that projects a fictional framework for the institution it houses.' 'Step into a building, be transported elsewhere', says Bressani, explaining that to enter a church is 'to cross the threshold between two worlds'.[13] *The MNI lobby feels like another world.*

The statue

The focus of the lobby is a marble statue of a female figure, unveiling herself. *She captures our attention right away.* This piece of sculpture has been well-studied already. *I've written about it myself in two other publications. This time, though,*

---

[13] Translated by myself with Martin Bressani's approval, from Martin Bressani and Marc Grignon, 'Une protection spéciale du ciel: Le décor de l'église de Saint-Joachim et les tribulations de l'Église catholique québécoise au début du XIXe siècle', *Journal of Canadian Art History*, 29 (2008): 8–49.

is different. There is much to say about 'Nature'.[14] It also might seem familiar because there are similar statues in important medical institutions in other places, such as Bordeaux, Paris and elsewhere. They are not identical but they bear a family resemblance. A mostly veiled female figure unveils herself, as if undressing privately. In the version at the Neuro, she uses her left hand to pull away the veil from her chest, shoulders and face. Including this statue, with its overt references to other institutions, thus established the Neuro as a node in a network of other, similar places, even though the architectural settings varied. *Art historian Mary Hunter says this, which makes total sense.* Having a copy of 'Nature', to Penfield, was thus something of a status symbol, visual evidence of belonging in an elite medical group, legible to those in the know. Some visitors might recognize that the MNI statue is a copy of the one in Paris. *Have a lot of Montrealers been to Paris? I think so. Recognizing its pedigree might make these viewers feel sophisticated or smart.*

The statue amplifies the meanings of the room. My movement upon entering the room is driven towards the statue, not only because it is a focus and destination but also because the shape of the room, the floor pattern and the furniture arrangement impel me to move towards it. It was undertaken by sculptor Adolphe Galli, copied by Louis-Ernest Barrias, under the watchful eye of American architect Welles Bosworth. *Funny to imagine today a doctor commissioning an architect to oversee an artist copy something. Penfield was obsessed with it.* For a while he even carried around a photo of the statue, *like others might carry a photo of a lover, or a spouse or a child.* In his autobiography, *No Man Alone*, he says, 'I even carried it in my pocket for a time.'[15] It was important to him, *I think*, because he believed it encapsulated his intentions for the MNI. That is, he thought the statue embodied his vision for the place better than anything else, better than the building, better than his writings. When he wrote to McGill University Principal Arthur Currie asking for the funding for statue, he said, 'this statue personifies the ideal of scientific investigation of the secrets of nature.'[16]

It is interesting that Penfield thought the statue communicated the mission more clearly than words, because Penfield was a prolific writer, both of medical papers and of letters. He also received many letters. *He liked words.* Architect Bosworth wrote to Penfield almost weekly with an account of progress made

---

[14] Adams, 'Designing Penfield', 234–9; 'Art Deco Medicine', 160–2.
[15] Wilder Penfield, *No Man Alone: A Neurosurgeon's Life* (Boston, MA: Little, Brown, 1977): 314.
[16] Letter from Wilder Penfield to Arthur Currie, 17 October 1932, Wilder Penfield Fonds, P 142, Osler Library of the History of Medicine, McGill University.

on the copying of the Paris model, undertaken by Barrias from November 1932 to April 1934. The Penfield-Bosworth correspondence reveals Penfield's strong feelings. The neurosurgeon said, for example, that 'the marble is so perfect'[17] and 'we are very much pleased with the statue', expressing his satisfaction.[18] 'The statue is lovely' tells us he liked how it looked.[19] *Could it mean otherwise? Other statements suggest he projected certain feelings on to others:* 'I think you [Bosworth] and Galli fell in love with it so that you could not bear to tint the draperies', he presumed.[20] *In love with it, the architect who designed MIT in love with a replicated statue. Seems unlikely to me. Penfield wants Bosworth and Galli to love Nature.*

Judging by his letters, Bosworth had a sharp sense of humour regarding the commission. *Bosworth is adorable.* When he asked Penfield for money, for example, he said, 'I haven't inquired at the bank, but I presume you have increased the amount so that I may now draw my first installment. I must hurry up and do it, as I have already given it away to my wife and mother-in-law for their Christmas presents.'[21]

As I rest in the lobby, staring at the statue, I consider my own feelings. As a woman, I'm slightly embarrassed that she is unclothed and on display in the lobby. Any shame I might feel, however, is quickly and effectively extinguished by a lifetime of conditioning. As a post-feminist, urban, North American woman, I am accustomed to seeing naked and semi-naked women depicted in public spaces. Sometimes they appear as symbols of societal values, such as justice and fertility. Sometimes they are enlisted to sell things, like cars. I learned decades ago from art historians like Marina Warner and John Berger that most images are produced for a male viewer.[22] I am over it. Because as a historian I know about Penfield's complicated feelings for the statue, I am somewhat entertained by Nature. It amuses me that a heroic figure in the history of medicine carried around a photo of a marble statue of a semi-naked woman and accused others of being in love with it. It feels like secret knowledge.

---

[17] Letter from Wilder Penfield to Welles Bosworth, 27 July 1933, Wilder Penfield Fonds, P 142, Osler Library of the History of Medicine, McGill University.
[18] Letter from Wilder Penfield to Welles Bosworth, 6 September 1934, Wilder Penfield Fonds, P 142, Osler Library of the History of Medicine, McGill University.
[19] Letter from Wilder Penfield to Welles Bosworth, 16 March 1934, Wilder Penfield Fonds, P 142, Osler Library of the History of Medicine, McGill University.
[20] Penfield to Bosworth, 16 March 1934, 2.
[21] Letter from Welles Bosworth to Wilder Penfield, 8 January 1933, Wilder Penfield Fonds, P 142, Osler Library of the History of Medicine, McGill University.
[22] Marina Warner, *Monuments & Maidens: The Allegory of the Female Form* (New York: Atheneum, 1985); John Berger, *Ways of Seeing* (London: Penguin, 1972).

I know from reading Penfield's letters how desperately he wanted the statue and even the exact moment when he thought it possible, which he expressed almost as an epiphany. In June 1932 Penfield wrote to his mother Jean Jefferson Penfield of the instance he first wanted 'Nature' for the MNI:

> There is a statue which stands at the foot of the stairway leading up the Medical Library in the University of Paris. It is done by a man named Barre [sic] in coloured marble. It is the figure of a young woman, heavily cloaked. Only her face and part of her breast can be seen. The gown seems to be held up to the white breasts by a scarab. At the base of the pedestal are the words in French – 'nature unveiling herself before Science'. I have always longed to have a copy. The other day in Cleveland it occurred to me while I was walking along the street, that we might have a copy made and placed in such a position in the entrance that it would suggest to one entering the ideal I have in mind for the whole Institute.[23]

Penfield longed for this statue. It was not until 12 October 1932 that Penfield wrote to Alan Gregg about the idea. Gregg was the head of the Rockefeller Foundation, the wealthy American foundation that paid for the construction of the MNI. Penfield asked for a personal meeting with Gregg, in a week. On the subject of feelings, he noted his anxiety over the statue:

> I am anxious to find out whether or not it would be possible to have the statue which stands at the entrance of the Ecole de medecin [sic] in Paris copied. You may remember it. It is by Barrias and says something about 'La Nature se Devoilant devant la Science'. If the statue is still as I remember it I would like to have it copied and placed in the Neurological Institute. What would your reaction to this be and how can such a thing be achieved?[24]

If the statue is still as he remembers it? Penfield already recognizes that his memory of the statue differs from reality.

Reading Penfield's letters also reveals feelings he had about real, *non-marble*, women too. For example, his wife Helen Penfield served as a sounding board for the famous doctor and was even cited now and then by Penfield to justify his own design decisions. *As if she is an authority*. For example, about the statue he said, 'The statue by Barrios [sic] seems to me altogether fitting and Helen feels so without question.'[25] By November 1932, when the commission to copy

---

[23] Letter from Wilder Penfield to Jean Jefferson Penfield, 17 July 1932, Wilder Penfield Fonds, P 142, Osler Library of the History of Medicine, McGill University.
[24] Letter from Wilder Penfield to Alan Gregg, 12 October 1932, Wilder Penfield Fonds, P 142, Osler Library of the History of Medicine, McGill University.
[25] Penfield to Jean Jefferson Penfield, 27 November 1932.

the statue was issued, his feelings of longing had changed to guilt: 'I have a sort of guilty feeling about this, as the statue is an early love of mine and it seems somehow wrong to have it now.'[26] *An early love of mine. Perhaps the wrongness he felt was linked to the fact that he had left behind his 'early love', that it was a mere copy, or that it cost money.* By 18 May 1934, however, he defended the expense to the university purchasing-department accountant, a Mr J. Finlay, who seemed to sense Penfield's strong feelings for 'Nature'. Penfield insisted, 'the statue is not my personal property or in any way a personal expenditure. It is being paid for out of funds set aside for that purpose from our budget, and it will be used solely as an artistic decoration in the entrance hall.'[27] *As an architectural historian, I am impressed that Penfield recognized 'decoration' as a 'use'. In my own experience working with doctors, I've noticed they use 'functional' as a stand-in for inexpensive.*

Furniture and decor

Let's now turn to the lobby furniture. *As you will recall, I am sitting on a settee, on the south wall of the lobby, which gives wide views of the entrance sequence from University Street to the left and allows me to glance at the marble statue now and then, to my right. Directly in front of me is the round, inlaid table. Let me ponder the round table.* Drawings at the CCA (33407, 2 April 1934) tell us it is 3 feet (91 cm) in diameter and 2'7" (79 cm) tall. At its centre, framed in a circle, is an inlaid depiction of a cross section of a brain. The framing circle is surrounded by eight triangulated segments. Another circle frames the eight segments. Here, at the centre of the lobby, in the centre of a round table, is an image of the organ that is the reason for this hospital: the brain. At the opening of the building on 27 September 1934, Penfield described the table inlay as 'the form of a cross-section of the human hemispheres'.[28] The table appears in dozens of archival photos, in different locations in the room. An extraordinary, large-scale drawing in the Canadian Centre for Architecture shows the table simultaneously in plan, section and elevation, revealing the materials to be maple and ash burl. When

---

[26] Penfield to Jean Jefferson Penfield, 27 November 1932.
[27] Letter from Wilder Penfield to J. Finlay, 18 May 1934, Wilder Penfield Fonds, P 142, Osler Library of the History of Medicine, McGill University.
[28] Wilder Penfield, 'The Significance of the Montreal Neurological Institute', *Neurological Biographies and Addresses: Foundation Volume* (London: Oxford University Press, 1936), 44.

I stand in front of the table, which is protected by glass, the reflection of 'Nature' appears exactly on the section of the brain (*I have a photo that shows exactly this*).

Also reflected in the glass top of the round table is the special ceiling design. The ram's head, Aries, is at the centre of the ceiling with four hieroglyphic figures that symbolize the brain. *I remember from previous research that these are drawn from the Edwin Smith papyrus of 3000 BC.*[29] Although our focus is on visual imagery, Penfield tells us that this choice relates to touch. He quotes medical librarian William Willoughby Francis: 'The papyrus states that when the surgeon probes with the finger he feels "a throbbing and a fluttering."'[30]

Archival documents show that the ceiling features the neuroglia cells within the cerebellum after a drawing by Camillo Golgi.[31] Penfield wrote about this image: 'The cells themselves with their sprawling expansions stand out black as when impregnated by Golgi's silver method. The nerve-cells are seen only faintly as rounded disks, while the tiny blood-vessels and coloured background complete the picture.'[32] *What I really like about the ceiling design is not the ram's head, or the hieroglyphics, or the quotes from Galen via W. W. Francis who invokes his famous second cousin, William Osler, but rather the repetitive, almost wallpaper-like background. Here is what Penfield says about it and about the nearby radiator covers, also in my scope from my comfortable position on the settee:*

> In the border about the ceiling in a repeated pattern is to be seen the outline of the fluid-filled cavities within the brain, the cerebral ventricles. The iron gratings used over the radiators in the alcove are from a drawing of a nerve fibre by the French neuro-anatomist Nageotte. The axone is shown with the radiating structure within the nerve sheath about it.[33]

Fascinated by how a neurological image could become such stunning ceiling decoration, I've looked around for drawings by Nageotte. Since I've never actually seen a brain, my references are to insects. I describe it to myself as about fifty black, spider-like forms overlaid on a network of greyish tunnels. I imagine this is how an ant farm might look in section or plan if a bunch of spiders invaded. And the radiator covers do not look to me at all like Nageotte's bug-like lexicon. Just for fun, I put Nageotte's name into the search engine in the Osler Library.

---

[29] Wilder Penfield and Montreal Neurological Institute, *Neurological Biographies and Addresses: Foundation Volume* (London: Oxford University Press, 1936), 42.
[30] Penfield, 'Significance of the Montreal Neurological Institute', 43.
[31] Penfield, 'Significance of the Montreal Neurological Institute', 6.
[32] Penfield, 'Significance of the Montreal Neurological Institute', 6.
[33] Penfield, 'Significance of the Montreal Neurological Institute', 7.

A typewritten essay from 1928 turns up: 'Impressions of Neurology, Neurosurgery, and Neurohistology in Central Europe' from 1928. Penfield writes:

> Professor J. Nageotte of the College de France holds the chair of Comparative Histology. His work has been largely upon peripheral nerves, however. Old, very deaf, and somewhat infirm, he is nevertheless fired with enthusiasm in his work and is mentally alert, still pursuing the subject of his discussions with Cajal upon the peripheral nerve. There is much to be learned in his laboratory in this particular field. He does not go into pathology.[34]

Old, deaf, infirm.

The ceiling must have been particularly important to Penfield, because in early November 1934, he sat down to write thank-you letters to colleagues who could not attend the celebratory opening on 27 September and he described the ceiling. Those who sent letters or telegrams that were read at the event merited these letters. For example, he wrote to Bernardus Brouwer, Jerzy Chorobski, Hugh Cairns, Otfrid Foerster, Walther Spielmeyer and others. To all he included a nearly identical paragraph, almost like a postscript:

> The picture on the front of the menu is a photograph of the ceiling of the entrance hall. The drawing of the neuroglia cells is from an original by Golgi. You will notice in the border of the ventricle, and the Greek legend 'Egkephalon de Trothenta Eidomen Iothenta' comes from Galen, and Francis has interpreted it as 'I have seen a severely wounded brain healed.' The hieroglyphics represent the word 'brain', being the first appearance of that word in literature; it was taken from the Smith papyrus. The ram, of course, symbolizes the head or the brain in astrology.[35]

In this set of nearly identical letters, Penfield describes the ceiling to them almost as a surrogate for the experience of seeing the decor. *Interesting he hardly ever mentions Nature in letters.* Also, a photo of the ceiling illustration constituted the front cover of the menu (Figure 13.4) for the exclusive dinner at the Mount Royal Club on the evening of the opening. The copy of the signed menu in the archives shows that forty-six individuals (*and their guests?*) were invited for

---

[34] Wilder Penfield, 'Neurology in the Scandinavian Countries' and 'Impressions of Neurology, Neurosurgery, and Neurohistology in Central Europe', 1928, Wilder Penfield Fonds, P 142, Osler Library of the History of Medicine, McGill University, 8–9. Typescript was undertaken for the Rockefeller Foundation while Penfield was in Europe in 1928.

[35] For example, see the letter from Wilder Penfield to Spielmeyer, 9 November 1934, Wilder Penfield Fonds, P 142, Osler Library of the History of Medicine, McGill University.

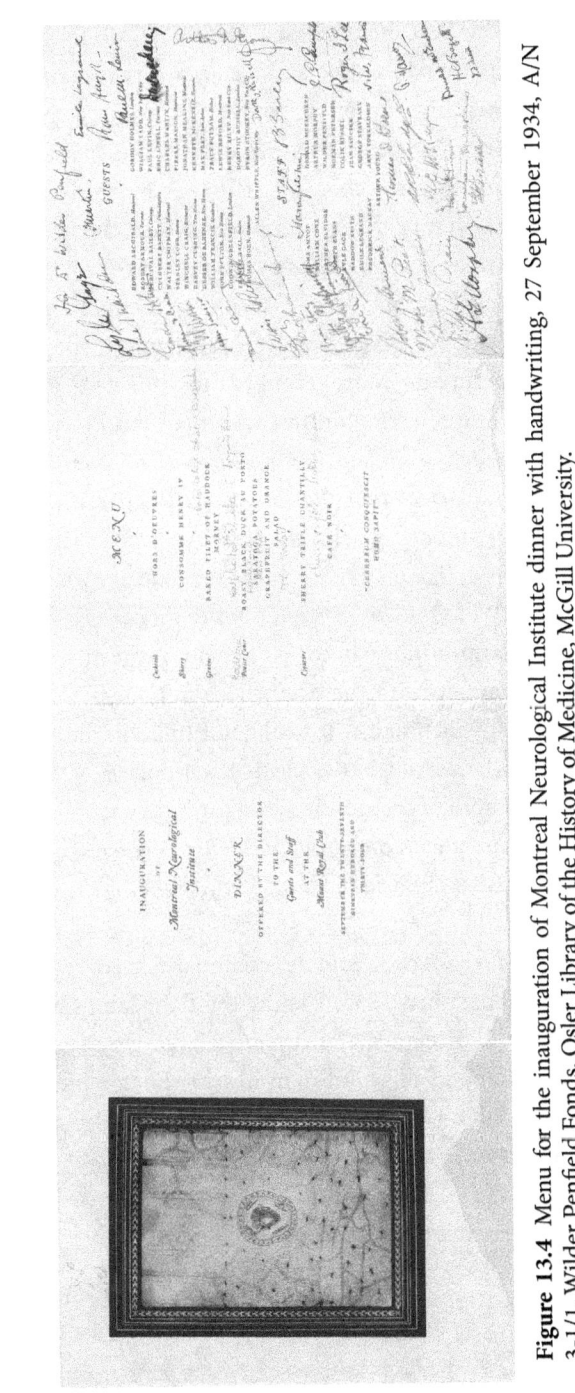

Figure 13.4 Menu for the inauguration of Montreal Neurological Institute dinner with handwriting, 27 September 1934, A/N 3-1/1, Wilder Penfield Fonds, Osler Library of the History of Medicine, McGill University.

consommé, haddock and duck *au porto*. Below the list of food appeared the Latin inscription: CEREBRUM CONQUIESCIT HOMO SAPIT.

Back to the lobby. Another incentive to look upwards is a ring of names of influential medical men high up on all four walls, even on the west wall, above the street entrance. This ring of names defines the space. It contains it. *It is like the fence around the schoolyard*. The location of the names can be somewhat confusing, even to those who have studied the architecture of the MNI, because the names change places over time. In the photo published in the *Journal of the Royal Architectural Institute of Canada* from October 1934, the names on the east wall, over 'Nature', are Victor Horsley, Hughlings Jackson and Charles Sherrington. More recent photos, however, show Thomas Willis, Wilder Penfield and Sherrington in this same location, with Penfield located directly over his beloved 'Nature'. *Email from Dr Richard Leblanc, 23 December 2020, 'You are correct that the names on the frieze were changed following Penfield's death and at Dr Feindel's initiative. I don't recall the exact date when this was done … Thomas Willis's name was added by Dr Feindel. He had a lifelong interest in Willis and his contributions to the cerebral circulation.'*[36] Thankfully, there is an extraordinary note by Penfield, suggesting which of his colleagues may have come up with the original names. Or perhaps it shows who Penfield 'paired' with each name. It is difficult to know, but in any case, an association with MNI neurologists is clear. Each doctor or scientist was somehow linked, in the mind of the author of the list, with a name in the lobby. *So they played musical chairs with the names but left no evidence of the change. It would appear to many that Penfield included himself among the other figures. More secret knowledge.*

The lamps. From my readings of primary material related to the opening of the building on 27 September, 1934, I know the floor lamps are based on drawings of the spine: 'The segmental structure of the lamp-stands betrays recent study of the anatomy of the spine.'[37] In historic photos these appear to be brass or metallic; in more recent photos they look black. *Are they painted? There is a splendid, large-scale (1 1/2" scale) drawing of the lamp at the CCA. Do these lamps look like spines to those of us who have never seen a spine? Or was the meaning only intended for experts?*

---

[36] Dr Richard Leblanc, email to Annmarie Adams, 23 December 2020.
[37] Penfield, 'Significance of the Montreal Neurological Institute', 8.

Control

Penfield sought absolute control of how the viewer would experience the room. For example, he insisted that the statue was in a proper position in the room to have the desired effect upon entry, where she appears to float just above the brain section depiction on the top of the round table. He managed this level of control by determining the statue's overall height and its effect on the viewer. *He must have been a control freak.* Writing to architect Macdonald in 26 May 1933, he said, 'In order to be seen properly the face of the statue must, of necessity, be slightly higher than the face of the observer but I should think it does not need to be more than eighteen inches about the observer's eye.'[38] *Penfield assumes everyone is the same height.* He reveals in this letter that the figure is 6'1" tall. Also remarkable in this letter is that it seems like Macdonald is only then learning about the plan to copy the statue. *This explains why the earlier plans have no niche.*

Penfield wanted visitors to get close to the statue. He compelled this by reducing the size of the lettering on the base of the statue. He wanted it 'just sufficient in size to be read when one stands before the statue.'[39] Additionally, since only one viewer can presumably occupy that ideal spot at a time, Penfield presumed viewers would take in 'Nature' one at a time. Not everyone agreed with Penfield's decisions, including the design experts. On seeing the photo of the lobby in the *Journal of the RAIC* (and months after the opening), Bosworth suggested to Penfield that the statue was too high in the niche, saying her head was a bit too crowded.[40] *Ross & Macdonald produced a splendid sheet of drawings in May 1934. Was this in response to Penfield's criticism, or was this the focus of his remarks? Hard to know.* There is also some discussion of whether the base should be black or white. Penfield told Macdonald to defer to Phillips and eventually they opted for Belgian black marble.[41] *When was Phillips hired?*

The timeline for Phillips's commission was surprisingly short, given the real and symbolic importance of the lobby. The MNI opened on 27 September 1934. Most of the extant correspondence between Penfield and Phillips is from March 1934, a short five months earlier. *Did somebody suggest to Penfield at this late date that he hire an interior designer? Maybe Bosworth? Did the space merit an interior designer because of the beloved statue?* Letters show that Phillips was working

---

[38] Letter from Wilder Penfield to Robert MacDonald [sic], 26 May 1933, Wilder Penfield Fonds, P 142, Osler Library of the History of Medicine, McGill University.
[39] Penfield to MacDonald [sic], 16 May 1934.
[40] Bosworth to Penfield, 13 November 1934.
[41] Penfield to MacDonald [sic], 16 May 1934.

on the space before the completion of *Nature* in Paris. Penfield reported to the New York designer on 16 March 1934 that the copying was complete.

My visit is drawing to a close. The lobby is a busy place. Penfield's feelings about the statue also impacted the building's exterior. When he told his mother that the statue suggested to visitors 'the ideal I have in mind for the whole Institute', he said 'there should be something more of course. The other thing has to do with pity for the suffering of our brothers. I don't know what to do about that. Perhaps that might be added in a further legend.'[42] *I bet that the inscription on the MNI's exterior is this legend he had in mind, this compensation for the limited message of the statue.* He even referred to it as a legend in a letter to his mother. In September 1933 he told her the story of the inscription for a stone slab outside the institution: 'At last, after much thought and consultation, have boiled it down to the simple and unpretentious legend: Dedicated to Relief of Sickness and Pain and to the study of Neurology.'[43] In the letter to his mother, Penfield took credit for the design, as if he were the architect, including his own qualms. He wrote, '[The architects] could not bring themselves to put a brain into stone until I brought them a drawing of one – done by Christopher Wren, and now they have sketched it for just over the door, and it is I who now hesitates [sic].'[44] *He finds, they sketch.*

Penfield's letters end in 1935, when Jean Jefferson Penfield died, essentially closing our window to the neurologist's private feelings on architecture and a host of other issues. *The letters are so precious. They allow us to assess a space through a figure other than the architect.* And even more, they reveal how Penfield's (ostensibly the client) architectural actions were motivated by feelings: powerful positive emotions and some anxieties. This view of Penfield flies in the face of the well-known image of him as a rather stoic, rational neurosurgeon. *I would suggest they show him as somewhat uncertain and domineering.* The letters also reveal the degree to which Penfield shaped his own legacy, 'by design', in both textual and architectural traces. *Channelling author William Goldman in* The Princess Bride, *'Me again, last time this chapter.*[45] *I rise to depart, buttoning up for the cold. University Street is quieter now. I exit the double doors, turning right under the overhead bridge. Fatigued by what Emily Robinson calls 'the intensity of the archival encounter',*[46] *I loop around the steep, snowy site of the empty Royal Victoria Hospital and head home to write this chapter.*

---

[42] Penfield to Jean Jefferson Penfield, 17 July 1932.
[43] Penfield to Jean Jefferson Penfield, 10 September 1933.
[44] Penfield to Jean Jefferson Penfield, 10 September 1933.
[45] Goldman, *Princess Bride*, 254.
[46] Robinson, 'Touching the Void', 503.

Select bibliography

The reproduction of all the primary and secondary works used in this book in a single list would, we feel, be unhelpful, given the wide range of specialist focus. Instead, we provide here a short list of secondary works that were influential in the writing of the various chapters in general terms, and that will provide the most coherent orientation for the reader who wishes to engage with the relevant literature. Specific references are, of course, given in full in each chapter.

Abel, Emily K., *Sick and Tired: An Intimate History of Fatigue* (Chapel Hill: University of North Carolina Press, 2021).

Ahmed, Sara, *The Cultural Politics of Emotion* (Edinburgh: Edinburgh University Press, 2004).

Banner, Olivia, *Communicative Biocapitalism: The Voice of the Patient in Digital Health and the Health Humanities* (Ann Arbor: University of Michigan Press, 2017).

Bates, Victoria, 'Sensing Space and Making Place: The Hospital and Therapeutic Landscapes in Two Cancer Narratives', *Medical Humanities*, 45 (2019): 10–20.

Baumann, Imanuel, *Dem Verbrechen auf der Spur: eine Geschichte der Kriminologie und Kriminalpolitik in Deutschland 1880 bis 1980* (Göttingen: Wallstein, 2006).

Biess, Frank, and Daniel M. Gross, eds, *Science & Emotions after 1945* (Chicago: University of Chicago Press, 2014).

Boddice, Rob, ed., *Pain and Emotion in Modern History* (Houndmills: Palgrave Macmillan, 2014).

Boddice, Rob, *The Science of Sympathy: Morality, Evolution and Victorian Civilization* (Urbana-Champaign: University of Illinois Press, 2017).

Boddice, Rob, *The History of Emotions* (Manchester: Manchester University Press, 2018).

Boddice, Rob, *A History of Feelings* (London: Reaktion, 2019).

Boddice, Rob, and Mark Smith, *Emotion, Sense, Experience* (Cambridge: Cambridge University Press, 2020).

Bonea, Amelia, Melissa Dickson, Sally Shuttleworth and Jennifer Wallis, eds, *Anxious Times: Medicine and Modernity in Nineteenth-Century Britain* (Pittsburgh: University of Pittsburgh Press, 2019).

Bourke, Joanna, 'Fear and Anxiety: Writing about Emotion in Modern History', *History Workshop Journal*, 55 (2003): 111–33.

Bourke, Joanna, *Rape: A History from the 1860s to the Present* (London: Little, Brown, 2007).

Bourke, Joanna, *The Story of Pain from Prayer to Painkillers* (Oxford: Oxford University Press, 2014).

Cabanas, Edgar, and Eva Illouz, *Manufacturing Happy Citizens: How the Science and Industry of Happiness Control Our Lives* (Cambridge: Polity, 2019).

Caduff, Carlo, *The Pandemic Perhaps: Dramatic Events in a Public Culture of Danger* (Oakland: University of California Press, 2015).

Caruth, Cathy, *Unclaimed Experience: Trauma, Narrative, and History* (Baltimore, MD: Johns Hopkins University Press, 1996).

Das, V., 'On Singularity and the Event: Further Reflections on the Ordinary', *Recovering the Human Subject: Freedom, Creativity and Decision* (Cambridge: Cambridge University Press, 2018), 53–73.

Dror, Otniel E., Bettina Hitzer, Anja Laukötter and Pilar León-Sanz, eds, 'History of Science and the Emotions', *Osiris*, 31 (2016).

Eghigian, Greg, *The Corrigible and the Incorrigible: Science, Medicine, and the Convict in Twentieth-Century Germany* (Ann Arbor: University of Michigan Press, 2015).

Elberfeld, Jens, *Anleitung zur Selbstregulation: Eine Wissensgeschichte der Therapeutisierung im 20. Jahrhundert* (Frankfurt: Campus, 2020).

Feder, Ellen K., 'Tilting the Ethical Lens: Shame, Disgust, and the Body in Question', *Hypatia*, 26 (2011): 633–50.

Fernandez, Luke, and Susan J. Matt, *Bored, Lonely, Angry, Stupid: Changing Feelings about Technology, from the Telegraph to Twitter* (Cambridge, MA: Harvard University Press, 2019).

Göbel, Hanna Katharina, and Sophia Prinz, eds, *Die Sinnlichkeit des Sozialen: Wahrnehmung und materielle Kultur* (Bielefeld: Transcript, 2015).

Hickman, Clare, *Therapeutic Landscapes: A History of English Hospital Gardens since 1800* (Manchester: Manchester University Press, 2013).

Hitzer, Bettina, *Krebs fühlen: Eine Emotionsgeschichte des 20. Jahrhunderts* (Stuttgart: Klett-Cotta, 2020).

Hitzer, Bettina, *Cancer and the Emotions in 20th-Century Germany* (Oxford: Oxford University Press, forthcoming).

Honigsbaum, Mark, *The Pandemic Century: One Hundred Years of Panic, Hysteria, and Hubris* (New York: W. W. Norton, 2020).

Hunt, Nigel, *Landscapes of Trauma: Psychology of the Battlefield* (London: Routledge, 2019).

Illouz, Eva, *Cold Intimacies: The Making of Emotional Capitalism* (Cambridge: Polity Press, 2007).

Kelly, A. H., F. Keck and C. Lynteris, *The Anthropology of Epidemics* (London: Routledge, 2019).

Kirby, Jill, *Feeling the Strain: A Cultural History of Stress in Twentieth-Century Britain* (Oxford: Oxford University Press, 2019).

Lakoff, Andrew, *Unprepared: Global Health in a Time of Emergency* (Oakland: University of California Press, 2017).

Lamb, Jonathan, *The Evolution of Sympathy in the Long Eighteenth Century* (London: Routledge, 2009).

Lars-Christer, Hydén, and Jens Brockmeier, eds, *Health, Illness and Culture: Broken Narratives* (New York: Routledge, 2008).
Lawlor, Clark, *Consumption and Literature: The Making of a Romantic Disease* (Houndmills: Palgrave Macmillan, 2007).
Loughran, Tracey, and Dawn Mannay, eds, *Emotion and the Researcher: Sites, Subjectivities and Relationships* (London: Emerald, 2018).
Lüdtke, Alf, *The History of Everyday Life: Reconstructing Historical Experiences and Ways of Life* (Princeton, NJ: Princeton University Press, 1995).
Lupton, Deborah, *Medicine as Culture: Illness, Disease and the Body* (3rd edition, London: Sage, 2012).
Meyers, Todd, and Stefanos Geroulanos, *The Human Body in the Age of Catastrophe: Brittleness, Integration, Science, and the Great War* (Chicago: University of Chicago Press, 2018).
Milnes, Christopher, *A History of Euphoria: The Perception and Misperception of Health and Well-Being* (New York: Routledge, 2019).
Newton, Hannah, *Misery to Mirth: Recovery from Illness in Early Modern England* (Oxford: Oxford University Press, 2018).
Reckwitz, Andreas, 'Affective Spaces: A Praxeological Outlook', *Rethinking History*, 16 (2012): 241–58.
Reckwitz, Andreas, 'How the Senses Organise the Social', *Praxeological Political Analysis*, ed. Michael Jonas and Beate Littig (New York: Routledge, 2017).
Rimmon-Kenan, Shlomith, 'What Can Narrative Theory Learn from Illness Narratives?', *Literature and Medicine*, 25 (2006): 241–5.
Robinson, Emily, 'Touching the Void: Affective History and the Impossible', *Rethinking History*, 14 (2010): 503–20.
Rosenberg, Charles E., *Explaining Epidemics and Other Studies in the History of Medicine* (Cambridge: Cambridge University Press, 1992).
Rosenberg, Charles E., and Janet Golden, eds, *Framing Disease: Studies in Cultural History* (New Brunswick: Rutgers University Press, 1992).
Scambler, Graham, 'Covid-19 as a "Breaching Experiment": Exposing the Fractured Society', *Health Sociology Review*, 29 (2020): 140–8.
Scheer, Monique, 'Are Emotions a Kind of Practice (and Is That What Makes Them Have a History? A Bourdieuian Approach to Understanding Emotion', *History and Theory*, 51 (2012): 193–220.
Schmidt, Nina, *The Wounded Self: Writing Illness in Twenty-First-Century German Literature* (Rochester, NY: Camden House, 2018).
Stenner, Paul, *Liminality and Experience: A Transdisciplinary Approach to the Psychosocial* (Houndmills: Palgrave Macmillan, 2017).
Viney, William, Felicity Callard and Angela Woods, 'Critical Medical Humanities: Embracing Entanglement, Taking Risks', *Medical Humanities*, 41 (2015): 2–7.

Index

Ahmed, Sara 127–8, 130–1, 135
Anderson, Benedict 6
animality 82, 119
Anthropocene 204–5, 211
anthropology 13, 45, 74, 143, 208
anxiety 4, 10, 27, 29, 49–51, 56–8, 69, 93–4, 96, 137, 139, 167, 204–5, 210, 272
   anxiety disorders 63, 148, 161, 243
   narratives of 126–30, 135, 265
   reduction of 193, 195, 198–9, 206, 211, 213–14
Art Deco 255, 257
artificial intelligence (AI) 86, 88, 91–2, 95–102
   algorithms 85, 88, 90–3, 95–7
   machine learning 88, 91
Ashrawi, Ilana 141
authority 3–4, 21, 151, 155, 216
autobiography 136–7, 255, 263
autopathography 128, 130, 133, 139

Barrias, Louis-Ernest 263–5
bed treatment 239–54
bioculture 4–5, 12–14, 17, 23
biophilia 207–10, 212, 214
bodies
   body history 4–5, 11–18, 220
   and climate/nature 197
   damaged 150–1, 198
   dangerous 44
   dead 37–40
   digital 88–90, 92
   diseased 37, 63, 78, 122, 127, 132, 138–9, 194
   emotional 122, 131, 127, 232
   examination of 162, 168–9
   and space 200, 238–41, 245–6, 249–52
Bosworth, Welles 263–4, 271
Buchan, William 219
Bude, Heinz 61
built environment 46–7, 57

Caduff, Carlo 74
cancer 9, 18, 78–9, 89, 121, 125, 129–38, 205
Carson, Rachel 204–5
Carter, Philippa 12
Caruth, Cathy 10
case-based knowledge 104–8
Centers for Disease Control and Prevention 25, 74
Charters, Erica 9
chatbot 95–8
Cheyne, George 217–19
cholera 63
chronic illness. *See also* pain, chronic 10, 16, 37, 76, 78, 82, 93, 100–1, 121, 221
chronic mental disease 183
civil war 22, 26–32, 34, 40, 47, 53, 58
class 4, 6, 169, 194, 219, 222–3, 229–32, 240, 254
contextualization 9–11, 14–15, 18, 22, 45, 57, 60, 84, 86, 105, 126, 142–3, 149–52
Covid-19 (coronavirus, SARS-CoV-2) 7–9, 21–2, 45–6, 61–2, 75, 81–2, 87–8, 206, 258
crime 160, 163, 176, 189, 192
criminal psychiatry 178, 191
criminal psychology 176, 184
criminal therapy 175, 183
criminology 177, 181, 191–2
crisis 8–9, 44–6, 48–53, 55–60, 61–2, 71, 73, 75, 82, 159, 173
Crosby, Alfred W. 64, 66

data 67–8, 74, 85–97, 100, 102
death. *See also* bodies, dead 44, 51, 205–6
   attitudes to 17, 130, 136, 148, 230
   burial 28, 38–40, 43–4, 50
   causes of 38, 49, 63, 77, 115
   cremation 39–40
   dying 25, 39, 54, 129–30, 133–5
   fear of 129, 139

funerals 37–9
  rituals surrounding 38, 57
  statistics 64–5, 68, 76, 81
desire 148, 181, 184, 203, 251–2
despair 16, 129, 131–2
diagnosis 74, 104, 113, 164, 177, 186–92, 232
  bureaucracy of 175
  categories of 3, 18
  changing 193–4, 215–16, 220–1
  response to 8–9, 17, 125, 128, 134, 137–8, 227–8, 254
  tools of 90–1, 149, 183–6, 231
Diagnostic and Statistical Manual (DSM) 122, 142
diarrhoea 35, 63
dichotomy 117–19, 173
digestion 132, 194, 217, 219–20, 224
digital biomarkers 85, 88–91, 95
disgust 9, 39, 82, 92, 138–9, 167, 173, 242
Diski, Jenny 125, 134–6, 139
disposability 151
distance 59, 80, 108, 115, 118, 120, 127, 131, 166
drawings 237–9, 241, 247–9, 252, 256, 261, 266–8, 272
Dross, Fritz 76

Eakin, Paul John 135
early detection 78–9
Ebola virus (EBV) 81
  'Ebola money' 44, 50, 55, 57–9
  in Liberia 18, 22, 25–9, 34–41
  in Sierra Leone 43–6
  symptoms of 35–6
ecology 203–4
Edgeworth, Maria 224, 229
ego documents 254
Eigen-Sinn 15
emotional commodities 193
emotional communities 6
emotional refuges 122
emotional regimes 69, 205
emotional styles 17, 86, 89, 92, 94, 102
emotive imagery 198–9
empathy 99–100, 133
encounter 3–4, 9–10, 126, 155, 171, 235–6, 272
epidemics. *See also* pandemics 4, 10, 22

Ebola. *See* Ebola
HIV 79, 81
influenza 66–7
polio 69
SARS 80
epidemiology 61, 63–4, 67, 72, 74–9, 81, 92
epigenetics 12
ethnography 46, 51, 144
evolution 6, 108, 112, 168–9, 207–8
experience
  collective 6, 9
  history of 7–19, 76, 194
  lived 3, 10, 21–2, 45, 85–6, 89, 139, 153, 168, 193–4, 215, 227–8, 231, 235

fashionable disease 18, 193–4, 215–33
fear
  of blood 27
  bodily signs of 91–2
  and civil war 27, 32–3
  of cremation 40
  of death 16, 129
  and Ebola 22, 27, 29, 36, 41, 46, 49–50, 52, 54–9
  and encounter 10
  of falling ill 4, 62, 129
  history of 11, 22–3
  and illness or disease 9, 36, 74–5, 77, 79–81, 110, 119, 126
  and landscape 204
  of masks 84
  of pain 205
  perception of 118
  societal 6, 32, 69–70, 74–5, 81
feminism 130, 157, 159, 169, 173, 264
forensic medical examiners 162
forensic medicine 155, 159, 162, 164–5, 182
framing 17, 22, 57, 80, 101, 170, 216
Framingham Heart Study 78
furniture 15, 236, 239, 248, 255, 259–60, 263, 266

Galli, Adolphe 263–4
Gate Control Theory 198
gender 4, 102, 135, 171, 173, 198, 216, 222, 254, 256
Ghebreyesus, Tedros Adhanom 75

gimmick, aesthetic of 211
Ginzburg, Carlo 15
global history 15
gout 194, 215, 219, 221–2, 225, 229–30, 233
Great Acceleration 204–5
grief 135
guided imagery 199–201, 207, 211–14
Guillain-Barré syndrome 66
guilt 169, 187, 204–5, 213, 266
gunshot wound 25, 27, 153

Happify, Happify Health 88–9, 92–102
healthcare worker 47, 51–3
hierarchy 106, 111, 119
history of emotions 3, 21, 76, 82, 95, 123
Hitchens, Christopher 131–4, 136–7, 139
HIV (Aids) 71, 79–81
Honigsbaum, Mark 61
hospital 34, 36–7, 53, 105, 113, 211, 223
    bed 4, 210
    design 255, 257, 259, 260–72
    emergency 28, 36
    experience 252
    furniture 266
    gardens 196
    psychiatric 237, 240–3, 245, 247
    rooms 206
    space 244
hysteria 18, 193

imaginary disease 215, 231
influenza 22, 65–77
International Health Regulations (IHR) 73
In the Shadow of Ebola 26–7
invalidity 16

Jay, Martin 8

Kaplan, Rachel and Stephen 201–2, 205

Labisch, Alfons 63
landscape 44–6, 49–50, 193–4, 195–214
Lawrence-Lightfoot, Sarah 122, 143–4
Lederberg, Joshua 71
Liberia Institute for Biomedical Research (LIBR) 35

life writing 122, 126, 135
lockdown 61, 75, 146, 206
Lock, Margaret 12

Macdonald, Robert 255, 261, 271
malaria 35, 37, 62, 71
McKay, Richard A. 9
medical humanities 21, 121, 126–7, 131, 143
medical jurisprudence 161–2, 165
Melzack, Ronald 198
memory 16, 22, 62, 65–8, 75, 136
    childhood 147, 150, 153
    collective 47, 77, 82
    cultural 22
    revised 74, 139
metaphor 11–12, 128, 144, 149–50, 210
methodology 5–11, 18, 104, 143–7
microhistory 15, 22, 144
Mitman, Gregg 22, 25
Montreal Neurological Institute 235, 255–72
mourning 70
movement (physical) 244, 251–2, 260–1, 263
music 201, 212, 224–5, 232, 256, 262

narrative (narration)
    and emotion 88, 109, 123, 131, 138
    expectation 133
    and experience 10, 17, 85, 96, 127, 151
    of illness 89, 92, 121, 125–7, 130, 132, 134–9
    and judgement 50
    and knowledge 22, 89, 108, 120, 121
    scripts 17, 86, 88, 100, 102
    strategies/styles/techniques 15, 18, 80, 83, 95, 108, 128–31, 133, 139, 187
    structure of 48, 89, 121, 253
    and suffering 29, 46, 121, 129, 150
    of time 8
nervousness 91, 219–20, 222, 224, 227, 232–3
neurasthenia 193, 233
neurology 256, 260–1, 268, 272
neuroscience 13, 128, 198
nursing 3, 34, 36, 46, 51–2, 58, 106, 114, 248

objectivity 90, 104–5, 114, 117–18, 120, 162, 247
oral history 26, 29, 143, 152–3

pain
  bodily 35, 151, 200, 227, 229
  chronic 16, 101
  emotional 155, 178, 192, 201, 130
  knowledge 197–8, 200, 272
  management 152, 195, 201, 206, 214
  and narration 126–7, 130–2, 134–5, 139
  perception of 195–198, 225
  politics of 156, 165, 176
  tolerance of 179, 193, 195–9, 201, 205, 213
painting 203–4, 206–7, 209–10, 212
Palsson, Gisli 12
pandemics. See also epidemics 7–8, 19, 21–2, 45, 61–77, 80–4, 87–8, 206
patient-centred perspective 3, 237–41, 247–52
Pear Therapeutics 91
Penfield, Wilder 235–6, 255–72
perception 13, 17–18, 108, 198, 235, 239–54
personality disorder 183–4, 188, 191
Phillips, Barnet 255
philosophy 7
photography 195, 209, 211–13
plasticity 12–14
police surgeons 159, 162–6
polio 49, 69, 77
political economy 55, 59
portraiture 122, 143–4, 149, 152
post-traumatic stress disorder (PTSD) 163–4
power. See also authority 10, 15, 21, 46–8, 117, 155–6, 159–69, 173, 220, 231, 239–40
preparedness 22, 70, 72, 74–5, 82
prevention 35, 44, 70, 72, 78–9, 105
prison 148–9, 151, 175–7, 180–1, 186–91
psychiatry 103–5, 109–12, 116, 122, 177–8, 235
psychology
  animal 86, 106, 109, 111, 119
  criminal 184
  evolutionary 6
  developmental 209

psychopathy 111, 155–6, 176–81, 191
psychotherapy 114–17, 176, 178–9, 182
public health 62, 64–70, 73, 79, 82, 159

rape 155, 157–73
rape myths 161, 165, 172
rape trauma syndrome (RTS) 163
Red Cross 40
Rengeling, David 66
repugnance. *See* disgust
resistance 48, 56, 59
right to maim 151
risk 50, 52, 78–80, 83, 89
ritual 4, 37–8, 41, 49, 52
Robert Koch Institute 73, 75, 77
Roper, Lyndal 11
Rosenberg, Charles 17
Rosenwein, Barbara 6
Ross, Bob 206–7

Sabrow, Martin 61
SARS 74, 80–2, 84
scandalized illness 63
Schlingensief, Christoph 129–31, 138–9
Schweikert, Ruth 136–9
Scott, Joan 144
script (cultural, emotional) 3, 9–11, 17–18, 155–6, 162, 164
sculpture 262–6, 271–2
security 27–8, 70–3, 75, 79, 81–3, 129
senses 3–4, 14, 18, 21, 91, 240–2, 25–3
  sense regime 240–1, 247, 249, 253–4
sensibility 197, 221, 223–5, 228, 243
sentiment analysis 97
sexual violence 155, 158–9, 161, 164, 166, 168, 173
Shalhoub-Kevorkian, Nadera 142, 151
shame 9, 119, 127, 137–9, 155, 157–73, 215, 243, 246
shell shock 193
Siemons, Mark 82
silence 10–11, 31, 172
Smail, Daniel Lord 11
Solastalgia 205
spa towns 225, 232
Stacey, Jackie 137
statistics 63, 67, 145, 158
subjectivity 6, 99–100, 119, 128, 144, 182, 216

Index

Taubenberger, Jeffrey K. 71
Taylor, Charles 29–34
tension (affective, emotional) 109–10, 180
therapeutic penology 176, 181, 184–5, 191
Thompson, E. P. 16
Tissot, S. A. D. 217–19
trauma
  bodily 122
  causes 153
  childhood 113, 121–2, 141–3, 149–51, 153
  chronic 121
  and context 151–2
  history 145, 151
  and memory 150, 153
  mental 18, 50, 122
  multigenerational 142, 150
  and rape 163, 170
  scripts of 164
  therapy 192
Trotter, Thomas 221
Trump, Donald 81

unchilding 142, 151, 153
universalism 12–14, 17, 168

vaccination 4, 7, 37, 44, 47, 65–70, 74–5, 77
violence 10, 45, 58–9, 149
  behaviour 107, 112, 146
  criminal 156
  sexual 155, 158–61, 164, 166, 168, 172–3
  State 141–2, 151
  and trauma 9, 143, 145, 153
virology 51, 61, 64, 68, 71–2, 74, 79, 81–2
virtual health 87–9, 92, 101–2
virtual landscape environments 195, 200, 211

Wahrman, Dror 11
Wall, Patrick 198
Weisser, Olivia 5
wellness 16, 93, 99, 235–6
wellness industry 193
West Bank 122, 145–6
Wilson, Edward O. 207–10
Woolf, Virginia 139
World Health Organization 35, 62, 70–1, 73, 75, 78, 82

www.ingramcontent.com/pod-product-compliance
Lightning Source LLC
Chambersburg PA
CBHW052214300426
44115CB00011B/1685